Practical Procedures in Implant Dentistry

Practical Procedures in Implant Dentistry

Edited by

Christopher C.K. Ho, *BDS Hons (SYD), Grad Dip Clin Dent (Oral Implants) (SYD), M Clin Dent (Pros) (LON), D Clin Dent (Pros) (SYD), MRACDS (Pros), FIADFE, FPFA, FACD*
Head of Post Graduate School of Dentistry, Australasian College of Dental Practitioners, Sydney, New South Wales, Australia

Clinical Lecturer, King's College London, Faculty of Dentistry Oral and Craniofacial Sciences, London, UK

Honorary Lecturer, Faculty of Dentistry, University of Sydney Sydney, New South Wales, Australia

Adjunct Associate Clinical Professor, Faculty of Dentistry University of Puthisastra, Phnom Penh, Cambodia

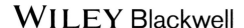

Registered Office(s)
John Wiley & Sons, Inc., 111 River Street, Hoboken, NJ 07030, USA
John Wiley & Sons Ltd, The Atrium, Southern Gate, Chichester, West Sussex, PO19 8SQ, UK

Editorial Office
9600 Garsington Road, Oxford, OX4 2DQ, UK

For details of our global editorial offices, customer services, and more information about Wiley products visit us at www.wiley.com.

Wiley also publishes its books in a variety of electronic formats and by print-on-demand. Some content that appears in standard print versions of this book may not be available in other formats.

Library of Congress Cataloging-in-Publication Data

Names: Ho, Christopher C. K. editor.
Title: Practical procedures in implant dentistry / edited by Christopher
   C.K. Ho.
Description: Hoboken, NJ : Wiley-Blackwell, 2022. | Includes
   bibliographical references and index.
Identifiers: LCCN 2021028071 (print) | LCCN 2021028072 (ebook) |
   ISBN 9781119399179 (paperback) | ISBN 9781119399162 (adobe pdf) |
   ISBN 9781119399193 (epub)
Subjects: MESH: Dental Implantation | Dental Implants
Classification: LCC RK667.I45 (print) | LCC RK667.I45 (ebook) | NLM WU
   640 | DDC 617.6/93–dc23
LC record available at https://lccn.loc.gov/2021028071
LC ebook record available at https://lccn.loc.gov/2021028072

Cover Design: Wiley
Cover Images: © Christopher C. K. Ho

Set in 10/12pt Warnock by Straive, Pondicherry, India

Printed in Singapore
M078420_060721

Contents

Foreword *xix*
List of Contributors *xxi*
About the Companion Website *xxiii*

1   Introduction *1*
Christopher C.K. Ho
References *4*

2   Patient Assessment and History Taking *5*
Christopher C.K. Ho
2.1   Principles *5*
2.1.1   Medical History *5*
2.1.2   Medications and Allergies *6*
2.1.3   Past Medical History *6*
2.1.3.1 Cardiovascular Disorders *6*
2.1.3.2 Diabetes Mellitus *7*
2.1.4   Age *7*
2.1.5   Smoking *7*
2.1.6   Osteoporosis and Bisphosphonate Therapy *8*
2.1.7   Radiotherapy *9*
2.1.8   Dental History *9*
2.1.9   Social History *10*
2.2   Tips *10*
References *10*

3   Diagnostic Records *13*
Aodhan Docherty and Christopher C.K. Ho
3.1   Principles *13*
3.1.1   Diagnostic Imaging and Templates *13*
3.1.1.1 Three-Dimensional Imaging *14*
3.1.1.2 Templates *14*
3.1.2   Guided Surgery *16*
3.1.3   Diagnostic Records *17*
3.1.3.1 Articulated Study Models *17*
3.1.3.2 Photographic Records *18*

3.2   Procedures   *18*
3.2.1   Template Design   *18*
3.2.1.1   Traditional Templates   *18*
3.2.1.2   Digital Templates   *18*
3.2.2   Photography   *19*
3.3   Tips   *23*
          References   *23*

4   Medico-Legal Considerations and Risk Management   *25*
          Christopher C.K. Ho
4.1   Principles   *25*
4.1.1   Informed Consent   *25*
4.2   Procedures   *26*
4.2.1   Dental Records   *26*
4.3   Tips   *28*
          Reference   *28*

5   Considerations for Implant Placement: Effects of Tooth Loss   *29*
          Kyle D. Hogg
5.1   Principles   *29*
5.1.1   Local Site Effects of Tooth Loss   *29*
5.1.2   Effects of Tooth Loss on the Individual Level   *32*
5.1.3   Effects of Tooth Loss on the Population Level   *32*
5.2   Procedures   *33*
5.3   Tips   *34*
          References   *34*

6   Anatomic and Biological Principles for Implant Placement   *37*
          Kyle D. Hogg
6.1   Principles   *37*
6.1.1   Osteology   *37*
6.1.2   Innervation and Vascular Supply   *40*
6.1.3   Musculature   *41*
6.2   Procedures   *41*
6.3   Tips   *47*
          References   *47*

7   Maxillary Anatomical Structures   *49*
          Kyle D. Hogg
7.1   Principles   *49*
7.2   Maxillary Incisive Foramen and Canal   *49*
7.2.1   Importance in Oral Implantology   *50*
7.3   Nasal Cavity   *50*
7.3.1   Importance in Oral Implantology   *51*
7.4   Infraorbital Foramen   *52*
7.4.1   Importance in Oral Implantology   *52*

7.5   Maxillary Sinus   *52*
7.5.1   Importance in Oral Implantology   *54*
7.6   Greater Palatine Artery and Nerve   *55*
7.6.1   Importance in Oral Implantology   *55*
         References   *56*

8   **Mandibular Anatomical Structures**   *59*
         Kyle D. Hogg
8.1   Principles   *59*
8.2   Mental Foramen and Nerve   *59*
8.2.1   Importance in Oral Implantology   *61*
8.3   Mandibular Incisive Canal and Nerve   *62*
8.3.1   Importance in Oral Implantology   *62*
8.4   Genial Tubercles   *63*
8.4.1   Importance in Oral Implantology   *63*
8.5   Lingual Foramen and Accessory Lingual Foramina   *63*
8.5.1   Importance in Oral Implantology   *63*
8.6   Sublingual Fossa   *64*
8.6.1   Importance in Oral Implantology   *65*
8.7   Submental and Sublingual Arteries   *65*
8.7.1   Importance in Oral Implantology   *65*
8.8   Inferior Alveolar Canal and Nerve   *65*
8.8.1   Importance in Oral Implantology   *67*
8.9   Lingual and Mylohyoid Nerves   *67*
8.9.1   Importance in Oral Implantology   *68*
8.10   Submandibular Fossa   *68*
8.10.1   Importance in Oral Implantology   *69*
8.11   Mandibular Ramus   *69*
8.11.1   Importance in Oral Implantology   *69*
         References   *69*

9   **Extraction Ridge Management**   *73*
         Tino Mercado
9.1   Principles   *73*
9.2   Osteoconductive Materials for Ridge Management   *74*
9.3   Biologically Active Materials for Ridge Management   *74*
9.4   Influence of Buccal Wall Thickness on Ridge Management   *82*
         References   *82*

10   **Implant Materials, Designs, and Surfaces**   *87*
         Jonathan Du Toit
10.1   Principles   *87*
10.2   Implant Bulk Materials   *87*
10.2.1   Pure Titanium Used for Implant Bulk Material   *88*
10.2.2   Titanium Alloys Used for Implant Bulk Material   *90*
10.2.3   Zirconia Used for Implant Bulk Material   *90*

10.2.4   Other Materials as Bulk Implant Material   *92*
10.3   Implant Surface Treatments   *92*
10.4   Implant Design   *95*
10.4.1   Implant Body Shape Design   *95*
10.4.2   Implant Thread Design   *96*
10.4.3   Implant Connection Designs   *96*
10.4.4   Which Implant Connections Are Better and Why?   *98*
10.5   Summary   *101*
          References   *101*

11   Timing of Implant Placement   *103*
          Christopher C.K. Ho
11.1   Principles   *103*
11.1.1   Classification for Timing of Implant Placement   *103*
11.1.2   Immediate Placement   *104*
11.1.3   Delayed Implant Placement   *107*
11.1.3.1 Resolution of Local Infection   *107*
11.1.3.2 Dimensional Changes of the Alveolar Ridge   *107*
11.2   Procedures   *108*
11.2.1   Systemic Risk Factors   *108*
11.2.2   Local Risk Factors   *108*
11.2.3   Biomaterials   *109*
11.2.4   Socket Morphology   *110*
11.2.5   Flapless Protocol   *111*
11.2.6   Clinician Experience   *112*
11.2.7   Adjunctive Procedures with Implant Placement   *112*
11.2.7.1 Simultaneous Bone Augmentation
          with Implant Placement   *112*
11.2.7.2 Adjunctive Soft Tissue Grafting   *112*
11.2.8   Selecting the Appropriate Treatment Protocol   *113*
11.3   Tips   *114*
          References   *114*

12   Implant Site Preparation   *117*
          Tom Giblin
12.1   Principles   *117*
12.2   Assessing Implant Sites and Adjacent Teeth   *118*
12.2.1   Periodontal Charting   *118*
12.2.2   Assessment of Gingival Biotype and Attached Mucosa   *118*
12.2.3   Photography   *118*
12.2.4   Aesthetic Assessment   *119*
12.2.5   Radiography   *119*
12.2.6   Occlusal Analysis   *120*
12.2.7   Endodontic Status of Adjacent Teeth   *120*
12.3   Site Preparation   *120*
12.3.1   Grafting – Sinus, Buccal, Soft Tissue   *121*

12.3.2   Occlusion   *121*
12.3.3   Adjacent and Opposing Teeth   *121*
12.3.4   Crown Lengthening and Gingivectomy   *122*
12.3.5   Orthodontics and Site Preparation   *122*
12.3.6   Provisional Phase   *124*
          References   *126*
          Further Reading   *126*

13   **Loading Protocols in Implantology**   *129*
          Christopher C.K. Ho
13.1   Principles   *129*
13.1.1   Definitions   *129*
13.1.2   Conventional Loading   *130*
13.1.3   Early Loading   *130*
13.1.4   Progressive Loading   *130*
13.1.5   Immediate Loading   *130*
13.2   Procedures   *131*
13.2.1   Selecting a Loading Protocol   *131*
13.2.2   Methods of Evaluation of the Primary Stability
          for Immediate Loading   *134*
13.3   Tips   *134*
          References   *135*

14   **Surgical Instrumentation**   *137*
          Christopher C.K. Ho
14.1   Principles   *137*
14.1.1   Mirror, Probe, and Tweezers   *137*
14.1.2   Scalpel Handles   *137*
14.1.3   Scalpel Blades   *138*
14.1.4   Curettes   *138*
14.1.5   Needle Holders   *138*
14.1.6   Periosteal Elevators   *139*
14.1.7   Retractors   *139*
14.1.8   Depth Probe   *139*
14.1.9   Tissue Forceps/Pliers   *139*
14.1.10   Mouth Props/Bite Blocks   *140*
14.1.11   Scissors   *140*
14.1.12   Extraction Forceps, Periotomes and Elevators   *140*
14.1.13   Kidney Dish   *140*
14.1.14   Surgical Kit, Electric Motor, 20:1 Handpiece,
          and Consumables   *140*
14.1.15   Grafting Well   *141*
14.2   Optional Instrumentation   *141*
14.2.1   Rongeurs   *141*
14.2.2   Benex   *141*
14.2.3   Bone Harvesters   *142*

14.2.4   Anthogyr Torq Control   *142*
14.2.5   Piezosurgery   *143*
14.3   Tips   *144*

15   Flap Design and Management for Implant Placement   *145*
Christopher C.K. Ho, David Attia, and Jess Liu
15.1   Principles   *145*
15.1.1   Neurovascular Supply to Implant Site   *145*
15.1.2   Flap Design and Management   *146*
15.1.3   Types of Flap Reflection   *146*
15.2   Procedures   *148*
15.2.1   Tissue Punch   *148*
15.2.2   Envelope Flap   *148*
15.2.3   Triangular (Two-Sided) and Trapezoidal (Three-Sided) Flap   *150*
15.2.4   Papilla-Sparing Flap   *151*
15.2.5   Buccal Roll   *152*
15.2.6   Palacci Flap   *152*
15.3   Tips   *152*
    References   *154*

16   Suturing Techniques   *155*
Christopher C.K. Ho, David Attia, and Jess Liu
16.1   Principles   *155*
16.1.1   Types of Sutures   *155*
16.1.1.1   Absorbable Sutures   *156*
16.1.1.2   Non-absorbable Sutures   *156*
16.1.2   Suture Adjuncts   *157*
16.1.3   Suture Size   *157*
16.1.4   Needle   *157*
16.2   Procedures   *158*
16.2.1   Simple/Interrupted Sutures   *158*
16.2.2   Continuous/Uninterrupted Suture   *159*
16.2.3   Mattress Sutures   *159*
16.2.3.1   Horizontal Mattress   *161*
16.2.3.2   Vertical Mattress   *161*
16.2.4   Suture Removal   *162*
16.3   Tips   *162*

**17   Pre-surgical Tissue Evaluation and Considerations
    in Aesthetic Implant Dentistry   *163***
Sherif Said
17.1   Principles   *163*
17.2   The Influence of Tissue Volume on Peri-implant 'Pink'
    Aesthetics   *163*
17.3   Tissue Volume Availability and Requirements   *165*
17.3.1   Hard Tissue Requirements   *165*

17.3.2   Soft Tissue Requirements   *166*
17.4   Pre-operative Implant Site Assessment   *166*
17.5   Key Factors in Diagnosis of the Surrounding Tooth Support
        Prior to Extraction   *167*
17.5.1   Integrity of the Interproximal Height
        of Bone   *168*
17.5.2   Essential Criteria Evaluation Prior to Extraction   *168*
17.5.3   Integrity of the Buccal Plate of Bone   *169*
17.6   Tips   *169*
17.7   Conclusion   *170*
        References   *170*

18   **Surgical Protocols for Implant Placement**   *173*
        Christopher C.K. Ho
18.1   Principles   *173*
18.1.1   Implant Positioning   *174*
18.2   Procedures   *176*
18.2.1   One-Stage versus Two-Stage Protocols   *177*
18.2.2   Post-operative Management Protocols   *177*
18.3   Tips   *179*
        References   *179*

19   **Optimising the Peri-implant Emergence Profile**   *181*
        David Attia and Jess Liu
19.1   Principles   *181*
19.1.1   The Peri-implant Emergence Profile   *181*
19.2   Procedures   *182*
19.2.1   Single-Stage versus Two-Stage Implant Surgery   *182*
19.2.2   Buccal Roll Flap   *183*
19.2.3   Pouch Roll Technique   *186*
19.2.4   Apically Repositioned Flap   *188*
19.2.5   Buccally Repositioned Flap   *191*
19.2.6   Free Gingival Graft   *193*
19.3   Tips   *196*
        References   *198*

20   **Soft Tissue Augmentation**   *199*
        Michel Azer
20.1   Principles   *199*
20.1.1   Types of Oral Soft Tissue   *199*
20.1.2   Anatomical Considerations for Harvesting Autogenous
        Soft Tissue Grafts   *200*
20.1.2.1   Hard Palate   *200*
20.1.2.2   Tuberosity   *200*
20.1.2.3   Buccal Attached Gingiva of Maxillary Molars   *201*
20.1.3   Soft Tissue Substitutes   *201*

20.1.3.1   Allogenic Origin   *201*
20.1.3.2   Xenograft Origin   *201*
20.1.4   Purpose of Soft Tissue Graft (Periodontal Plastic Surgery)   *201*
20.1.4.1   Aesthetic Purpose   *201*
20.1.4.2   Functional Purpose   *201*
20.2   Procedures   *201*
20.2.1   Techniques   *201*
20.2.1.1   Harvesting the Palatal Tissue Graft as a Free Gingival Graft
            and Connective Tissue Graft   *201*
20.2.1.2   Root Coverage   *202*
20.2.1.3   Soft Tissue Augmentation Prior to Bone
            Grafting   *202*
20.2.1.4   Soft Tissue Graft to Gain Keratinised Tissue   *203*
20.3   Tips   *209*
            References   *209*
            Further Reading   *210*

**21   Bone Augmentation Procedures   *211*
            Michel Azer
21.1   Principles   *211*
21.1.1   Why is Bone Grafting Necessary?   *211*
21.1.2   Defect Topography Classification   *211*
21.1.3   Requirements for Successful Tissue Grafting   *212*
21.1.4   Materials Used for Augmentation   *212*
21.1.4.1   Autogenous Bone   *212*
21.1.4.2   Membranes   *212*
21.1.4.3   Membrane Fixation Systems   *213*
21.2   Procedures   *213*
21.2.1   Bone Graft with Non-resorbable Membrane   *213*
21.2.2   Autogenous Bone Graft   *215*
21.3   Tips   *217*
            References   *217*

**22   Impression Taking in Implant Dentistry   *219*
            Christopher C.K. Ho
22.1   Principles   *219*
22.1.1   Impression Techniques Used in Implant Dentistry   *220*
22.1.1.1   Abutment Level Impressions   *220*
22.1.1.2   Implant Level Impressions   *220*
22.1.2   Customised Impression Copings   *222*
22.1.3   Multiple Unit Impressions   *222*
22.2   Procedures   *224*
22.2.1   Implant Level Impression   *224*
22.2.2   Digital Impressions   *225*

22.3   Tips   *225*
          References   *226*

23   Implant Treatment in the Aesthetic Zone   *227*
          Christopher C.K. Ho
23.1   Principles   *227*
23.1.1   General Considerations   *227*
23.1.1.1 Lip Contour and Length   *228*
23.1.1.2 Tooth Display at Repose and in Broad Smile   *228*
23.1.1.3 Smile Line   *228*
23.1.1.4 Teeth Length, Shape, Alignment, Contour, and Colour   *229*
23.1.1.5 Gingival Display, Gingival Zeniths, and Papillae of Maxillary
          Anterior Teeth   *229*
23.1.1.6 Width of Edentulous Space   *230*
23.1.1.7 Gingival Biotype   *230*
23.1.2   Major Deficiencies in Hard and Soft Tissues   *230*
23.2   Procedures   *232*
23.2.1   Assessment of Gingival Biotype   *232*
23.2.2   Clinical Management   *232*
23.2.3   Timing of Implant Placement   *233*
23.2.4   Thickness of Soft Tissues   *234*
23.3   Tips   *234*
          References   *235*

24   The Use of Provisionalisation in Implantology   *237*
          Christopher C.K. Ho
24.1   Principles   *237*
24.1.1   Prosthetically Guided Tissue Healing   *237*
24.2   Procedures   *240*
24.2.1   Direct Techniques   *240*
24.2.2   Indirect Techniques   *240*
24.3   Tips   *241*
          Reference   *242*

25   Abutment Selection   *243*
          Christopher C.K. Ho
25.1   Principles   *243*
25.1.1   Custom Abutments   *245*
25.1.2   Prefabricated (Stock) Abutments   *245*
25.1.3   Material Selection   *247*
25.1.4   Abutment Design   *249*
25.2   Procedures   *250*
25.3   Tips   *250*
          References   *251*

26   **Screw versus Cemented Implant-Supported Restorations**   *253*
Christopher C.K. Ho
26.1   Principles   *253*
26.1.1   Retrievability   *253*
26.1.2   Aesthetics   *254*
26.1.3   Passivity   *254*
26.1.4   Hygiene (Emergence Profile)   *255*
26.1.5   Reduced Occlusal Material Fracture   *255*
26.1.6   Inter-arch Space   *256*
26.1.7   Occlusion   *256*
26.1.8   Health of Peri-Implant Tissue   *256*
26.1.9   Provisionalisation   *256*
26.1.10   Clinical Performance   *256*
26.2   Procedures   *257*
26.2.1   Screw-Retained Restoration   *257*
26.2.2   Cement-Retained Restoration   *260*
26.2.3   Lateral Set-Screw (Cross-Pinning)   *261*
26.2.4   Angle Screw Correction/Bi-axial Screws   *262*
26.3   Tips   *263*
     References   *264*

27   **A Laboratory Perspective on Implant Dentistry**   *265*
Lachlan Thompson
27.1   The Shift from Analogue to Digital   *265*
27.2   Standards in Manufacturing Today   *265*
27.3   The Importance of Implant Planning for the Laboratory   *267*
27.4   Digital Planning to Manage Aesthetic Cases   *268*
27.5   Scanning for Implant Restorations   *268*
27.6   Digital Data Acquisition for Full Arch Cases   *271*
27.7   Inserting Full Arch Cases at Surgery   *272*
27.8   Tips   *275*

28   **Implant Biomechanics**   *277*
Tom Giblin
28.1   Principles   *277*
28.1.1   Forces and their Nature   *277*
28.1.1.1   Pressure = Force/Area   *278*
28.1.1.2   Impulse = Force/Time   *278*
28.1.1.3   Compressive, Tensile, and Shear Forces   *279*
28.1.1.4   Application to Materials and Occlusion   *279*
28.1.1.5   Incline Plane Mechanics (Normal Force)   *280*
28.1.2   Beams   *280*
28.1.3   Levers   *281*
28.1.4   Cantilevers   *282*
28.1.5   Bone   *283*
     Reference   *285*
     Further Reading   *285*

29   **Delivering the Definitive Prosthesis**   *289*
        Aodhan Docherty and Christopher C.K. Ho
29.1   Principles   *289*
29.1.1   Soft Tissue Support   *289*
29.1.2   Occlusal Verification   *290*
29.1.3   Aesthetic Evaluation   *290*
29.1.4   Torque Requirement for Delivery   *292*
29.1.5   Cementation Technique and Material Selection – Cemented
         Crowns   *292*
29.1.6   Screw Access Channel Management – Screw-Retained
         Crowns   *294*
29.1.7   Pink Porcelain   *295*
29.2   Procedures   *296*
29.2.1   Delivering a Cement-Retained Crown – Chairside
         Copy Abutment Technique   *296*
29.2.1.1 Creating a Polyvinyl Siloxane Copy Abutment   *296*
29.2.1.2 Delivering a Cement-Retained Crown Using a Copy
         Abutment Technique   *296*
29.3   Tips   *298*
         References   *298*

30   **Occlusion and Implants**   *299*
        Christopher C.K. Ho and Subir Banerji
30.1   Principles   *299*
30.1.1   Excessive Forces on Dental Implants   *301*
30.1.2   Bruxism and Implants   *301*
30.2   Procedures   *302*
30.2.1   Clinical Occlusal Applications   *303*
30.3   Tips   *305*
         References   *305*

31   **Dental Implant Screw Mechanics**   *307*
        Christopher C.K. Ho and Louis Kei
31.1   Principles   *307*
31.1.1   Factors Affecting Implant Screw Joint Stability   *308*
31.1.1.1 Preload   *308*
31.1.1.2 Embedment Relaxation (Settling Effect)   *308*
31.1.1.3 Screw Material and Coating   *308*
31.1.1.4 Screw Design   *309*
31.1.1.5 Abutment/Implant Interface Misfit   *309*
31.1.1.6 Abutment/Implant Interface Design   *309*
31.1.1.7 Functional Forces   *310*
31.1.1.8 Number of Implants   *310*
31.1.1.9 Torque Wrench   *310*
31.2   Procedures   *311*
31.2.1   Techniques for Retrieving a Fractured Screw   *311*
31.2.1.1 The Ultrasonic Scaler Technique   *311*

31.2.1.2   Screwdriver Technique   *312*
31.2.1.3   Manufacturer Rescue Kits   *312*
31.3   Tips   *312*
            References   *313*

32   Prosthodontic Rehabilitation for the Fully Edentulous Patient   *315*
            Christopher C.K. Ho
32.1   Principles   *315*
32.1.1   Number of Implants for Full Arch Implant Rehabilitation   *317*
32.1.1.1   Removable Overdenture   *317*
32.1.2   Fixed Implant-Supported Bridgework   *319*
32.2   Procedures   *320*
32.2.1   Occlusal Vertical Dimension   *320*
32.2.2   Phonetics   *321*
32.2.3   Swallowing   *322*
32.2.4   Facial Appearance   *322*
32.2.5   Impression Taking   *322*
32.2.6   Abutment Selection   *322*
32.2.7   Prosthodontic Options for Fixed Bridgework   *323*
32.2.8   Occlusion   *323*
32.3   Tips   *323*
            References   *326*

33   Implant Maintenance   *327*
            Kyle D. Hogg and Christopher C.K. Ho
33.1   Principles   *327*
33.1.1   Radiographic Analysis   *328*
33.2   Procedures   *330*
33.3   Tips   *333*
            References   *333*

34   The Digital Workflow in Implant Dentistry   *335*
            Andrew Chio and Anthony Mak
34.1   Components and Steps of the Digital Implant Workflow   *336*
34.1.1   Digital Diagnostic Impression   *336*
34.1.2   Cone Beam Computed Tomography   *337*
34.1.3   Digital Implant Treatment Planning   *337*
34.1.4   The Digital Surgical Guide   *338*
34.1.5   Pre-surgical Fabricated Temporary Prosthesis   *342*
34.1.6   Guided Implant Surgery   *342*
34.1.7   Implant Digital Impressions   *343*
34.1.8   Manufacturing of the Customised Prosthesis   *343*
            References   *347*

35   Biological Complications   *351*
            Christopher C.K. Ho
35.1   Principles   *351*
35.1.1   Attachment Differences   *352*

35.1.2   Crestal Bone Loss *353*
35.1.3   Peri-implant Disease *353*
35.1.3.1 Prevalence of Peri-implant Diseases *354*
35.1.3.2 Risk Factors in Peri-implant Disease *354*
35.2   Procedures *357*
35.2.1   Treatment of Peri-implant Disease *357*
35.2.1.1 Methods of Decontamination *358*
35.2.2   Treatment of Peri-implant Mucositis *360*
35.2.3   Treatment of Peri-implantitis *361*
35.2.3.1 Non-surgical Therapy for Peri-implantitis *361*
35.2.3.2 Surgical Therapy for Peri-implantitis *361*
35.2.4   Recommendations *364*
35.2.5   Supportive Care *365*
35.3   Tips *366*
          References *367*

36   **Implant Prosthetic Complications** *371*
          Christopher C.K. Ho and Matthew K. Youssef
36.1   Principles *371*
36.1.1   Incidence of Prosthetic Complications *372*
36.1.1.1 Implant-Supported Single Tooth Crowns and Implant-Fixed
          Dental Prostheses *372*
36.1.1.2 Full Arch Implant-Fixed Dental Prostheses *373*
36.1.2   Aetiology of Prosthetic Complications *374*
36.1.2.1 Mechanical Overloading *374*
36.1.2.2 Cement Excess *374*
36.1.2.3 Proximal Contact Loss *374*
36.2   Procedures *374*
36.2.1   Occlusion *374*
36.2.2   Unfavourable Implant Position *375*
36.2.3   Anterior Implants *375*
36.2.4   Implant Fracture *375*
36.2.5   Screw Loosening *377*
36.2.6   Abutment Screw Fracture *377*
36.2.7   Stripped Screw Head *377*
36.2.8   Passive Fit *378*
36.2.9   Mechanical and Biological Complications of Framework Misfit *380*
36.2.10   Impression Technique *381*
36.2.11   Gingival Fistula *381*
36.2.12   Prevention of Prosthetic Complications *382*
36.3   Tips *383*
          References *383*

          Index *387*

Foreword

It is a true pleasure to be invited to write a foreword for this comprehensive new textbook on implant dentistry, a fast evolving discipline ranging from basic biological fundamentals to advanced clinical principles. The responsibility is large to write a new book on dental implants and to cover in detail topics such as digital planning, patient selection, implant and regenerative biomaterials, surgical and restorative steps, oral maintenance, follow-up, and the diagnoses of implant problems. The Editor has successfully managed to do so and has compiled a clear and practical guide for the clinician.

I welcome his timely efforts as the implant field has developed so rapidly that it is hard for any clinician, young or old, to stay abreast of new developments and not to forget the foundations that made this field possible. The master clinician behind the book is one of the true experts in implant dentistry. Dr. Chris Ho gained his extensive clinical and evidence-based experience over many years practising and teaching the field. He completed basic implant training as a general practitioner, then moved to advanced restorative training as a prosthodontist, and advanced surgical training with global experts in implant, bone, and soft tissue surgery. It takes that kind of discipline and devotion to master a complex field and enjoy the day-to-day implant practice, treating patients without stress and with consistent success. This book documents the task and will be a reference for many years to come.

I have gotten to know Chris as a dedicated and passionate clinician, educator, author, and friend over the many years that he has been vital to the gIDE Master Clinician Program. It is important for every dentist, from young graduate to experienced practitioner, to understand that it takes that kind of devotion to master a technique and become an implant expert. Many years of learning and training bring good and bad days, with learning curves that range from easy to steep, but the passion and discipline never disappears in the journey to become a Master Clinician in implant dentistry.

I believe that this book will be part of the journey for any dentist interested in improving and mastering their dental implant therapy.

Enjoy, train hard, and don't forget to have fun while learning.

Sascha Jovanovic, DDS, MS
Specialist in Periodontics (UCLA)
Specialist in Implant Therapy (Loma Linda University)
Specialist in Prosthodontics (Univ. of Aachen)
Master of Science in Oral Biology (UCLA)
Academic Chairman, gIDE Institute
Periodontist/Implant Surgeon, gIDE Dental Center
Assistant Professor, LLU School of Dentistry
Past-co-director, UCLA Implant Center
Past-president, European Association for Osseointegration (EAO)

List of Contributors

David Attia, *BOH (DentSci) (Griffith), GradDipDent (Griffith), MSc (Oral Implantology) (Goethe), PGDipClin (Orth) (CoL)*
Clinical Lecturer
Australasian College of Dental Practitioners, Sydney, New South Wales, Australia

Michel Azer, *DDS (MIU), MS CAGS (BU)*
Former Clinical Assistant Professor
Henry M. Goldman School of Dental Medicine, Advanced Education Program Department of Periodontology, Boston, MA, USA

Subir Banerji, *BDS, MClinDent (Prostho), PhD, MFGDP(UK), FDS RCPS (Glasg), FICOI FICD, FIADFE*
Programme Director, MSc Aesthetic Dentistry
Senior Clinical Lecturer
King's College London, Faculty of Dentistry, Oral and Craniofacial Sciences, London, UK
Associate Professor
University of Melbourne Dental School, Melbourne, Victoria, Australia

Andrew Chio, *BDS (Melb)*
Private practice, Melbourne, Victoria, Australia

Aodhan Docherty, *BMedSci, BDent (Hons) (SYD), Grad Dip Clin Dent (Oral Implants) (SYD), PGDipClin (Orth) (CoL)*
Clinical Lecturer
Australasian College of Dental Practitioners, Sydney, New South Wales, Australia

Jonathan Du Toit, *BChD (UWC), MSc (Wits), Dip Oral Surg (CMFOS), Dipl Implantol (Frankfurt), MChD (OMP) (UP), FCD(SA) OMP*
Specialist in Periodontics and Oral Medicine
Senior Lecturer
Implant and Aesthetic Academy, Cape Town, South Africa

Tom Giblin, *BSc (Syd) BDent (Hons) (Syd) CertPros (Texas), DICOI*
Clinical Lecturer
Australasian College of Dental Practitioners
Private practice, Sydney, New South Wales, Australia

Christopher C.K. Ho, BDS Hons (SYD), Grad Dip Clin Dent (Oral Implants) (SYD), M Clin Dent (Pros) (LON), D Clin Dent (Pros) (SYD), MRACDS (Pros), FIADFE, FPFA, FACD
Head of Post Graduate School of Dentistry, Australasian College of Dental Practitioners, Sydney, New South Wales, Australia
Clinical Lecturer
Faculty of Dentistry, Oral and Craniofacial Sciences, King's College London, London, UK
Honorary Lecturer
Faculty of Dentistry, University of Sydney, New South Wales, Australia
Adjunct Associate Clinical Professor
Faculty of Dentistry, University of Puthisastra, Phnom Penh, Cambodia

Kyle D. Hogg, DDS (Univ. of Michigan), AEGD (Univ. of Florida), MClinDent Prosthodontics (Lon)
Post-graduate Tutor and Clinical Lecturer
King's College London, Faculty of Dentistry, Oral and Craniofacial Sciences, London, UK

Louis Kei, BDSc Hons (Qld), MRACDS (GDP), DClinDent (Pros) (USyd), MRACDS (Pros)
Clinical Lecturer
Faculty of Dentistry,
University of Sydney, New South Wales, Australia

Jess Liu, DDS (NYUCD), MS (BU)
Clinical Assistant Professor
Director of the Implant Fellowship
Henry M. Goldman School of Dental Medicine, Advanced Education Program Department of Periodontology, Boston, MA, USA

Anthony Mak, BDS (SYD), Grad Dip Clin Dent (Oral Implants) (SYD))
Private practice, Sydney, New South Wales, Australia

Tino Mercado, DMD, GCClinDent (Oral Path) (Qld), MDSc (Perio) (Qld), MRACDS (Perio), PhD, FPFA, FICD
Associate Professor
School of Dentistry, University of Queensland, Brisbane, Queensland, Australia

Sherif Said, BDS, MSD, CAGS, FRCD(C)
Diplomate of the American Board of Periodontics
Clinical Assistant Professor
Department of Periodontology
Henry M. Goldman School of Dental Medicine, Boston University
Private practice, Toronto, Canada

Lachlan Thompson,
Dip. Dental Technology (Perth)
Perth, Australia

Matthew K. Youssef, BHSc MDent (LaTrobe), PG Dip Implants (CSU)
Private practice, Melbourne, Victoria, Australia

About the Companion Website

Don't forget to visit the companion website for this book:

www.wiley.com/go/ho/implant-dentistry

There you will find valuable material designed to enhance your learning, including:

- Videos demonstrating clinical techniques and procedures.

Scan this QR code to visit the companion website.

1

Introduction
Christopher C.K. Ho

The phenomenon of osseointegration has allowed for major improvements in both oral function and the psychosocial well-being of edentulous patients. The improvement in quality of life may be life-changing, allowing patients fixed replacement of teeth or, in cases of removable dental prostheses, significant improvement in retention and stability. In the 1950s, Swedish physician Per-Ingvar Brånemark conducted *in vivo* animal experiments studying revascularisation and wound healing using optical titanium chambers in rabbit tibia. On removal of the titanium chambers it was discovered that bone was attached to the titanium. Subsequently, Brånemark dedicated his research to the study of bony integration. He defined osseointegration as 'the direct structural and functional contact between ordered living bone and the surface of a load carrying implant' [1].

Since those early days, progress in implant treatment has been remarkable, with many innovative and technological advances, including three-dimensional (3D) imaging and computer-aided design/computer-aided manufacturing (CAD/CAM), new biomaterials, advances in implant configuration and connections, with surface modifications that have allowed improved surface reactivity for better bone–implant contact. Historically, specialist teams of surgeons and prosthodontist/restorative dentists undertook this therapy and achieved very high levels of success. However, with increasing numbers of implants and time *in situ*, as well as treatment by less-experienced clinicians, there has been an increase in the number of complications encountered.

When implant treatment fails or a complication arises it can be extraordinarily disheartening for patients and clinicians alike. As well as significant costs there is the surgical morbidity of carrying out implant insertion with considerable time involvement. This leads to disappointment if treatment fails and may even lead to medico-legal repercussions. No treatment is immune to failure, but proper management through comprehensive evaluation, diagnosis, and planning is paramount to success and minimising any complications. Along with careful case selection and planning, treatment should be performed with high levels of evidence-based protocols and professional excellence and followed up with regular continuing care.

Practical Procedures in Implant Dentistry, First Edition. Edited by Christopher C.K. Ho.
© 2022 John Wiley & Sons Ltd. Published 2022 by John Wiley & Sons Ltd.
Companion website: www.wiley.com/go/ho/implant-dentistry

Since the introduction of moderately roughened implant surfaces and tapered, threaded implants the success of implants has become predictable, with very few failures occurring. The early failures are most likely due to surgical error, such as overheating of bone or not attaining sufficient primary stability due to over-preparation. Most late failures occur as a result of peri-implant infection or implant overload, and in the aesthetic zone due to insufficient soft or hard tissues around the implant. Extensive research has been conducted, combined with long-term patient experience, allowing us to refine and improve the treatment protocols. There have been major developments in knowledge that have allowed significant improvements, including the following:

- *A prosthetically driven approach*: Historically, a surgically driven approach was used in which implants were placed in the bony anatomy available. However, in cases of deficiency this resulted in final restorations that were compromised. A prosthetically driven approach is referred to as 'backwards planning'; the final ideal tooth position is planned, and augmentation may need to be performed to allow the final implant to be in the optimal position.
- *Radiographic imaging*: Cross-sectional imaging with cone beam computed tomography (CBCT) scans in combination with the use of planning software allows 3D positioning for the prosthetically planned approach. Improved safety and predictability in implant insertion has resulted. The use of surgically guided templates to provide precise implant placement with alignment in the correct axis enhances predictability and reliability in placing implants that are bodily within bone, and with access alignment that may allow screw retention. It also allows the clinician to diagnose whether augmentation may need to be undertaken in either a simultaneous or staged approach with implant placement.
- *Importance of the soft tissue interface*: It is now understood that the peri-implant soft tissues are paramount for long-term stability and predictability. The soft tissue interface is similar to that of natural teeth and a barrier to microbial invasion. Histologically, peri-implant tissues possess a junctional epithelium and supracrestal zone of connective tissue. This connective tissue helps seal off the oral environment, with the fibres arranged parallel to the implant surface in a cuff-like circular orientation. This arrangement may impact how the tissue responds to bacterial insult or cement extrusion into the sulcus. Natural teeth have gingival fibres inserting into cementum tissues, but because of the parallel arrangement of fibres around implants the tissues are more easily detached from the implant surface. This may lead to breakdown such as that seen in peri-implantitis or cement extrusion. This inflammatory breakdown is often seen at an accelerated rate compared to that of periodontitis. Literature has also demonstrated the presence of a 'biologic width' around dental implants, and understanding the influence of thick tissue will help prevent bone loss and provide improved stability [2, 3].
- *Implant design*: Both macrostructure and microstructure of implants have undergone continuous development to attain better primary stability, quicker osseointegration, and increased bone–implant contact. Micromotion may disturb tissue healing and vasculature, with micromotion greater than 100–150 µm

detaching the fibrin clot from the implant surface. Modern implant designs have focused on achieving enhanced primary stability, with manufacturers developing a tapered implant that allows for the widest part of the implant to engage the cortical bone at the crest, while the apical portion is tapered to allow the trabecular bone to be compressed. The original implant connections were an external hex, however modern implant designs have focused on platform-switched internal connections. These are often conical connections, with several manufacturers' designs approaching a Morse taper. This creates significant friction through the high degree of parallelism between the two structures within the connection. It has been shown to reduce the microgap size and distribute stress more evenly; there is also increasing evidence that it helps to preserve peri-implant bone and stabilise soft tissues. Extensive research into implant microstructure has established the optimal environment for bone–implant contact, with both additive and subtractive techniques used to develop moderately rough surfaces (Sa 1–2 μm). Most implant manufacturers produce this surface by using acid etching, grit blasting, or anodic oxidation. This roughness improves the osteoconductivity of the surface.

- *Digital implant dentistry – computer-aided design (CAD), computer-aided manufacturing (CAM), chairside intra-oral scanning, and 3D printing*: This area has undergone significant technological improvements in recent years, with implant planning software allowing accurate planning of dental implants using CBCT. The ability to print surgical guides through 3D printing is now commonplace, with many dental practices able to access this technology due to the reduced cost of printing. CAD/CAM fabrication of prosthetic abutments and implant bars allows customised designs that are passively fitting, economic, and homogeneous, with no distortion compared to that of cast metal frameworks. The many different materials dental clinicians have available to mill nowadays, including zirconia, ceramics, hybrid ceramics, cobalt-chrome, and titanium, allow the modern clinician to select appropriate materials for both aesthetics and strength when required.

- *Loading protocols*: The original protocols demanded an unloaded period of healing after implant surgery that ranged from three to six months. With the improved designs possessing better primary stability and roughened surface implants, these delayed loading protocols have been challenged, with immediate loading of implants providing immediate function in the first 48 hours. This has led to better acceptance of treatment, with reduced numbers of appointments and intervention. Survival rates are high for immediate loaded and conventional loaded implants, however immediate loading may pose a greater risk for implant failure if there is the possibility of micromotion.

- *Complications and long-term maintenance*: Because the original implant patients were treated over 50 years ago now, many patients have had implants for multiple decades. Complications are known. These can be mechanical in nature, such as screw loosening/fracture, veneering material fractures and wear, or biological complications with peri-implantitis and inflammation. Proper planning minimises such failure and complications. Patients should still understand that regular continuing care is required and that their implant treatment may require servicing and may even need replacement in the future.

We hope that this book provides the reader with information that allows their practice of implant dentistry to be successful and predictable, ultimately improving a patient's quality of life. The book has been formatted to ensure that the reader has access to relevant information in a recognisable format under the headings 'Principles, Procedures, and Tips'. This will give practising clinicians accessible information to learn new skills, and provides a continual reference for revision prior to performing procedures. We hope this will ensure that the clinician undertakes best practice within their dental office in the field of implant dentistry.

References

1 Brånemark, P.-I., Hansson, B.O., Adell, R. et al. (1977). *Osseointegrated Implants in the Treatment of the Edentulous Jaw*, 132. Stockholm: Almqvist and Wiksell.
2 Linkevicius, T., Apse, P., Grybauskas, S., and Puisys, A. (2009). The influence of soft tissue thickness on crestal bone changes around implants: a 1-year prospective controlled clinical trial. *Int. J. Oral Maxillofac. Implants* 24 (4): 712–719.
3 Tomasi, C., Tessarolo, F., Caola, I. et al. (2014). Morphogenesis of peri-implant mucosa revisited: an experimental study in humans. *Clin. Oral Implants Res.* 25 (9): 997–1003.

2

Patient Assessment and History Taking

Christopher C.K. Ho

2.1 Principles

Careful patient selection, evaluation, and treatment planning are fundamental to the success of implant therapy and will help to avoid future complications or failures. Since Brånemark et al. [1] published research documenting successful osseointegration on endosseous titanium implants in 1969, the use of osseointegrated dental implants has increasingly become the treatment option for the replacement of missing teeth. Despite the predictability of dental implants, a small but significant number of patients continue to experience implant failure, and it is important to understand the risk factors involved. Informed consent is the process of communication between a clinician and a patient whereby a patient grants permission for the proposed treatment based on understanding the nature of the problem, the risks, and the benefits of the procedure and treatment alternatives, including no treatment.

The first objective is to gather all relevant information to plan treatment. It is essential to obtain appropriate information about the patient's dental and medical history, and to conduct a comprehensive examination in conjunction with diagnosis from radiographic imaging and study casts.

2.1.1 Medical History

The general health status of a patient should always be assessed prior to any surgical procedure. Although there is minimal association between general health status and implant survival [2], there are certain situations where implant procedures may risk the health of a patient or possibly be associated with higher failure rates of osseointegration.

Medical questionnaires are routinely used and, in addition, it is best practice to verbally ask specific questions about the health of patients. There are two basic questions that a clinician should ask prior to implant surgical procedures:

1) Is the patient fit medically to have the procedure done?
2) Is there anything in their history that would interfere with healing and the normal osseointegrative process?

Table 2.1 Relative contraindications to implant surgery.

Diabetes
Tobacco use
Uncontrolled cardiovascular disease/hypertension
Cancer/leukaemia
Renal/liver problems
Bisphosphonate medications
Blood disorders/anticoagulant therapy
HIV/immunosuppression
Alcohol abuse
Psychological disorders
Pregnancy
Irradiation

These two simple questions should form the basis of your questioning as to whether patients are able to undergo a surgical procedure and determine any risk factors with the healing process. There are very few absolute contraindications to implant surgery, however there are certain conditions which may increase the risk of complications with the surgical procedure or wound healing. The conditions listed in Table 2.1 have been suggested as possible contraindications to implant treatment and should be carefully managed.

2.1.2 Medications and Allergies

A list of medications (including any herbal preparations or medications taken on as-needed basis) along with the dosage and indications for the medication should be recorded. Patients should be asked whether they take any over-the-counter medications such as aspirin on a regular basis as they often forget to mention this when recording medications prescribed. Any allergies should be documented to preclude any reaction.

2.1.3 Past Medical History

Several conditions are discussed below, however further investigation is required if there is any uncertainty as to the prognosis.

2.1.3.1 Cardiovascular Disorders
- Uncontrolled hypertension (blood pressure above 160/90 mmHg) places the patient at greater risk of stroke, heart failure, myocardial infarction, and renal failure. Implant surgery may therefore pose a risk to potential adverse cerebrovascular and cardiovascular events.
- Patients who have had a cardiac infarction within the previous six months should not undergo surgery, and patients with a history of angina should have

glyceryl trinitrate tablets/sublingual sprays available when undergoing implant surgery.

- The use of antibiotic prophylaxis may be required for patients with a history of prosthetic valves, infective endocarditis, or rheumatic fever.
- Anticoagulant therapy may cause extended bleeding post-operatively, and patients taking warfarin or heparin should have an International Normalised Ratio (INR) of less than 2.5 prior to the surgical procedure. Consultation with the patient's physician is recommended to determine whether the patient should cease anticoagulant therapy such as aspirin.

2.1.3.2 Diabetes Mellitus

- Diabetes mellitus is a common endocrine disorder affecting the metabolism of glucose. Patients with diabetes may experience increased susceptibility to wound-healing complications and increased inflammatory destruction. Furthermore, they possess altered bone and mineral metabolism which may interfere with bone metabolism [3]. A prospective study of 89 patients with well-controlled type 2 diabetes found an early failure rate of 2.2% in implants placed in edentulous mandibles. This increased to 7.3% after one year when the implants were loaded with overdentures [4]. The five-year results of this study revealed a survival rate of 90% [5]. Diabetes mellitus is not a barrier to successful osseointegration provided the implants are placed in patients with well-controlled diabetes.

2.1.4 Age

- Placement of implants in younger patients that are skeletally immature is contraindicated. Implants act like ankylosed teeth and hence lack the ability to erupt and compensate for changes in growth. This may lead to the implant submerging over time and may also interfere with the normal growth of the jaw. Individual assessment by serial cephalometric radiographs, one year apart, is needed to confirm that growth has truly ceased [6] prior to implant placement.
- In the elderly patient, there is no upper age limit contraindication for implant therapy. However, the elderly patient may not be able to undergo prolonged surgical procedures, is likely to possess more systemic health factors and have decreased ability to adapt to new prostheses, may have poorer oral hygiene practices, and may require longer healing times due to changes in bone and calcium metabolism which can potentially affect osseointegration.
- Nevertheless, the literature suggests that age does not have an impact on osseointegration of implants, nor survival of the implants after osseointegration.

2.1.5 Smoking

- It has been documented that smoking may impair wound healing through the vasoconstrictive effects of nicotine, which may compromise tissue perfusion and vascularity. This also may reduce the tissue capacity to combat infection.
- Multiple studies demonstrate a significant relationship between smoking and higher failure rates of implants [2, 7, 8]. Bain and Moy [8] revealed that

smokers had more than twice the percentage of implant failures when compared to non-smokers (11.3 versus 4.8%). Two studies investigated the effect of smoking on initial healing of the implant [7, 9]. They showed smokers had a higher failure rate than non-smokers, particularly in the maxilla.

- Bain [7] found a statistically significant difference between smokers and non-smokers, as well as between smokers and those who underwent a protocol of cessation of smoking during the period of implant placement and initial healing. Under the protocol suggested by Bain, patients are advised to cease smoking for a minimum of one week prior to and at least eight weeks after implant surgery. The short-term implant success rates were similar to those who had never smoked. However, long-term heavy smokers should be informed about the reduced success rate, especially for maxillary implants.

2.1.6 Osteoporosis and Bisphosphonate Therapy

- Osteoporosis has been defined as a decrease in bone mass and bone density with an increased risk and/or incidence of fracture. Currently there is no evidence to suggest that clinical diagnosis of osteoporosis affects all parts of the skeleton uniformly. Thus, a diagnosis of osteoporosis in other parts of the skeleton does not presume that the maxilla and mandible are affected. A systematic review [10] reports no evidence for a higher failure rate of dental implants in the osteoporotic patient.
- The mode of action of bisphosphonate and other osteoporosis-related medications is to disrupt osteoclastic-mediated bone resorption, and this may reduce bone deposition by osteoblasts with a reduction in bone resorption and bone turnover.
- Medication-related osteonecrosis of the jaw is a potential complication with long-term use of bisphosphonates and complex surgeries. The impaired bone healing may leave exposed bone uncovered by mucosa resulting in chronic pain, infection, bone loss, and possible pathologic jaw fracture. The risk is increased in IV infusion therapy of these medications, other comorbidities, duration of medication usage, and the complexity of surgery.
- In a postal survey, Mavrokokki et al. [11] estimated the risk of osteonecrosis of the jaw after dental extraction to be 0.09–0.34% with weekly oral alendronate (Fosamax) and 6.7–9.1% with IV formulations used for bone malignancy.
- The American Association of Oral and Maxillofacial Surgeons updated position paper (2014) on bisphosphonate-related osteonecrosis of the jaws listed additional risk factors of corticosteroid use, diabetes, smoking, poor oral hygiene, and chemotherapy [12]. Their recommendations are as follows:
  - For individuals on oral bisphosphonate for less than four years with no clinical risk factors, no alteration or delay in the planned surgery is necessary. It is suggested that if dental implants are placed, informed consent should be provided related to possible long-term implant failure and the low risk of developing osteonecrosis of the jaws if the patient continues to take an antiresorptive agent.
  - For those patients who have taken an oral bisphosphonate for less than four years and have also taken corticosteroids or anti-angiogenic medications

concomitantly, the prescribing provider should be contacted to consider discontinuation of the oral bisphosphonate (drug holiday) for at least two months prior to oral surgery, if systemic conditions permit. The antiresorptive should not be restarted until osseous healing has occurred.
  – For those patients who have taken an oral bisphosphonate for more than four years with or without any concomitant medical therapy, the prescribing provider should be contacted to consider discontinuation of the antiresorptive for two months prior to oral surgery, if systemic conditions permit. The bisphosphonate should not be restarted until osseous healing has occurred.
- Current management is based on minimal evidence and expert opinion with an emphasis on prevention. Informed consent must be attained on possible risks and complications. Ongoing careful monitoring is essential when considering implant treatment for these patients.

2.1.7 Radiotherapy

- Radiation treatment may lead to oral effects such as xerostomia, hypovascularity, mucositis, fibrosis, and osteoradionecrosis.
- A systematic review by Colella et al. [13] reported similar failure rates for implants placed pre-radiotherapy compared with those placed post-radiotherapy: 3.2 and 5.4%, respectively. Implant failure rate was significantly higher in the maxilla (17.5%) compared with the mandible (4.4%), with all implant failures occurring within three years after radiotherapy and most within 1–12 months. No implant failures were reported when radiation dose was less than 45 Gy.
- The adjunctive use of hyperbaric oxygen therapy (HBO) has been suggested in the treatment of irradiated patients. HBO increases the blood-to-tissue oxygen gradient, improving the healing capacity of irradiated tissue by stimulating capillary growth and osteogenesis. Treatment consists of breathing 100% pressurised oxygen for approximately 90 minutes for about 20 sessions pre-surgery and 10 post-surgery. Esposito et al. [14] in a Cochrane review of HBO and implant treatment failed to show any appreciable clinical benefits.
- Ihde et al. [15] reported in a systematic review that implants placed in irradiated bone exhibited a two to three times greater failure rate compared with non-irradiated bone, with doses above 50 Gy having a higher failure rate. No significant differences in failure rate were found with implants placed at various intervals, either before or after radiotherapy for a clinical recommendation to be made. However, implants placed in the maxilla were at least twice as likely to fail and no specific implant could be recommended based on survival data.

2.1.8 Dental History

Questioning on past history of dental treatment is helpful to understand the reason for tooth loss and to identify any risk factors that the patient may present with. The aetiology for tooth loss may be congenitally missing, periodontal disease, fractured or carious tooth beyond restoration, endodontic complications, along with other reasons. Patients that present with a history of periodontal disease may have lost significant amounts of alveolar bone, complicating implant treatment with the need for bony augmentation, as well as being in the higher risk category of peri-implantitis. Questions about how the tooth was removed or if there was difficulty in removal of the tooth may provide useful information, as surgical removal of the tooth and difficulty in extraction resulting in bone removal may indicate a need for future hard or soft tissue augmentation. Valuable information is gathered in the history that may enlighten the clinician as to what progressed prior to their visit to the practice.

Determining the level of the patient's expectations is important to assess whether it will be possible to achieve the desired result, or whether they may need to be referred to a more experienced colleague for assistance. In cases of deficient soft tissue, it may be virtually impossible to recreate perfect soft tissue aesthetics with natural dental papilla, and discussions on the use of pink replacement with porcelain may be necessary.

Excellent patient compliance is necessary for long-term success of dental implants, with regular dental attendance providing continual assessment, occlusal verification, and reinforcement of correct hygiene techniques. This provides the supportive care that a patient requires and at initial consultation it is necessary to advise the patient on the need for continual care. Regular oral hygiene with excellent plaque control will provide the environment for healthy peri-implant tissues, and implant therapy should only be initiated once this has been achieved.

2.1.9   Social History

A social history may include aspects of the patient's developmental, family, and medical history, as well as relevant information about life events, social class, race, religion, and occupation.

Asking the patient about any environmental influences such as alcohol, tobacco (amounts and durations), and drug use (including illicit drugs), along with the frequency, will assist in a complete history.

2.2   Tips

- A systematic and repeatable approach should be adopted, consulting with patients to ensure that a comprehensive history is taken.
- Documents and checklists may be used to ensure that clinicians do not miss critical information when taking history and examining patients. These may provide prompts when questioning patients on relevant information required.

References

1 Brånemark, P.-I., Adell, R., Breine, U. et al. (1969). Intra-osseous anchorage of dental prostheses: I. Experimental studies. *Scand J Plast Reconstr Surg* 3 (2): 81–100.

2 Chuang, S.K., Wei, L.J., Douglass, C.W., and Dodson, T.B. (2002 Aug). Risk factors for dental implant failure: a strategy for the analysis of clustered failure-time observations. *J Dent Res* 81 (8): 572–577.

3 Wood, M.R. and Vermilyea, S.G. (2004). A review of selected dental literature on evidence-based treatment planning for dental implants: report of the Committee on Research in Fixed Prosthodontics of the Academy of Fixed Prosthodontics. *J Prosthet Dent* 92 (5): 447–462.

4 Shernoff, A.F., Colwell, J.A., and Bingham, S.F. (1994 Oct). Implants for type II diabetic patients: interim report. VA implants in diabetes study group. *Implant Dent* 3 (3): 183–187.

5 Olson, J.W., Shernoff, A.F., Tarlow, J.L. et al. (2000 Nov). Dental endosseous implant assessments in a type 2 diabetic population: a prospective study. *Int J Oral Maxillofac Implants* 15 (6): 811–818.

6 Westwood, R.M. and Duncan, J.M. (1996 Nov). Implants in adolescents: a literature review and case reports. *Int J Oral Maxillofac Implants* 11 (6): 750–755.

7 Bain, C.A. (1996). Smoking and implant failure--benefits of a smoking cessation protocol. *Int J Oral Maxillofac Implants* 11 (6): 756–759.

8 Bain, C.A. and Moy, P.K. (1993 Nov). The association between the failure of dental implants and cigarette smoking. *Int J Oral Maxillofac Implants* 8 (6): 609–615.

9 De Bruyn, H. and Collaert, B. (1994 Dec). The effect of smoking on early implant failure. *Clin Oral Implants Res* 5 (4): 260–264.

10 Mombelli, A. and Cionca, N. (2006 Oct). Systemic diseases affecting osseointegration therapy. *Clin Oral Implants Res* 17 (S2): 97–103.

11 Mavrokokki, T., Cheng, A., Stein, B., and Goss, A. (2007 Mar). Nature and frequency of bisphosphonate-associated osteonecrosis of the jaws in Australia. *J Oral Maxillofac Surg* 65 (3): 415–423.

12 Ruggiero, S.L., Dodson, T.B., Fantasia, J. et al. (2014 Oct). American Association of Oral and Maxillofacial Surgeons position paper on medication-related osteonecrosis of the jaw—2014 update. *J Oral Maxillofac Surg* 72 (10): 1938–1956.

13 Colella, G., Cannavale, R., Pentenero, M., and Gandolfo, S. (2007 Jul). Oral implants in radiated patients: a systematic review. *Int J Oral Maxillofac Implants* 22 (4): 616–622.

14 Esposito, M., Grusovin, M.G., Patel, S. et al. (2008 Jan). Interventions for replacing missing teeth: hyperbaric oxygen therapy for irradiated patients who require dental implants. *Cochrane Database Syst Rev* 1: CD003603.

15 Ihde, S., Kopp, S., Gundlach, K., and Konstantinović, V.S. (2009 Jan). Effects of radiation therapy on craniofacial and dental implants: a review of the literature. *Oral Surg Oral Med Oral Pathol Oral Radiol Endod* 107 (1): 56–65.

3

Diagnostic Records
Aodhan Docherty and Christopher C.K. Ho

3.1 Principles

3.1.1 Diagnostic Imaging and Templates

Prosthodontically driven treatment planning is the objective of implant therapy, and imaging is an essential component of diagnosis and treatment planning. The use of radiographic imaging and templates (guides/stents) allow correct three-dimensional positioning of implants as well as avoiding any critical anatomical zones which may lead to neurovascular injury or damage to other structures.

Diagnostic imaging provides information about:

- The quantity of bone
- The quality of bone
- Relationships to critical anatomical structures such as the inferior alveolar nerve, nasopalatine canal, mental foramen, maxillary sinus, and other teeth
- The presence of disease and pathology.

Radiographic imaging is used in pre-surgical planning to determine the length and width of the proposed dental implant, and the position within the alveolus. Modern implant dentistry requires accuracy of implant positioning to attain natural aesthetics with correct emergence and proper contours of the final restorations. The use of imaging and surgical guides can facilitate proper 3D placement. Poor implant placement can lead to soft tissue deficiencies with loss of papilla, recession, or damage to other anatomical structures.

Historically, clinicians were limited to using conventional two-dimensional imaging for dental implant treatment planning. The main drawbacks of 2D imaging are the lack of cross-sectional information and precise location of anatomical structures [1]. These 2D imaging techniques include the following:

- *Intra-oral periapical radiographs*: Using a parallel technique, this image provides high-resolution information and any potential associated pathology and disease in the local region; however, it is limited in the physical size of the film and being a single plane.

- *Occlusal radiographs*: These provide an overall view of the patient's bony anatomy, but they provide limited information due to superimposition of structures and magnification.
- *Lateral cephalometric radiographs*: These provide the mid-sagittal jaw width as well as the maxillo-mandibular jaw relationship.
- *Panoramic radiographs*: These provide an overview of vital structures and quantity of bone. However, magnification and distortion are a major limitation, and the panoramic view provides no cross-sectional information. It is still widely used during the diagnostic phase as an initial screening record.

3.1.1.1 Three-Dimensional Imaging

Computed tomography (CT) has revolutionised treatment planning for dental implants. It provides a vast array of images in high resolution, such as panoramic, cross-sectional, axial, and 3D. The major drawbacks are cost, accessibility, and higher radiation dosage. With radiation dosage in mind, the advent of cone beam computed tomography (CBCT) scanners in the late 1990s have been designed for the maxillofacial region. CBCT imaging reduces the radiation exposure to the patient and is also more accessible as many dental offices and radiology centres possess these machines. CBCT provides high-resolution images allowing visualisation of anatomical structures and identification of local pathology, and provides multiplanar views of the tissue volume to be investigated. CBCT utilises a cone-shaped X-ray beam with both the source and detector rotating around the patient. It is currently the recommended comprehensive diagnostic method to obtain a comprehensive analysis for implant placement. The American Academy of Oral and Maxillofacial Radiology consider the CBCT as a standard of care examination for dental implant planning [2].

Radiographic imaging aims to follow the ALARA principle, which is to use a dose that is as low as reasonably achievable. Intra-oral radiographs and orthopantomograms typically deliver dosage equivalent to days of background radiation, while the CBCT emits dosages of a week or more of additional background radiation. CT imaging is equivalent to several weeks of background radiation. The CBCT allows selection of smaller field of view (FOV) and by restricting it to the region of interest (ROI) there is a reduction in the effective dose of radiation (Table 3.1).

The limitation with CBCT is in assessment of soft tissue volume and the use of CT imaging is preferred if an assessment of soft tissue volumes is needed. A further limitation for both CT and CBCT is artefacts from the presence of radiopaque restorations and implants. This can be seen as cupping (distortion of metallic objects), beam hardening (dark streaks between dense objects), scatter, and motion artefacts (longer exposure times are vulnerable to patient movement).

3.1.1.2 Templates

Radiographic templates can be used in diagnostic imaging, and these are based on desired tooth positions, and accordingly planned with correct spacing and biomechanical principles. These guides are used to determine if the desired implant prosthesis is possible and can assist the surgeon in determining if augmentation is required at the surgical site. They must replicate the desired final tooth position and must be stable during the process of taking the CBCT. There

Table 3.1 Ionising radiation dosage chart: comparing background radiation to both dental, medical and the yearly Australian safety limit.

Procedure	Effective dose (μSv)	Dose as days of equivalent background radiation
1 day of background radiation (sea level)	7–8	1
1 dental PA radiograph	6	1
Kodak CBCT focused field anterior	4.7	0.71
Kodak CBCT focused field maxillary posterior	9.8	1.4
Kodak CBCT focused field mandibular posterior	38.3	5.47
Chest X-ray	170	25
Medical CT (head)	2000	1515
Federal occupational safety limit per year (Australia)	The current legal limit of radiation exposure for Australian workers is 20 000 μSv/y averaged over 5 years, and not more than 50 000 μSv received in any 1 year for effective (whole-body) dose	

Sources: Ludlow, J.B., Davies-Ludlow, L.E., Brooks, S.L. et al. (2006). Dosimetry of 3 CBCT devices for oral and maxillofacial radiology. *Dentomaxillofac. Rad.* 35: 219–226; White, S.C. and Pharaoh, M.J. (2009). *Oral Radiology: Principles and Interpretation.* St. Louis, MO: Mosby Elsevier; Australian Radiation Protection and Nuclear Safety Agency (2016). *Radiation Protection in Planned Exposure Situations.* ARPANSAR.

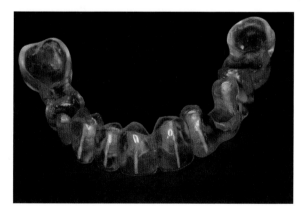

Figure 3.1 Analogue/traditional radiographic template.

are various methods for creating radiographic guides including conventional analogue and more recent digital techniques:

- The analogue technique traditionally starts from waxing up the desired teeth on articulated study models, creating a vacuum-formed retainer or acrylic template, then filling the desired positions with a radiopaque material (Figure 3.1).

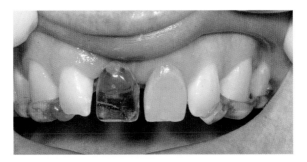

Figure 3.2 Acrylic radiographic/surgical guide.

- Digital techniques begin with intra-oral scans and the desired tooth position is planned. The radiographic guide can then be milled or 3D printed.

Templates (guides/stents) have various functions:

- They simulate prescribed teeth in the intended implant sites. These are positioned according to prosthodontic planning with the numbers of implants as well as the position of the teeth for best aesthetics, function, and phonetics. The implants are positioned so that they are 1.5 mm away from teeth and 3 mm from adjacent implants.
- They indicate any need to replace soft and/or hard tissues.
- They are used in surgical site assessment, radiographic assessment, and surgical placement of implants. This may also allow visualisation to see whether screw retention is possible.

Radiographic templates constructed during the initial prosthetic work-up may be used in conjunction with the CBCT, allowing the clinician to determine whether bone grafting will be needed and also to guide the clinician in choosing an appropriate prosthesis [3].

Various methods have been used to allow imaging with the use of gutta percha markers, radiopaque teeth, or barium sulfate in acrylic. The use of radiopaque gutta percha markers have been used to simulate the alignment of the implants which provide information about the intended placement on the cross-sectional imaging. These gutta percha markers are then removed, and the radiographic templates can further be modified to become a surgical template (Figure 3.2). These templates indicate teeth position but are not precisely defined due to the fact that the surgeon may have to manually correct the placement of implants.

The templates can be supported by teeth, implants, mucosa, and bone. They need to be stable, retentive, and to fit accurately as poor fit may lead to poor positioning of the template, leading to errors in the implant position. Furthermore, they should be rigid and not easily distorted when inserting.

3.1.2 Guided Surgery

Prosthetic planning has evolved to allow virtual implant planning. CT and CBCT imaging have facilitated advances in the treatment planning of dental implants as the information can now be transferred to implant-planning software to digitally

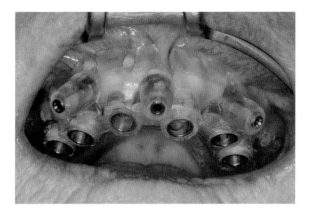

Figure 3.3 Guided surgery in a full arch implant rehabilitation.

plan the case. This is achieved by merging CBCT and intra-oral scans, allowing clinicians to perform virtual tooth and implant placement, and even to perform guided surgery (Figure 3.3). These computer-aided design (CAD) programs are used to fabricate surgical templates which are manufactured by either stereo-lithography (SLA) or 3D printing. In a recent systematic review, Tahmaseb et al. [4] identified 24 clinical and preclinical accuracy studies involving nine different static surgical guidance systems. Meta-analysis of the accuracy related a total mean error of 1.12 mm (maximum of 4.5 mm) at the entry point of the osteotomy and 1.39 mm at the apex (maximum of 7.1 mm). The angular difference between planned and obtained position was 3.53 degrees (maximum of 21.16 degrees). Although the average accuracy was quite acceptable it was reported that there were significant errors as demonstrated by the maximum errors. These are mainly due to the potential for the templates to not fit correctly or move during placement. The use of guided surgery should therefore be attempted with care, with special attention to accurate template fitting prior to use. The most accurate templates have been tooth-supported templates, whereas bone-supported templates have been reported to have the highest inaccuracy [4]. Further development is required to improve the accuracy of static surgical guidance systems.

Further technological advances have led to the launch of dynamic surgical navigation (e.g. X-Guide™; X-Nav Technologies) in which real-time surgery is guided using computer software and delivers interactive information to improve the precision and accuracy of implant positioning.

3.1.3 Diagnostic Records

3.1.3.1 Articulated Study Models
Study models that have been articulated with a facebow transfer record and a maxillo-mandibular relationship (MMR) record allow the clinician to measure and analyse occlusal relationships and spatial considerations, and to manufacture templates. The casts can be used to create a diagnostic set-up of the proposed prosthesis using wax and/or denture teeth. This set-up may then be transferred to

the mouth to be evaluated, used as a radiographic guide or a surgical guide, and potentially transformed into a provisional restoration. More recently, the use of chairside intra-oral scanning, DICOM data files from CBCT, and STL files from 3D optical scanning are merged to allow planning with interactive 3D software. The proposed virtual set-up of teeth allows visualisation of the planned restoration in relation to the bone and soft tissue architecture. This allows analysis of the bony ridge in relation to the planned tooth position, so that the length, diameter, position, and alignment of implants can be determined accurately.

3.1.3.2 Photographic Records

Photography is an essential diagnostic and communication tool for the implant clinician. Comprehensive treatment planning takes time and deliberation, hence photographs are an essential step in the process as they allow the clinician to view both the intra-oral and extra-oral clinical situation when the patient is not in the dental practice. Photographs can be used to educate patients, helping them to understand the proposed treatment, and are important clinical records and aids in the treatment planning process.

3.2 Procedures

3.2.1 Template Design

3.2.1.1 Traditional Templates

Various methods have been used in imaging, including the use of gutta percha markers, radiopaque teeth, or barium sulfate in acrylic resin. The use of radiopaque gutta percha markers have been used to simulate the alignment of the implants, providing information about the intended placement on the cross-sectional imaging. These gutta percha markers are then removed, and the radiographic templates further modified to become a surgical template. These templates indicate teeth position but are not precisely defined because the surgeon may have to manually correct the placement of implants upon assessing the imaging.

3.2.1.2 Digital Templates

More recently, digital scanning has allowed us to 'digitally' wax up the tooth in the gap, design a template, and then either mill or 3D print this in acrylic. The design of the digital template should ensure that there is adequate support from hard tissues such as teeth adjacent to the gap, and the missing tooth is included in the template, so the doctor may drill through it to prepare space for the radiographic markers. Some doctors prefer to have 'windows' cut out of the acrylic to visually ensure seating of the template.

Although the digital workflow is constantly evolving, historically it began with this approach:

1) Intra-oral scanning (or conventional impressions)
2) Construction of digital radiographic guides with radiopaque marker

3) CBCT (small FOV)
4) Conversion of radiographic guide to surgical guide based on the findings of the CBCT.

Modern digital workflows involve a streamlined approach which allows creation of the surgical guide being designed and milled from an initial intra-oral scan and CBCT:

1) Intra-oral scanning (or conventional impressions)
2) CBCT (small FOV)
3) Merging the intra-oral scan with the CBCT, design and construction of a surgical guide.

3.2.2 Photography

The following sets of photographs are a minimum standard:

- *Full face (frontal)*: This image is shot at the same level as the patient and should cover their whole head. This vertical angle is important for majority of the images taken in dental photography. The interpupillary line and long axis of teeth is used to align the camera (Figure 3.4).
- *Full smile – frontal, right, and left lateral view*: This view shows the lips as well as the teeth visible for this angle. The upper lateral incisor is centred on the slide. The contralateral central incisor should be visible and possibly the lateral incisor and canine (Figures 3.5–3.7).

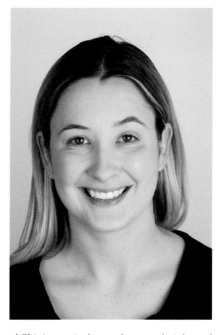

Figure 3.4 Full face frontal. This image is shot at the same height as the patient, including their whole head, and can be taken with lips at rest and also in broad smile.

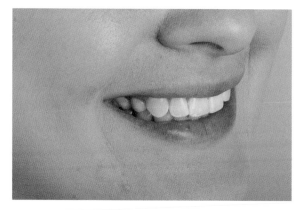

Figure 3.5 Right lateral smile.

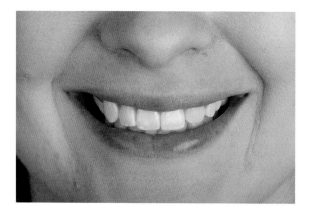

Figure 3.6 Frontal smile.

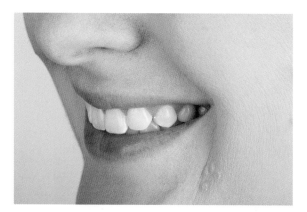

Figure 3.7 Left lateral smile.

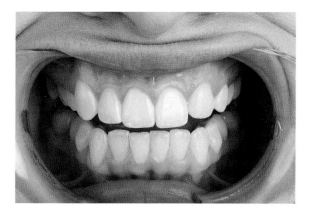

Figure 3.8 Retracted frontal shot with teeth apart.

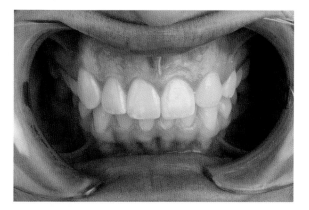

Figure 3.9 Retracted frontal shot with teeth in maximum intercuspation.

- *Retracted anterior view*: This is an intra-oral photograph using retractors held by the patient, with the teeth together or slightly apart (Figures 3.8 and 3.9).
- *Upper and lower right and left lateral retracted view*: The image is centred on the lateral incisor so that it is in the centre of the picture. The retractor is pulled to side that the picture is being taken of, while the contralateral retractor is loosely held which allows the photograph to extend further posteriorly to capture the posterior teeth (Figures 3.10 and 3.11).
- *Upper and lower occlusal retracted view (use mirror)*: This is a reflected view from a high-quality mirror, with as many teeth as possible included. Keep the mirror clear of fogging by warming it or using an air–water syringe. The mouth should be opened as wide as possible to allow the best mirror position. In the lower jaw is exactly the same as with the upper teeth but the patient needs to be asked to keep their tongue back so that is does not obscure the teeth (Figures 3.12 and 3.13).

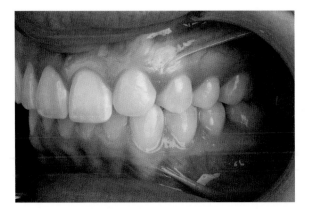

Figure 3.10 Retracted left photograph displaying left side of teeth. The left lateral incisor should be in the centre of the photograph.

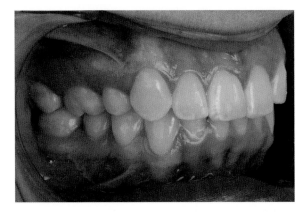

Figure 3.11 Retracted right photograph displaying right side of teeth. The right lateral incisor should be in the centre of the photograph.

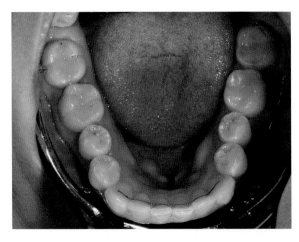

Figure 3.12 Occlusal photograph of mandibular teeth using a photographic mirror.

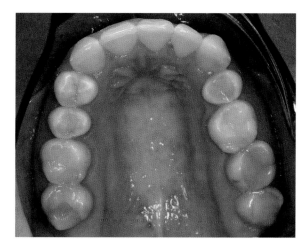

Figure 3.13 Occlusal photograph of maxillary teeth using a photographic mirror.

3.3 Tips

- Conventional periapical and panoramic imaging is still very useful for treatment planning. Although CBCT is essential in planning, it can be difficult to appreciate the crown and root position of teeth adjacent to the planned site, because any given slice will vary. Clinicians who rely upon one slice during placement may encounter issues with proximity of the implant to the adjacent teeth.
- When using surgical templates, ensure windows are cut out of the template adjacent to the implant sites to allow the clinician to visualise that the template fits accurately. These windows can be located in different parts of the template as well as in close proximity to the osteotomy site.
- Practise the ALARA principle in radiographic imaging and, when possible, reduce the FOV to the ROI. Most modern CBCT machines are able to reduce FOV, thus lowering any dosage to patients.

References

1 Fortes, J., de Oliveira-Santos, C., Matsumoto, W. et al. (2018). Influence of 2D vs 3D imaging and professional experience on dental implant treatment planning. *Clin. Oral Investig.* 23: 929–936.
2 Harris, D., Horner, K., Gröndahl, K. et al. (2012). E.A.O. guidelines for the use of diagnostic imaging in implant dentistry 2011. A consensus workshop organized by the European Association for Osseointegration at the Medical University of Warsaw. *Clin. Oral Implants Res.* 23: 1243–1253.
3 Tischler, M. (2010). Treatment planning implant dentistry: an overview for the general dentist. *Gen. Dent.* 58 (5): 368–374.
4 Tahmaseb, A., Wismeijer, D., Coucke, W., and Derksen, W. (2014). Computer technology applications in surgical implant dentistry: a systematic review. *Int. J. Oral Maxillofac. Implants* 29 (Suppl): 25–42.

4

Medico-Legal Considerations and Risk Management

Christopher C.K. Ho

4.1   Principles

As dental professionals we possess a duty of care to exercise appropriate knowledge, skill, and care to our patients. There are ethical obligations attached to membership of the profession to provide an optimal level of care. The doctor/patient relationship is underpinned by two fundamental principles: 'beneficence', doing good and acting in the patient's best interests, and 'non-maleficence', doing no harm [1]. The Latin phrase *primum non nocere*, or first do no harm, is one of the fundamental principles in healthcare practice. It is important to gain the necessary informed consent for patients so that they not only understand the advantages and disadvantages of treatment, but also any risks or inadvertent outcomes that may occur.

There are different laws and regulations in each country that may impact dental practice and these are present to ensure the safety of patient care. This may involve having evidence of competency for the intended treatment, and infection control, workplace safety, continuing education requirements, and materials that can be used in practice.

It is important to only provide treatment for which you have appropriate training within your scope of practice. A clinician should be able to demonstrate the experience and education undertaken, completing a logbook of all continuing professional development attended. Furthermore, a clinician will need to record all aspects of the examination, assessment, and treatment, as well as consent attained, in a neat and legible manner. With the advent of digital records this has improved record keeping, helping legibility and avoiding any deterioration in radiographic records, such as happened in the past with dental film. The increasing use of digital impressions and scanning has taken away the onerous task of storing physical models, allowing data storage in the cloud and giving the ability to access the virtual models relatively easily.

4.1.1   Informed Consent

Informed consent is permission granted in full knowledge of the possible consequences, typically that which is given by a patient to a doctor for treatment with

Practical Procedures in Implant Dentistry, First Edition. Edited by Christopher C.K. Ho.
© 2022 John Wiley & Sons Ltd. Published 2022 by John Wiley & Sons Ltd.
Companion website: www.wiley.com/go/ho/implant-dentistry

knowledge of the possible risks and benefits. As implant treatment is an elective treatment it should involve a two-way communication between patient and clinician that provides an unbiased and objective view of the treatment. This includes the intended outcome, alternatives to treatment, and an understanding of treatment difficulty and risk of complications or failure. It is customary that this is conveyed to the patient verbally; many clinicians also provide informed consent forms and other literature that clearly document treatment for patients.

4.2 Procedures

4.2.1 Dental Records

Dental records are important medical and legal records documenting all aspects of treatment along with information on what biomaterials, hardware, and implant systems were used. They should be complete, accurate, and legible. If a complaint is encountered in relation to treatment the records are your only defence if the patient proceeds with legal action.

The records should include:

- Reason for attendance (chief complaint)
- Medical history
- Dental history
- Social and family history
- Clinical assessment – extra-oral and intra-oral examination
- Diagnostic records, including photographs, radiographs, study models, diagnostic wax-up, etc.
- Surgical phase of treatment:
  - Medications administered or prescribed, including local anaesthetics, sedation, and antibiotics, with their dosage
  - Surgical flap design and wound closure, including suture size and type
  - Implant components with type of implant system and the lot numbers
  - Biomaterial usage, including bone graft, membranes, tacks
  - Primary stability and insertion torque, implant stability quotient (ISQ) values
  - Post-operative instructions and management
- Prosthodontic phase:
  - Implant integration assessment
  - Impression technique and materials
  - Shade selection and photography
  - Laboratory prescription
  - Insertion of prosthesis with components used, abutment screw torque, type of retention (screw/cement) and screw access closure
  - Radiographs to document baseline radiographs
  - Oral hygiene instruction and continuing care frequency
- Continuing care:
  - Assess prosthesis integrity
  - Assess occlusion

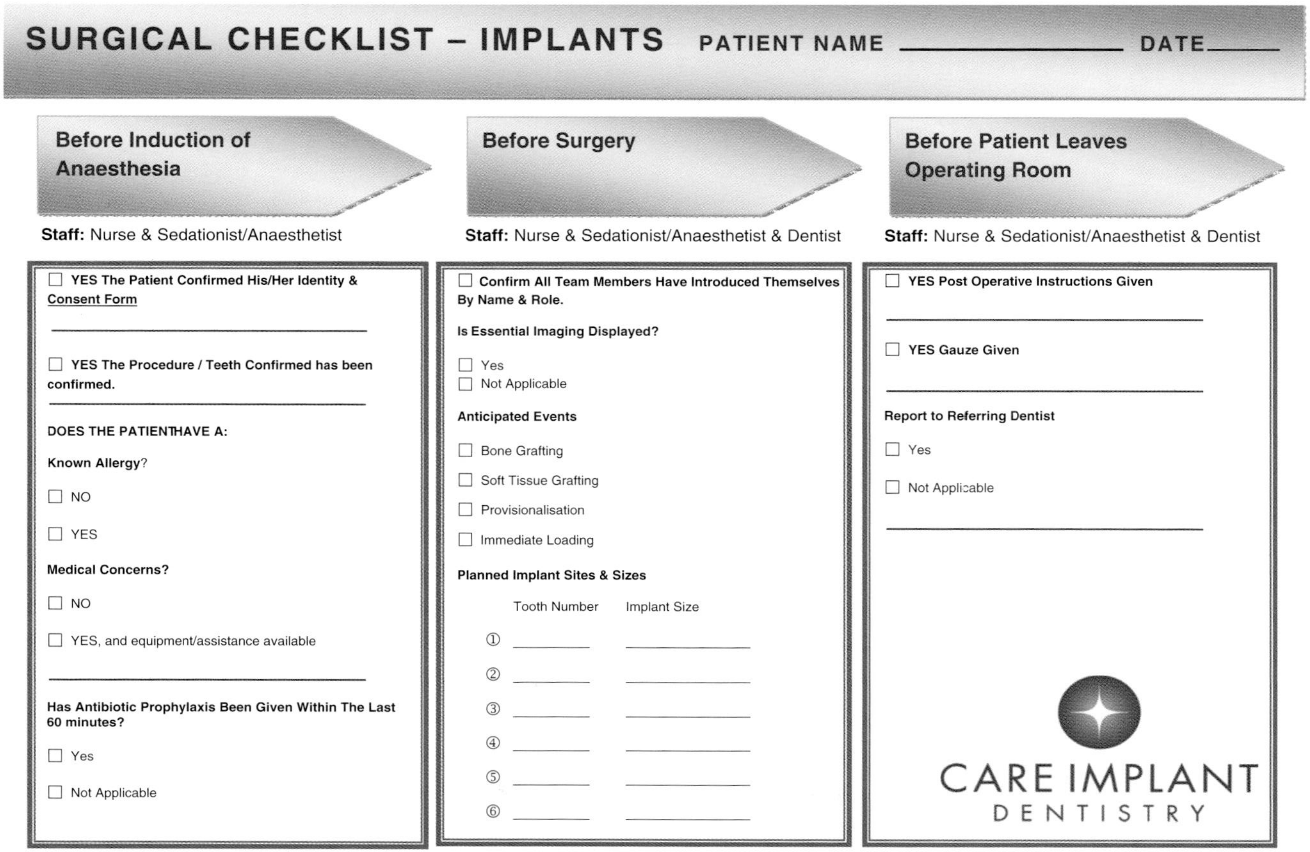

SURGICAL CHECKLIST – IMPLANTS   PATIENT NAME _____   DATE _____

Before Induction of Anaesthesia

Staff: Nurse & Sedationist/Anaesthetist

☐ YES The Patient Confirmed His/Her Identity & Consent Form

☐ YES The Procedure / Teeth Confirmed has been confirmed.

DOES THE PATIENT HAVE A:

Known Allergy?

☐ NO

☐ YES

Medical Concerns?

☐ NO

☐ YES, and equipment/assistance available

Has Antibiotic Prophylaxis Been Given Within The Last 60 minutes?

☐ Yes

☐ Not Applicable

Before Surgery

Staff: Nurse & Sedationist/Anaesthetist & Dentist

☐ Confirm All Team Members Have Introduced Themselves By Name & Role.

Is Essential Imaging Displayed?

☐ Yes

☐ Not Applicable

Anticipated Events

☐ Bone Grafting

☐ Soft Tissue Grafting

☐ Provisionalisation

☐ Immediate Loading

Planned Implant Sites & Sizes

	Tooth Number	Implant Size
①	_____	_____
②	_____	_____
③	_____	_____
④	_____	_____
⑤	_____	_____
⑥	_____	_____

Before Patient Leaves Operating Room

Staff: Nurse & Sedationist/Anaesthetist & Dentist

☐ YES Post Operative Instructions Given _____

☐ YES Gauze Given _____

Report to Referring Dentist

☐ Yes

☐ Not Applicable _____

CARE IMPLANT
DENTISTRY

Figure 4.1 Example of a surgical checklist. Source: Care Implant Dentistry.

 – Assess peri-implant tissue health with probing depths and bleeding on probing
 – Radiographs to monitor bone levels.

4.3 Tips

- *Checklists*: A checklist is a type of aid used to reduce failure by compensating for potential limits of human memory and attention (Figure 4.1). It helps to ensure consistency and completeness in carrying out a task. It is good practice to have a checklist summary to provide consistency of care because clinicians and their teams often lull themselves into skipping steps after performing procedures multiple times as it becomes familiar and repetitive. A checklist may aid in protecting against such failure and remind the team of the steps and procedures required. The author likes to work with checklists both at consultation and treatment procedures. At the time of consultation a checklist ensures everything is explained to the patient, with written documentation of what was communicated. Moreover, this is carried through into clinical practice, with checklists on what is required for procedures, as well as a pre-surgical checklist to confirm that patients are ready for their surgical procedure. An example of what may be included in this pre-surgical checklist includes:
  – Patient confirmation of procedure
  – Medical history update, including any medications taken and allergies
  – Pre-operative antibiotics and pain medications
  – Planned implant and components in stock
  – Anticipated events, e.g. soft tissue or hard tissue grafting, provisionalisation, and immediate loading.
- Make sure you have explained all treatment options, even those you may not consider within your area of expertise. This should include all advantages and disadvantages as well as any risks of treatment.
- Be prepared to refer the patient if the treatment is beyond your area of expertise or experience.
- It is good practice to conduct a consultation with your patient and provide a written treatment plan. Time must be allowed for the patient to have opportunity to discuss and ask any questions pertaining to their intended treatment.
- The patient needs to be informed of all likely costs and time for treatment. This should also include any future costs of treatment including any maintenance required.

Reference

1 Banerji, S., Mehta, S., and Ho, C. (2017). *Practical Procedures in Aesthetic Dentistry*, 3–5. Chichester: Wiley.

5

Considerations for Implant Placement

Effects of Tooth Loss

Kyle D. Hogg

5.1 Principles

Tooth extractions are among the most commonly performed dental procedures worldwide, with the wound created in the form of the extraction socket typically healing in a routine and uneventful manner. The effects of tooth loss in humans can perhaps best be understood when viewed at three related levels, namely: local site effects, effects on the individual, and effects on the population (Figure 5.1). The effects of tooth loss on the site, individual, and population levels have a profound influence on clinical decision-making and treatment strategies. While the site of the extraction heals in a predictable manner, the impact of the loss of the tooth on the individual can be quite variable. There is considerable evidence relating tooth loss to diminished oral health-related quality of life at the population level, and in addition a more heterogeneous experience can be found at the individual level [1].

5.1.1 Local Site Effects of Tooth Loss

The loss of a tooth or teeth initiates a dynamic sequence of events resulting in marked changes to the surrounding alveolar process of the jaw, largely a tooth-dependent structure [2], while causing little change to the underlying basal bone. The gradual pattern of bone resorption in the mandible is depicted in Figure 5.2, which shows the contour changes from the dentate state (image on lower left) to advanced alveolar bone loss (image on upper right).

Immediately following tooth extraction, the residual socket fills with blood and a clot is formed [3, 4]. The blood clot occupying the volume of the socket is rapidly remodelled within the first week following extraction, with granulation tissue rich in vascular structures, fibroblasts, and inflammatory cells beginning to fill the socket [3, 5]. Connective tissue begins to replace granulation tissue between the first and third weeks post-extraction [3, 5, 6]. The epithelium then migrates across the underlying connective tissue at this time, soon closing the orifice of the extraction socket. The granulation tissue and connective tissue is

Practical Procedures in Implant Dentistry, First Edition. Edited by Christopher C.K. Ho.
© 2022 John Wiley & Sons Ltd. Published 2022 by John Wiley & Sons Ltd.
Companion website: www.wiley.com/go/ho/implant-dentistry

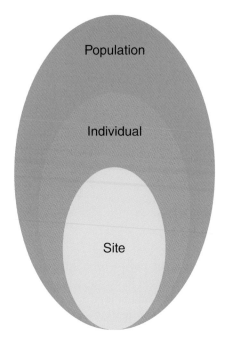

Figure 5.1 Tripartite effect of tooth loss.

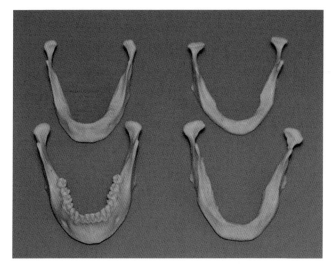

Figure 5.2 Resorption patterns of the mandibular edentulous ridge (note the significant reduction of the alveolar process with lesser change of the underlying basal bone).

gradually replaced by a primary matrix and woven bone at approximately six weeks post-extraction, with the socket predominantly containing primary matrix and woven bone by weeks 12–24 [3, 5]. While initial tissue modelling in the extraction socket is a relatively rapid process, remodelling of woven bone into lamellar bone requires more time, with little observation of the lamellar bone

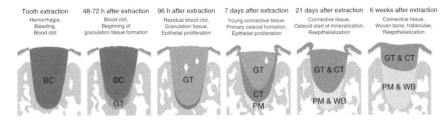

Tooth extraction	48-72 h after extraction	96 h after extraction	7 days after extraction	21 days after extraction	6 weeks after extraction
Hemorrhagia, Bleeding, Blood clot	Blood clot, Beginning of granulation tissue formation	Residual blood clot, Granulation tissue, Epithelial proliferation	Young connective tissue, Primary osteoid formation, Epithelial proliferation	Connective tissue, Osteoid start of mineralization, Reepithelialization	Connective tissue, Woven bone, trabeculae, Reepithelialization

Figure 5.3 Progressive healing of extraction socket. BC, blood clot; GT, granulation tissue; CT, connective tissue; PM, provisional matrix; WB, woven bone.

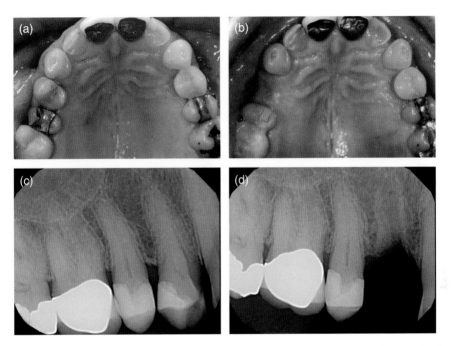

Figure 5.4 Hard and soft tissue healing of a single tooth extraction. (a) Clinical photograph of UR4 prior to atraumatic extraction and (b) four months following extraction. (c) Radiographic image of UR4 prior to extraction, and (d) four months following extraction.

being present at 12–24 weeks post-extraction [5]. Figure 5.3 depicts how the healing process of the extraction socket evolves over time.

This return to tissue homeostasis does not prevent alterations to the local hard and soft tissue contours following healing, as the resulting residual ridge architecture is diminished in both horizontal and, to a lesser degree, vertical dimensions (Figure 5.4). The clinical reduction of alveolar ridge width upon healing was found to be 3.87 mm on average, while the clinical vertical reduction was 1.67 mm [7]. The alteration of the residual ridge width is most pronounced on the buccal aspect [8, 9]. This observed pattern of resorption often results in a narrower and shorter ridge that is relocated to a more palatal or lingual position relative to its pre-extraction condition [10]. This pattern of bone loss may have a direct influence over the subsequent positioning of any replacement teeth proposed, both for functional and aesthetic purposes.

The alteration of soft tissue dimension following tooth extraction happens more rapidly than that of the hard tissue, with more than 50% of the changes observed in the first two weeks following extraction [11]. In the pre-extraction condition, no significant correlation has been observed between soft tissue thickness and the buccal bony wall thickness under the tissue [12]. Soft tissue thickness generally tends to increase, sometimes quite substantially, following tooth extraction in subjects with the more common thin buccal bony wall phenotypes [11, 13]. This thickening of the soft tissues may mask an underlying deficient bony ridge. Conversely, subjects exhibiting thicker bony wall phenotypes do not exhibit changes in the facial soft tissue thickness from the pre-extraction condition [11].

Changes in hard and soft tissues following extraction of a tooth may be further exacerbated by systemic factors such as smoking [14]. Local site-specific factors include the pre-existing condition of the tooth and surrounding tissue, the number and proximity of teeth being extracted, the number and proximity of teeth remaining, the condition of the extraction socket after tooth removal, the influence of hard and soft tissue biotype, and the use of an interim prosthesis [15].

5.1.2   Effects of Tooth Loss on the Individual Level

There is variability not only in the way which individuals heal from an extraction of a tooth, but also how the individual responds to the loss of the tooth from a functional, emotional, and quality of life perspective. While initial soft tissue healing occurs consistently during the first few weeks post-extraction in almost all individuals, there is a greater variability in the period of time during which mineralised bone is formed in the socket [5]. Tooth loss in general can be the cause of functional or aesthetic impairment, creating difficulties in chewing efficiency, phonetics, or aesthetic challenges, depending upon the location and number of teeth lost (Figure 5.5). Notably there is strong evidence that the distribution and location of tooth loss has an impact on the oral health-related quality of life. Oral health-related quality of life scores tend to drop sharply when lacking a minimum number of occluding pairs of teeth (10 occluding pairs) or total remaining teeth (20 teeth) [1], consistent with the concept of a shortened dental arch [16]. Studies on the impact of tooth loss on an individual's quality of life consist of pooled data reported at the population level and thus may mask heterogeneous data at the individual level. There appears to be wide variation in the emotional response to tooth loss among individuals that cannot be linked closely to the distribution or number of teeth lost [17].

5.1.3   Effects of Tooth Loss on the Population Level

Rates of complete edentulism have been decreasing, particularly in the past few decades, in a number of countries [18]. However, considerable variation exists in the rate of edentulism in many populations, with no simple observable relationship between socio-economic and socio-demographic indicators and complete edentulism rates, nor enhanced access to care and complete

(a)

(b)

(c)

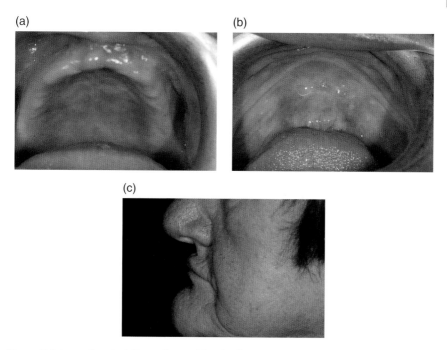

Figure 5.5 Loss of vertical dimension and facial soft tissue support. (a, b) Clinical image of patient's edentulous maxilla (a) and mandible (b). (c) Resulting effect on patient's facial profile, vertical dimension, and soft tissue support without prosthetic replacement of teeth.

edentulism rates [19]. There is a growing trend towards retention of teeth longer into life, leading to increased rates of partial edentulism, particularly in middle-aged populations and older [20]. Partially dentate individuals appear to have changing expectations and preferences to treatment strategies focused on conservation and restoration of missing teeth by fixed prostheses [21].

5.2 Procedures

Discussion of both short- and long-term effects of tooth loss should be a part of establishing meaningful informed consent for extraction of a tooth or teeth. During the pre-surgical consultation a thorough medical history should be taken with special consideration given to aspects which may be indicative of contraindications to surgical treatment or influence effective wound healing. A comprehensive extra- and intra-oral examination should be conducted and informed consent to the planned treatment and extractions should be obtained. Previous extraction sites should be examined closely as well, discussing the history and reason for extraction while evaluating the healing response to the extraction. An evaluation of the patient's temporomandibular joint and occlusal stability may help determine if the individual is a candidate for a shortened dental arch. Lastly, an open discussion on the anticipated effect of tooth loss on patient function, aesthetics, and phonetics should be conducted.

5.3 Tips

- Evaluate the pre-extraction hard and soft tissue contours at the site of anticipated tooth loss. Carefully consider how the mean horizontal and vertical (3.87 and 1.67 mm, respectively) reduction of the ridge might influence the planned surgical and restorative treatment.
- Utilise conventional radiography and, where indicated, three-dimensional imaging via cone beam computed tomography (CBCT) to assess the condition of the alveolar process, the buccal plate thickness, presence or absence of periapical pathology, and the proximity of important anatomical features prior to tooth extraction.
- Extract the tooth in an atraumatic manner in order to preserve the bone of the residual extraction socket and avoid iatrogenic trauma to the bone or soft tissues, which may lead to increased dimensional changes of the healed ridge.
- Upon removal of the tooth, thoroughly debride and explore the socket. Eliminate any soft tissue remnants and determine the relative continuity of the bony walls of the socket. Consider the benefits of no intervention versus ridge preservation versus ridge augmentation on the site of tooth loss and any future restorative treatment.
- The bone biotype can be estimated by running a gloved finger across the buccal surfaces of the maxillary and mandibular arches, feeling for root prominences. A smooth ridge may indicate a favourable bony contour following extraction, whereas a ridge which has significant bony prominences may result in considerable buccal bone loss following exodontia.

References

1 Gerritsen, A., Allen, P., Witter, D. et al. (2010). Tooth loss and oral-health related quality of life: A systematic review and meta-analysis. *Health and Quality of Life Outcomes* 8: 126–136.

2 Schroeder, H. (1986). The periodontium. In: *Handbook of Microscopic Anatomy*, vol. 5 (eds. A. Oksche and L. Vollrath), 233–246. Berlin: Springer.

3 Amler, M. (1969). The time sequence of tissue regeneration in human extraction wounds. *Oral Surgery Oral Medicine Oral Pathology* 27: 309–318.

4 Cardaropoli, G., Araujo, M., and Lindhe, J. (2003). Dynamics of bone tissue formation in tooth extrtaction sites. *Journal of Clinical Periodontology* 30: 809–818.

5 Trombelli, L., Farina, R., Marzola, A. et al. (2008). Modeling and remodeling of human extraction sockets. *Journal of Clinical Periodontology* 35: 630–639.

6 Evian, C., Rosenberg, E., Coslet, J., and Corn, H. (1982). The osteogenic activity of bone removed from healing extraction sites in humans. *Journal of Periodontology* 53: 81–85.

7 Van der Weijden, F., Dell'Acqua, F., and Slot, D. (2009). Alveolar bone dimensional changes of post-extraction sockets in humans: A systematic review. *J Clin Periodontol* 36: 1048–1058.

8 Lekovic, V., Camargo, P., Klokkevold, P. et al. (1998). Preservation of alveolar bone in extraction sockets using bioabsorbable membranes. *Journal of Periodontology* 69: 1044–1049.

9 Lekovic, V., Kenney, E., Weinlaender, M. et al. (1997). A bone regenerative approach to alveolar ridge maintenance following tooth extraction. Report of 10 cases. *Journal of Periodontology* 68: 563–570.

10 Pinho, M., Roriz, V., Novaes, A. Jr. et al. (2006). Titanium membranes in prevention of alveolar collapse after tooth extraction. *Implant Dentistry* 15: 53–61.

11 Chappuis, V., Engel, O., Shahim, K. et al. (2015). Soft tissue alterations in esthetic post-extraction sites: A three dimensional analysis. *Journal of Dental Research* 94 (Suppl): 187–193.

12 Zweers, J., Thomas, R., Slot, D. et al. (2014). Characteristics of periodontal biotype, its dimensions, associations, and prevalence: A systematic review. *J Clinical Periodontology* 41: 958–971.

13 Farmer, M. and Darby, I. (2014). Ridge dimensional changes following single-tooth extraction in the aesthetic zone. *Clinical Oral Implant Research* 25: 272–277.

14 Saldanha, J., Casati, M., Neto, F. et al. (2006). Smoking may affect the alveolar process dimensions and radiographic bone density in maxillary extraction sites: A prospective study in humans. *Journal of Oral and Maxillofacial Surgery* 63: 1359–1365.

15 Chen, S., Wilson, T. Jr., and Hammerle, C. (2004). Immediate or early placement of implants following tooth extraction: review of biological basis, clinical procedures, and outcomes. *Int J Oral Maxillofacial Implants* 19: 12–25.

16 Kayser, A. (1981). Shortened dental arches and oral function. *Journal of Oral Rehabilitation*: 457–462.

17 Davis, D.F., Scott, B., and Redford, D. (2000). The emotional effects of tooth loss: A preliminary quantitative study. *British Dental Journal* 188 (9): 503–506.

18 Osterberg, T. and Carlsson, G. (2007). Dental state, prosthodontic treatment and chewing ability - A study of five cohorts of 70 year-old subjects. *J Oral Rehabilitation* 34: 553–559.

19 Mojon, P. (2003). The world without teeth: Demographic trends. In: *Implant Overdentures: The standard of care for edentulous patients* (eds. J. Feine and G.E. Carlsson), 3–14. Chicago: Quintessence.

20 Marcus, S., Drury, T., Brown, L., and Zion, G. (1996). Tooth retention and tooth loss in the permanent dentition of adults: United States 1988 - 1991. *J Dent Research* 75: 684–695.

21 Cronin, M., Meaney, S., Jepson, N., and Allen, P. (2009). A qualitative study of trends in patient preferences for the management of the partially dentate state. *Gerodontology* 26: 137–142.

6

Anatomic and Biological Principles for Implant Placement
Kyle D. Hogg

6.1 Principles

Possessing a thorough knowledge of oral and maxillofacial anatomical structures is a prerequisite to providing safe, effective, and predictably successful implant surgery. Accurate assessment of a patient's anatomy during a pre-surgical evaluation is vitally important not only to develop a comprehensive plan of treatment, but also to limit the potential risks of surgical complications. Comprehensive medical histories, patient interviews, and clinical exams should be supplemented by conventional two-dimensional radiography and three-dimensional imaging, where indicated, to provide the surgeon with sufficient information regarding pertinent anatomy. This chapter will provide an overview of important anatomical structures of the head and neck, focusing on the osteology, vascularity, innervation, and musculature of the region. (For more information on the placement of dental implants in proximity to specific vital anatomical structures please refer to Chapters 7 and 8.)

6.1.1 Osteology

The skull is the skeletal structure of the head that serves to protect the brain and support the face. In the adult, the skull consists of 22 individual bones (8 paired bones, 6 single bones), 21 of which are immobile and combined into a single unit. The 22nd bone is the mandible, which, uniquely, is the only moveable bone of the skull. The skull can be further subdivided into the cranial bones (numbering 8) and facial bones (numbering 14). The cranial bones collectively form the cranial vault, which protects the brain and houses both middle and inner ear structures. The facial bones support the facial structures, form the nasal cavity and the orbit, and house the teeth. The facial bones are of particular importance in relation to dentofacial aesthetics and implantology, with the paired bones of the maxilla, palatine, and zygomatic arches as well as the single bone of the mandible routinely involved in implant treatment. Table 6.1 gives a summary of the bones comprising the skull [1]. Figures 6.1–6.3 show for skull osteology schematics and articulation.

Practical Procedures in Implant Dentistry, First Edition. Edited by Christopher C.K. Ho.
© 2022 John Wiley & Sons Ltd. Published 2022 by John Wiley & Sons Ltd.
Companion website: www.wiley.com/go/ho/implant-dentistry

Table 6.1 Osteology summary.

Bone	Paired	Single	Cranial/Facial	Articulation
Frontal		X	Cranial	Maxilla, zygomatic, sphenoid, parietal, ethmoid, nasal, lacrimal
Parietal	X		Cranial	Temporal, frontal, parietal, occipital, sphenoid
Temporal	X		Cranial	Mandible, zygomatic, sphenoid, parietal, occipital
Occipital		X	Cranial	Temporal, atlas (C1), parietal, sphenoid
Sphenoid		X	Cranial	Maxilla, ethmoid, palatine, vomer, frontal, parietal, temporal, occipital, zygomatic
Ethmoid		X	Cranial	Maxilla, palatine, vomer, nasal, lacrimal, inferior nasal concha, frontal, sphenoid
Zygomatic	X		Facial	Maxilla, frontal, temporal
Maxilla	X		Facial	Maxilla, zygomatic, frontal, sphenoid, ethmoid, palatine, vomer, nasal, lacrimal, inferior nasal concha
Palatine	X		Facial	Maxilla, palatine, vomer, inferior nasal concha, ethmoid, sphenoid
Vomer		X	Facial	Maxilla, palatine, ethmoid, sphenoid
Nasal	X		Facial	Maxilla, nasal, frontal
Lacrimal	X		Facial	Maxilla, frontal, ethmoid, inferior nasal concha
Inferior nasal concha	X		Facial	Maxilla, palatine, lacrimal, ethmoid
Mandible		X	Facial	Temporal

Source: Norton, N. (2007). *Netter's Head and Neck Anatomy for Dentistry.* Philadelphia: Saunders Elsevier. ©2007, Elsevier.

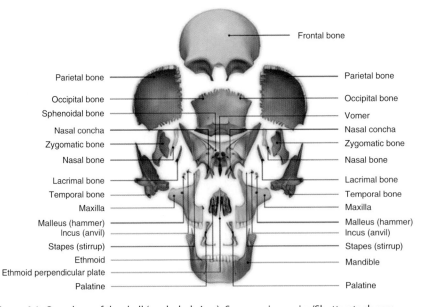

Figure 6.1 Osteology of the skull (exploded view). *Source:* sciencepics/Shutterstock.com.

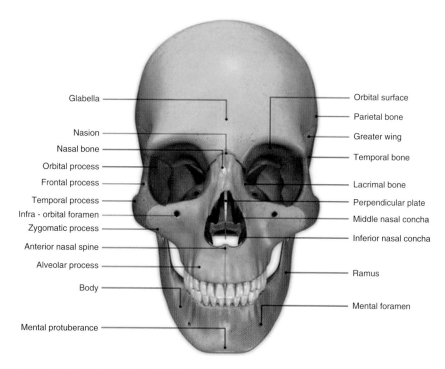

Glabella
Nasion
Nasal bone
Orbital process
Frontal process
Temporal process
Infra - orbital foramen
Zygomatic process
Anterior nasal spine
Alveolar process
Body
Mental protuberance

Orbital surface
Parietal bone
Greater wing
Temporal bone
Lacrimal bone
Perpendicular plate
Middle nasal concha
Inferior nasal concha
Ramus
Mental foramen

Figure 6.2 Osteology of the skull (frontal view). *Source*: sciencepics/Shutterstock.com.

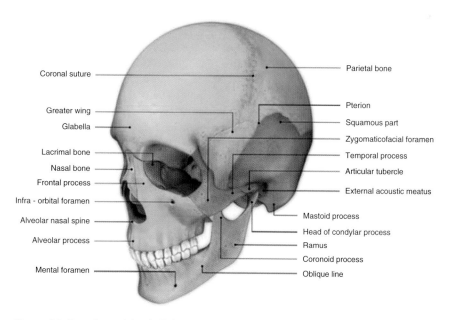

Coronal suture
Greater wing
Glabella
Lacrimal bone
Nasal bone
Frontal process
Infra - orbital foramen
Alveolar nasal spine
Alveolar process
Mental foramen

Parietal bone
Pterion
Squamous part
Zygomaticofacial foramen
Temporal process
Articular tubercle
External acoustic meatus
Mastoid process
Head of condylar process
Ramus
Coronoid process
Oblique line

Figure 6.3 Osteology of the skull (lateral view). *Source*: sciencepics/Shutterstock.com.

6.1.2 Innervation and Vascular Supply

The innervation and vascular supply of the maxillary and mandibular dentition are reliant upon the nerves and blood vessels that supply the bones in which they are housed, namely the paired bones of the maxilla and the singular mandible. The maxilla is an immobile part of the midface, with a neurovasculature separate from that of the mobile mandible, which is considered part of the lower face.

The second division of the trigeminal nerve (cranial nerve V division II, CN V2) is called the maxillary nerve, which is responsible for the sensory innervation of the maxillary dentition. It branches off the trigeminal nerve at the trigeminal ganglion and exits the skull via the foramen rotundum. It then branches into four major divisions: the posterior superior alveolar nerve (PSA), the infraorbital nerve, the zygomatic nerve, and branches to the pterygoid plexus. The infraorbital nerve further branches into the middle superior alveolar nerve (MSA) and the anterior superior alveolar nerve (ASA) [1].

The PSA, MSA, and ASA form the superior dental plexus. The PSA innervates the maxillary molars and posterior aspect of the maxillary sinus. The MSA innervates the premolars, the medial and lateral aspects of the maxillary sinus, and sometimes the mesiobuccal root of the first molar. The ASA innervates the incisors, canines, and the anterior aspect of the maxillary sinus.

The infraorbital nerve also exits the infraorbital foramen before branching off into the nasal, inferior palpebral, and superior labial nerves. These branches supply the cartilaginous ala of the nose, the dermal surface of the lower eyelid, and the upper lip, respectively.

Both maxillary and mandibular dentitions derive their blood supply from the external carotid artery via its maxillary artery branch. The maxillary arch is supplied by a plexus of three arteries: the PSA artery, the MSA artery, and the ASA artery. The PSA artery supplies the maxillary molars, premolars, and posterior maxillary sinus. The MSA artery (when present) and ASA artery both branch off of the infraorbital artery, and supply the premolar/canine region with medial and lateral aspects of the maxillary sinus, and anterior dentition with anterior aspects of the maxillary arch and sinus, respectively [2].

Venous drainage of the maxilla occurs via the PSA vein, the MSA vein, and the ASA vein, which converge to form the pterygoid venous plexus. The pterygoid venous plexus is drained via the relatively short maxillary vein to the retromandibular vein [1].

The third and largest division of the trigeminal nerve (cranial nerve V division III, CN V3) is called the mandibular nerve and is responsible for both sensory and motor innervation of the mandible after branching off the trigeminal ganglion and exiting the skull via the foramen ovale. The mandibular nerve then further divides into a meningeal branch, followed by another split into the anterior division and posterior division.

The anterior division is the smaller of the two divisions and mainly motor in function, with the exception of the buccal branch which remains sensory in nature. The other branches of the anterior division are the masseteric nerve, the anterior and posterior deep temporal nerves, the medial pterygoid nerve, and finally the lateral pterygoid nerve.

The larger posterior division conversely is mainly sensory in function, with the exception of the mylohyoid branch which remains motor in nature. The other branches of the posterior division are the auriculotemporal nerve, the lingual nerve, and the inferior alveolar nerve. The lingual nerve supplies sensory innervation to the mucous membranes of the anterior two-thirds of the tongue and the gingiva on the lingual aspect of the mandibular teeth. The inferior alveolar nerve is the largest branch of the mandibular nerve, running between the sphenomandibular ligament and mandibular ramus before entering the mandible at the mandibular foramen. The inferior alveolar nerve emerges from the mandible in the vicinity of the second premolar via the mental foramen. It provides sensory innervation to all mandibular teeth, associated periodontal ligaments, and the gingiva from the premolars anteriorly to the midline. The inferior alveolar nerve terminates into the mental and incisive nerves at the approximate level of the second premolar. The mental nerve supplies the chin, lip, facial gingiva, and mucosa from the second premolar anteriorly to the midline. The incisive nerve continues anteriorly supplying the teeth and periodontal ligaments from approximately the first premolar to the midline, depending on the location of where the branching of the inferior alveolar nerve into the mental and incisive nerves occurs [1].

The mandibular arch is supplied by a single branch of the maxillary artery called the inferior alveolar artery. It mirrors the path of the inferior alveolar nerve through the mandible via the mandibular foramen. Likewise, it terminates into the branches of the mental and incisive arteries at approximately the level of the second premolar. The mental and incisive arteries supply the labial gingiva of the anterior dentition and the anterior dentition themselves, respectively. Venous drainage of the mandible occurs via the singular inferior alveolar vein, which drains into the pterygoid venous plexus. Figures 6.4–6.6 give a detailed overview of the innervation and vascular supply of the skull.

6.1.3   Musculature

The muscles of the head and neck relevant to oral implantology can be categorised as muscles of mastication, which are paired muscles that aid in the process of grinding and chewing food and turning it into a bolus, and muscles of facial expression, which are generally flat paired muscles that enable movements of the face and facial expression. All muscles of mastication are innervated by branches of the mandibular division of the trigeminal nerve (CN V3), while all muscles of facial expression are innervated by branches of the facial nerve (CN VII). Tables 6.2 and 6.3 give summaries of key facts [1, 2] and Figure 6.7 shows an anatomical rendering.

6.2   Procedures

Begin the patient assessment with some light conversation with your patient comfortably seated in the dental chair. Discuss the patient's chief complaint and motivations for seeking treatment. Observe the functionality of the muscles of

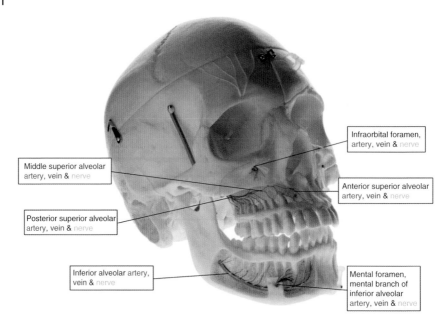

Infraorbital foramen, artery, vein & nerve

Middle superior alveolar artery, vein & nerve

Anterior superior alveolar artery, vein & nerve

Posterior superior alveolar artery, vein & nerve

Inferior alveolar artery, vein & nerve

Mental foramen, mental branch of inferior alveolar artery, vein & nerve

Figure 6.4 Innervation and vascular supply of the maxillary and mandibular dentition.

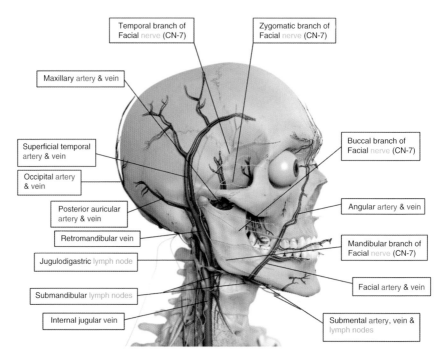

Temporal branch of Facial nerve (CN-7)

Zygomatic branch of Facial nerve (CN-7)

Maxillary artery & vein

Buccal branch of Facial nerve (CN-7)

Superficial temporal artery & vein

Occipital artery & vein

Posterior auricular artery & vein

Angular artery & vein

Retromandibular vein

Mandibular branch of Facial nerve (CN-7)

Jugulodigastric lymph node

Submandibular lymph nodes

Facial artery & vein

Internal jugular vein

Submental artery, vein & lymph nodes

Figure 6.5 Anatomical rendering of head and neck – lateral view. *Source*: SciePro/Shutterstock.com.

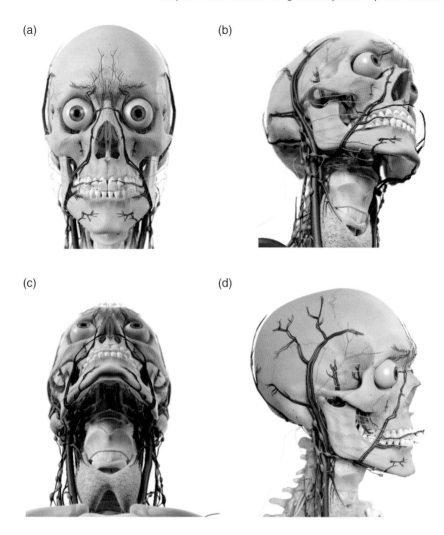

(a) (b) (c) (d)

Figure 6.6 Anatomical rendering of head and neck (structures unlabeled). (a) Frontal view. (b) Oblique view. (c) Inferior view. (d) Lateral view. *Source*: SciePro/Shutterstock.com.

facial expression during your exchange, being sure to note any perceived abnormalities as well as the patient's smile dynamics and dentofacial aesthetics.

Initiate the clinical exam by confirming the presence of typical anatomical features by performing a thorough extraoral and intraoral examination, further investigating any deviation from normal. Assess the stability of the temporomandibular joint, checking for repeatability of occlusion and an absence of pain upon loading the temporomandibular joint. Be sure to palpate the muscles of mastication and associated local lymph nodes, checking for any swelling or tenderness. Additionally, record the patient's maximum pain-free opening, assessing the range of motion and determining if there is sufficient room for any required surgical instrumentation and access.

Table 6.2 Muscles of mastication summary.

Muscle	Origin	Insertion	Action	Innervation
Masseter	Zygomatic arch and maxillary process of zygomatic bone	Lateral surface of ramus of mandible	Elevation and retraction of mandible	Masseteric nerve (CN V3)
Temporalis	Temporal fossa	Coronoid process and anterior margin of the ramus of the mandible	Elevation and retraction of the mandible	Deep temporal nerve (CN V3)
Medial pterygoid	Medial surface of lateral plate of pterygoid process, pyramidal process of palatine bone (deep head); maxillary tuberosity, pyramidal process of palatine bone (superficial head)	Medial surface of mandible	Elevation and side-to-side movements of mandible	Medial pterygoid nerve (CN V3)
Lateral pterygoid	Roof of infratemporal fossa (superior head), lateral surface of the lateral pterygoid plate (inferior head)	Pterygoid fovea of mandible and temporomandibular joint articular disc (superior head) and condylar process (inferior head)	Protrusion and side-to-side movements of mandible	Lateral pterygoid nerve (CN V3)

Sources: Al-Faraje, L. (2013). *Surgical and Radiologic Anatomy for Oral Implantology.* Chicago: Quintessence Publishing Co.; Norton, N. (2007). *Netter's Head and Neck Anatomy for Dentistry.* Philadelphia: Saunders Elsevier.

Table 6.3 Muscles of facial expression summary.

Muscle	Origin	Insertion	Action	Innervation
Orbicularis oris	Deep surface of the skin of the maxilla and mandible	Mucous membranes of the lips	Closes or purses the lips	Buccal and mandibular branches of CN VII
Buccinator	Molar areas of the alveolar processes of maxilla and mandible	Orbicularis oris, lips, and submucosal surfaces of lips and cheeks	Keeps bolus out of vestibule, expels air from oral cavity	Buccal branch of CN VII
Levator labii superiorus	Frontal process of the maxilla and the infraorbital margin	Skin of the upper lip	Elevates upper lip	Buccal and zygomatic branches of CN VII
Depressor labii inferioris	Anterior area of oblique line of mandible	Middle of lower lip	Pulls lower lip inferiorly and laterally	Mandibular branch of CN VII
Levator labii superioris alaeque nasi	Frontal process of maxilla	Alar cartilage and upper lip muscles (levator labii superioris and orbicularis oris)	Elevates the upper lip and dilates nostrils	Buccal and zygomatic branches of CN VII

Table 6.3 (Continued)

Muscle	Origin	Insertion	Action	Innervation
Mentalis	Frenulum of lower lip	Skin of the chin	Elevates and protrudes the lower lip	Mandibular branch of CN VII
Risorius	Fascia superficial to the masseter muscle	Skin of the angle of the mouth	Retracts the corners of the mouth during smiling broadly and laughing	Buccal branch of CN VII
Depressor anguli oris	Mandible below canines, premolars, and first molars	Skin of corner of mouth and orbicularis oris	Pulls the angle of the mouth inferiorly and laterally	Buccal and mandibular branches of CN VII
Levator anguili oris	Canine fossa of maxilla inferior to infraorbital foramen	Angle of the mouth	Elevates the angle of the mouth	Zygomatic and buccal branches of CN VII
Zygomaticus major	Zygomatic bone (lateral and posterior surfaces)	Muscles of the angle of the mouth	Pulls corner of the mouth laterally and superiorly	Zygomatic branch of CN VII
Zygomaticus minor	Zygomatic bone (lateral and posterior surfaces)	Corner of the upper lip	Pulls upper lip superiorly	Zygomatic branch of CN VII
Nasalis	Transverse part on maxilla	Transverse on aponeurosis at bridge of nose	Compress nostrils	Buccal and zygomatic branches of CN VII
	Alar part on maxilla	Ala nasi	Open nostrils	
Procerus	Facial aponeurosis of the lower nasal bone	Skin between eyebrows	Pulls eyebrows medially and inferiorly	Temporal and zygomatic branches of CN VII
Orbicularis oculi	Medial orbital margin, medial palpebral ligament, and lacrimal crest	Close muscles occipitofrontalis, corrugator supercilia, eyelids	Closes eyelid	Temporal and zygomatic branches of CN VII
Corrugator supercili	Frontal bone supraorbital ridge	Middle of the eyebrow	Draws the eyebrows medially and inferiorly	Temporal branch of CN VII
Platysma	Skin over lower neck and upper lateral thorax	Inferior border of mandible, skin over lower face, angle of mouth	Wrinkles skin of lower face and neck	Cervical branch of CN VII

Sources: Al-Faraje, L. (2013). *Surgical and Radiologic Anatomy for Oral Implantology.* Chicago: Quintessence Publishing Co.; Norton, N. (2007). *Netter's Head and Neck Anatomy for Dentistry.* Philadelphia: Saunders Elsevier.

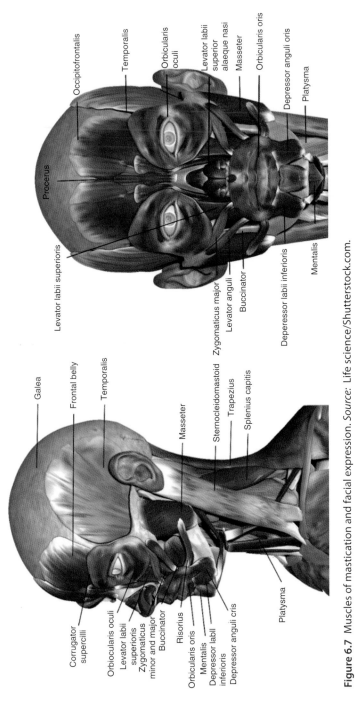

Figure 6.7 Muscles of mastication and facial expression. *Source:* Life science/Shutterstock.com.

Once this has been completed, begin your focused exam pertaining to the patient's chief complaint. Identify local or regional anatomical structures that may become involved in the course of surgical or prosthetic treatment being planned for the individual. Consider appropriate pain management techniques for the planned surgery via delivery of local anaesthetic to the local innervation. Carefully plan any incisions required for surgical access with respect to any local vital structures.

6.3   Tips

- Conduct your patient assessment in an organised fashion, starting externally and then working your way to the oral cavity and site in question.
- Develop an organised approach to patient anatomical assessment to increase efficiency and repeatability.
- Pay particular attention to the patient's ability to open, and their ability to stay open during a potentially longer procedure, to determine if the patient is a candidate for surgery or if other accommodations may be required.
- Develop a surgical plan for local anaesthetic and incision design. Familiarise yourself with the local vital structures that may be encountered during surgery.
- Determine if any specialised testing, imaging, or additional referrals are required to confirm patient suitability for implant surgery.

References

1 Norton, N. (2007). *Netter's Head and Neck Anatomy for Dentistry*. Philadelphia: Saunders Elsevier.
2 Al-Faraje, L. (2013). *Surgical and Radiologic Anatomy for Oral Implantology*. Chicago: Quintessence Publishing Co.

7

Maxillary Anatomical Structures

Kyle D. Hogg

7.1 Principles

An understanding of the anatomical structures of the maxilla relevant to oral implantology is a prerequisite for providing safe and predictable surgical treatment. Thorough pre-operative planning and review of important regional anatomy in should be performed at the treatment planning stage in advance of implant placement to avoid both surgical and prosthetic complications.

Anterior Maxilla
- Maxillary incisive foramen and canal
- Nasal cavity
- Infraorbital foramen

Posterior Maxilla
- Maxillary sinus
- Greater palatine artery and nerve.

7.2 Maxillary Incisive Foramen and Canal

The maxillary incisive foramen is located at the midline of the inferior surface of the maxillary palatal process approximately 10 mm behind the mesial incisal edges of the central incisor clinical crowns. This foramen is the opening to the incisive canal, which carries bundles of the nasopalatine nerve and the anterior branches of the greater palatine artery, both sourced bilaterally [1]. The incisive canal is approximately 11 mm long, with the incisive foramen located inferiorly possessing a mean diameter of 4.5 mm that tapers to about 3.4 mm at the level of the nasal floor superiorly [2].

The nasopalatine nerve is a branch of the posterior superior nasal nerves arising from the pterygopalatine ganglion branch of the maxillary nerve (CN V2). This nerve courses inferiorly and anteriorly, passing through the incisive foramen, where it supplies innervation to the anterior part of the palate, before ultimately communicating with the greater palatine nerve. Thus, local anaesthesia

Practical Procedures in Implant Dentistry, First Edition. Edited by Christopher C.K. Ho.
© 2022 John Wiley & Sons Ltd. Published 2022 by John Wiley & Sons Ltd.
Companion website: www.wiley.com/go/ho/implant-dentistry

delivered to the incisive foramen may be utilised when performing surgical procedures or operative dentistry in the region of the anterior maxilla.

The anterior branch of the greater palatine artery branches off the greater palatine artery after it emerges from the greater palatine foramen in the posterior palate and runs anteriorly across the hard palate towards the incisive foramen. Once it passes through the incisive canal, the anterior branch of the greater palatine artery anastomoses with the sphenopalatine artery on the nasal septum or in the region of the canal itself.

7.2.1 Importance in Oral Implantology

While the incisive foramen and canal are seldom selected as a site for placement of a dental implant these anatomical features can limit the bone volume available for implant placement in the anterior maxilla, specifically the central incisors. This can be a common occurrence in patients with a resorbed maxillary alveolar process secondary to tooth loss. In these individuals the distance in the sagittal plane between the anterior border of the incisive foramen and canal and the buccal plate of the anterior maxilla is often reduced in comparison with subjects that are dentate in this region. The incisive foramen and canal are positioned proximal to the confluence of the nasal septum, nasal floor, anterior nasal spine, and hard palate when viewed from the frontal plane. The complex bony architecture in this region limits the effectiveness of pre-operative evaluation using traditional two-dimensional periapical radiographs. Three-dimensional imaging via cone beam computed tomography (CBCT) scans provide more accurate assessment of both foramen and canal morphology, which can vary significantly [3], and allow for evaluation of available bone volume.

At times, the location and morphology of the incisive foramen and canal may prevent placement of dental implants in the position of the maxillary central incisors, as seen in the clinical case highlighted in Figure 7.1. If the proposed treatment does not permit the selection of alternative suitable sites for dental implant placement guided bone regeneration (GBR) techniques may be required to augment the bone volume anterior to the border of the canal to facilitate implant placement in that area. The incisive canal itself can be grafted in a procedure called incisive canal deflation to provide further bone volume for subsequent implant placement. This technique can be performed under local anaesthetic with reflection of a full-thickness flap raised, permitting access for complete removal of canal contents via rotary curettage. The canal can then be grafted with particulate bone without long-term ill-effects to the patient [4, 5]. While a transient loss of sensation in the anterior maxillary palatal area is possible, the revascularisation and reinnervation of the region due to the anastomoses with the greater palatine artery and nerve typically return sensation within several months.

7.3 Nasal Cavity

The inferior border of the nasal cavity is relevant to oral implantology due to its proximity to the oral cavity and tooth root apices. It consists of the anterior nasal spine and the maxillary alveolar process located anterior to the incisive canal and the hard palate or palatine process of the maxilla and horizontal plate of the

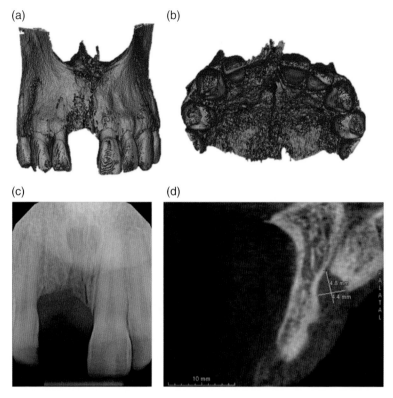

Figure 7.1 Three-dimensional versus two-dimensional view of incisive foramen. A CBCT scan can provide invaluable information about the true anatomical relationship between the incisive foramen and the proposed site for a dental implant. The 3D reconstruction from the CBCT scan depicted in (a) and (b) allows for a more accurate assessment of the edentulous site when compared to the 2D periapical radiograph (c). The sagittal slice (d) shows the enlarged foramen.

palatine bone posterior to the incisive canal, when viewed sagittally through the midline. The nasal cavity provides the superior limit to the volume of the maxillary alveolar process available in the anterior region for implant placement, with the buccal plate providing the anterior limit while the palatal plate or incisive canal provides the posterior limit.

The nasal cavity is very well vascularised, with the sphenopalatine artery, a branch of the internal maxillary artery, providing the largest contribution of arterial supply. It is a branch of the sphenopalatine artery that anastomoses with the greater palatine artery via the incisive canal. The nasopalatine nerve, a branch of the maxillary division of the trigeminal nerve (CN V2), provides sensory input for the nasal cavity and follows the path of the sphenopalatine artery through the incisive canal where it anastomoses with the greater palatine nerve.

7.3.1 Importance in Oral Implantology

Dental implant placement in the anterior maxilla may be limited by the position of the anterior portion of the nasal cavity, particularly when the vertical height of the residual alveolar process is reduced. In such instance, penetration of the inferior border of the nasal cavity may occur. Nasal floor augmentation (NFA) techniques utilising autogenous bone grafts, allografts, xenografts, and combination grafts have been described in the literature [6–9] as methods for managing the atrophic maxilla. Although more clinical research is needed to fully evaluate the predictability of NFA, it may provide a viable and less invasive option than a traditional Le Fort 1 osteotomy [10].

7.4 Infraorbital Foramen

The infraorbital foramen is located immediately below the inferior border of the orbit and contains the infraorbital artery and infraorbital nerve (Figure 7.2). The infraorbital artery originates as a branch of the maxillary artery and anastomoses with the facial artery following its emergence through the infraorbital foramen. The infraorbital nerve is a terminal branch of the maxillary nerve (CN V2). It resides beneath the quadratic labii superioris and provides sensory innervation to the lower portion of the eyelid, the upper lip, and the lateral portion of the nose.

7.4.1 Importance in Oral Implantology

Due to its superior location relative to the position of the alveolar process, the infraorbital foramen is not typically encountered in the surgical placement of dental implants. The infraorbital nerve can, however, be damaged by flap reflection and the use of retractors when performing a lateral window technique sinus lift and/or in cases of extensive maxillary ridge atrophy. Pulpal and soft tissue anaesthesia of the maxillary premolars, canine, and incisors may be achieved via the infraorbital block, which delivers anaesthetic to the infraorbital foramen as referenced 1 cm below the inferior orbital margin.

7.5 Maxillary Sinus

The maxillary sinuses are among the four pairs of paranasal sinuses (frontal sinuses, sphenoid sinuses, ethmoid sinuses, and maxillary sinuses), and the only sinuses relevant to oral implantology. The maxillary sinus expands throughout

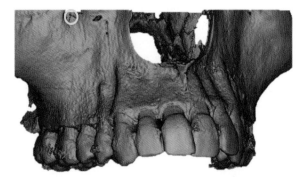

Figure 7.2 Location of the infraorbital foramen. The location of the infraorbital foramen is circled in yellow and can be found far superior to the maxillary occlusal plane.

childhood, with continued inferior expansion resulting in close approximation of the sinus floor to the root apices of the maxillary premolars and molars [11]. In the event of the loss of a maxillary posterior tooth, continued sinus pneumatisation inferiorly can result in inadequate bone volume for placement of a dental implant in the alveolar process or basal bone (Figure 7.3) [12].

The maxillary sinus in adults is a hollow pyramidal shaped space in the maxilla approximately 15 mL in volume [13], roughly 3.5 cm high × 2.4 cm wide × 3.5 cm antero-posteriorly [14]. The sinus communicates with the nasal cavity via an opening high on the medial wall of the sinus called the ostium, which is an opening approximately 3 mm in diameter [15] in the middle meatus or space located just superior to the inferior concha.

(a)

(b)

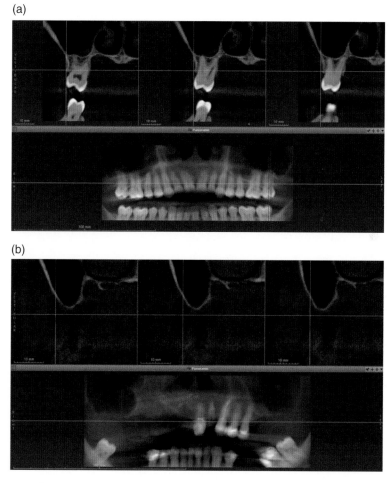

Figure 7.3 Changes in the presentation of the maxillary sinus. (a) In the dentate subject depicted in these panoramic and cross-sectional CBCT scan views, a significant volume of bone is maintained in the alveolar process buccally, lingually, superiorly, and even inter-radicularly. (b) In the partially edentulous subject similarly depicted, a marked loss of the alveolar process and pneumatisation of the maxillary sinus can be observed. This has resulted in an almost uniform, eggshell-thin layer of bone separating the maxillary sinus from the oral cavity.

The anterior wall of the maxillary sinus is formed by the canine fossa and is close to the infraorbital foramen. The lateral wall of the sinus is formed by the zygoma. The superior wall of the sinus is the orbital floor. The posterior wall of the sinus separates the space from the structures of the infratemporal fossa and the pterygomaxillary fossa. The inferior wall or floor of the sinus is created by the alveolar process and basal bone, as well as the hard palate.

The pyramidal shape of the maxillary sinus may be further complicated or compartmentalised by the presence of bony septa, which can cause partial division of the sinus. These septa are very common and may be found in 25–33% of sinuses [16, 17]. Although numerous variations, shapes, sizes, and locations [18] may be encountered, septa tend to have a wider base inferiorly and converge to a sharp edge superiorly.

The maxillary sinus derives its sensory innervation from branches of the maxillary nerve (CN V2) via the anterior, middle, and posterior superior alveolar nerve branches as well as the infraorbital nerve. Blood supply to the sinus stems from branches of the maxillary artery, namely the infraorbital and posterior superior alveolar arteries with some contribution additionally from the sphenopalatine and posterior lateral nasal arteries. Venous drainage of the maxillary sinus occurs via the facial vein, the pterygoid plexus, and the sphenopalatine vein.

The lining of the maxillary sinus consists of a specialised pseudostratified ciliated columnar epithelium and is called the Schneiderian membrane, which in health is usually less than 1 mm thick [19]. This complex respiratory mucosa contains specialised beaker (goblet) cells that produce mucus. The mucus traps inhaled particles, keeps the surface of the membrane moist, and serves to humidify inhaled air. The ciliated columnar epithelium provide a means of transport for the produced mucus. As a functional unit, the muco-ciliary escalator lifts the mucus secretions and small particles up to the ostium and out to the nose.

7.5.1 Importance in Oral Implantology

A frequently encountered challenge when treating the edentulous posterior maxilla with dental implants is insufficient bone volume in an area with poor bone quality [20]. The bone volume of the residual alveolar ridge available for implant placement in this region may be limited by the presence of the maxillary sinus with or without pneumatisation, the loss of alveolar bone height following tooth loss, or a combination of both [21]. Bone volume may be increased via augmentation procedures of the maxillary sinus utilising a variety of surgical techniques and grafting materials in a predictable fashion [22–24].

Current evidence suggests that both lateral sinus floor elevation (SFE) and crestal SFE techniques are both predictably successful and safe, resulting in good long-term implant survival rates [25, 26]. Examples of lateral sinus floor elevation are depicted in Figure 7.4. The clinician may utilise parameters including residual bone height, residual bone width, length of edentulous span, and residual bone quality to help guide the selection of a lateral versus crestal SFE, as well as determining whether a simultaneous or delayed implant placement is indicated. Future research on the long-term viability of short implants (4–6 mm) may show a decrease in the need for SFE altogether [27].

(a)

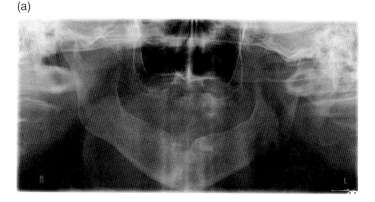

(b)

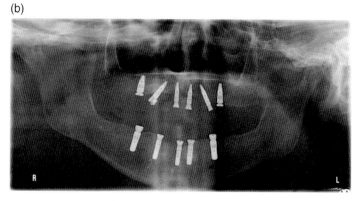

Figure 7.4 Implant placement following maxillary sinus augmentation in a staged approach. Sinus floor elevation (SFE) via a lateral window approach was performed on both the right and left posterior edentulous segments, as the bone quality and residual bone height as shown in the panoramic radiograph (a) were not favourable for a simultaneous implant placement in conjunction with the grafting procedure. Following sinus graft consolidation over a period of six months, implants were placed in the posterior segments uneventfully as shown in the panoramic radiograph (b).

7.6 Greater Palatine Artery and Nerve

Upon exiting the greater palatine foramen located medial and slightly distal to the maxillary third molar, the greater palatine artery and nerve run anterior along the hard palate to the incisive foramen as described earlier. The greater palatine neurovascular bundle is typically located at the junction of the vertical and horizontal palatal walls of the palatal vault (Figure 7.5).

7.6.1 Importance in Oral Implantology

When creating an incision in the region of the greater palatine artery a zone of safety should be maintained to avoid injury to the artery with potential resulting bleeding and soft tissue necrosis. This zone of safety will often depend on the anatomical variation of the individual patient. Although the greater palatine

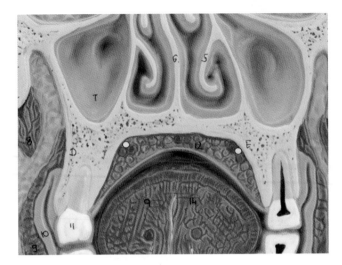

Figure 7.5 Position of the greater palatine artery and nerve. The greater palatine neurovascular bundle is outlined in purple in the frontal section of the skull at the level of the premolars. Individuals with higher palatal vaults exhibit greater distances from the lingual gingival margin to the neurovascular bundle than lower palatal vaults.

neurovascular bundle is typically located at the junction of the vertical and horizontal palatal walls, significant variations in palatal vault depth mean the neurovascular bundle could be as close as 7 mm from the lingual gingival margin at the first molar site in low palatal vault phenotypes to as much as 17 mm in high palatal vault phenotypes [28]. The harvest of connective tissue grafts and free gingival grafts is routinely performed in the maxillary posterior palatal tissues from the first molar site forward to the canine. In most dentate patients without significant periodontal disease it is possible to harvest connective tissue and free gingival grafts up to 8 mm in height without injury to the neurovascular bundle [29].

References

1 Song, W., Jo, D.I., Lee, J.Y. et al. (2009). Microanatomy of the incisive canal using three-dimensional reconstruction of microCT images: an ex vivo; study. *Oral Surg. Oral Med. Oral Pathol. Oral Radiol. Endod.* 108 (4): 583–590.

2 Friedrich, R., Laumann, F., Zrnc, T., and Assaf, A. (2015). The nasopalatine canal in adults on cone beam computed tomograms – a clinical study and review of the literature. *in vivo;* 29 (4): 467–486.

3 Mraiwa, N., Jacobs, R., and Van Cleynenbreugel, J. (2004). The nasopalatine canal revisited using 2D and 3D CT imaging. *Dentomaxillofac. Radiol.* 33: 396–402.

4 Marcantonio, E.J. (2009). Incisive canal deflation for correct implant placement: case report. *Implant Dent.* 18: 473–479.

5 Rosenquist, J. and Nystrom, E. (1992). Occlusion of the incisal canal with bone chips. A procedure to facilitate insertion of implants in the anterior maxilla. *Int. J. Oral Maxillofac. Surg.* 21: 210–211.

6 Garg, A. (1997). Nasal sinus lift: an innovative technique for implant insertions. *Dent. Implantol. Update* 8: 49.

7 Garg, A. (2008). Subnasal elevation and bone augmentation in dental implantology. *Dent. Implantol. Update* 19: 17.

8 Hising, P., Bolin, A., and Branting, C. (2001). Reconstruction of the severely resorbed alveolar ridge crests with dental implants using bovine bone mineral for augmentation. *Int. J. Oral Maxillofac. Implants* 16: 90.

9 Mazor, Z., Lorean, A., and Mijiritsky, E. (2012). Nasal floor elevation combined with dental implant placement. *Clin. Implant Dent. Relat. Res.* 14 (5): 768–771.

10 El-Ghareeb, M., Pi-Anfruns, J., Khosousi, M. et al. (2012). Nasal floor augmentation for the reconstruction of the atrophic maxilla: a case series. *J. Oral Maxillofac. Surg.* 70 (3): 235–241.

11 Sicher, H. and DuBrul, E. (1975). The viscera of the head and neck. In: Oral Anatomy, 7e, 418–424. St. Louis: Mosby.

12 Mehra, P. and Murad, H. (2004). Maxillary sinus disease of odontogenic origin. *Otolaryngol. Clin. North Am.* 37: 347–364.

13 Sahlstrand-Johnson, P., Jannert, M., Strombeck, A., and Abul-Kasim, K. (2011). Computed tomography measurements of different dimensions of maxillary and frontal sinuses. *BMC Med. Imaging* 11: 8.

14 Sharma, S., Jehan, M., and Kumar, A. (2014). Measurements of maxillary sinus volume and dimensions by computed tomography scan for gender determination. *J. Anat. Soc. India* 63: 36–42.

15 El-Anwar, M., Raafat, A., Mostafa, R. et al. (2018). Maxillary sinus ostium assessment: a CT study. *Egypt. J. Radiol. Nucl. Med.* 49 (4): 1009–1013.

16 Kim, M., Jung, U., and Kim, C. (2006). Maxillary sinus septa: prevalence, height, location, and morphology. A reformatted computed tomography scan analysis. *J. Periodontol.* 77: 903–908.

17 Velasquez-Plata, D., Hover, L., Peach, C., and Adler, M. (2002). Maxillary sinus septa: a 3-dimensional computerized tomographic scan analysis. *Int. J. Oral Maxillofac. Implants* 17: 854–860.

18 McGowan, D., Baxter, P., and James, J. (1993). The Maxillary Sinus and its Dental Implications. Oxford: Butterworth-Heinemann.

19 Mogensen, C. and Tos, M. (1977). Quantitative histology of the maxillary sinus. *Rhinology* 15: 129–140.

20 Cawood, J. and Howell, R. (1988). A classification of the edentulous jaws. *Int. J. Oral Maxillofac. Surg.* 17: 232–236.

21 Garg, A. (1999). Augmentation grafting of the maxillary sinus for placement of dental implants: anatomy, physiology, and procedures. *Implant Dent.* 8: 36–46.

22 Del Fabbro, M., Wallace, S., and Testori, T. (2013). Long-term implant survival in the grafted maxillary sinus: a systematic review. *Int. J. Periodontics Restorative Dent.* 33: 773–783.

23 Jensen, O., Shulman, L., Block, M., and Iacono, V. (1998). Report of the sinus consensus conference of 1996. *Int. J. Oral Maxillofac. Implants* 13 (Suppl): 11–45.

24 Seong, W.J., Barczak, M., Jung, J. et al. (2013). Prevalence of sinus augmentation associated with maxillary posterior implants. *J. Oral Implantol.* 39: 680–688.

25 Esposito, M., Felice, P., and Worthington, H.V. (2010). Interventions for replacing missing teeth: augmentation procedures for the maxillary sinus. *Cochrane Database Syst. Rev.* 3.

26 Felice, P., Pistilli, R., Piattelli, M. et al. (2014). 1-stage versus 2-stage lateral sinus lift procedures: 1-year post-loading results of a multicentre randomised controlled trial. *Eur. J. Oral Implantol.* 7 (1): 65–75.

27 Esposito, M., Felice, P., and Worthington, H. (2014). Interventions for replacing missing teeth: augmentation procedures of the maxillary sinus. *Cochrane Database Syst. Rev.* 13 (5).

28 Reiser, G., Bruno, J., Mahan, P., and Larkin, L. (1996). The subepithelial connective tissue graft palatal donor site: anatomic considerations for surgeons. *Int. J. Periodontics Restorative Dent.* 16: 130–137.

29 Monnet-Corti, V., Santini, A., and Glise, J. (2006). Connective tissue graft for gingival recession treatment: assessment of the maximum graft dimensions at the palatal vault as a donor site. *J. Periodontol.* 77: 899–902.

8

Mandibular Anatomical Structures

Kyle D. Hogg

8.1 Principles

An understanding of the anatomical structures of the mandible relevant to oral implantology is a prerequisite for providing safe and predictable surgical treatment. Thorough pre-operative planning and review of important regional anatomy in should be performed at the treatment planning stage in advance of implant placement to avoid both surgical and prosthetic complications.

Anterior Mandible
- Mental foramen and nerve
- Mandibular incisive canal and nerve
- Genial tubercles
- Lingual foramen and accessory lingual foramina
- Sublingual fossa
- Submental and sublingual arteries

Posterior Mandible
- Inferior alveolar canal and nerve
- Lingual and mylohyoid nerves
- Submandibular fossa
- Mandibular ramus.

8.2 Mental Foramen and Nerve

The mental nerve exits the buccal surface of the body of the mandible through the mental foramen, with the emergence pattern of the foramen most commonly directed posteriorly [1]. The mental foramen is routinely located between the root apices of the mandibular first and second premolars (Figure 8.1) [2]; however, a review of the literature has shown that the location of the mental foramen is not constant among individuals in either the horizontal or vertical planes [3]. Advanced alveolar ridge atrophy may result in the mental foramen being present in rather superior locations near the crest of the ridge.

Practical Procedures in Implant Dentistry, First Edition. Edited by Christopher C.K. Ho.
© 2022 John Wiley & Sons Ltd. Published 2022 by John Wiley & Sons Ltd.
Companion website: www.wiley.com/go/ho/implant-dentistry

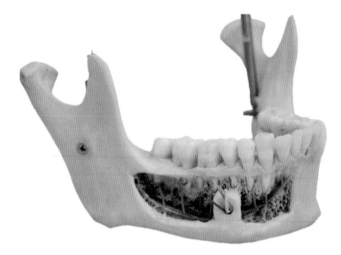

Figure 8.1 Mental foramen and neurovascular bundle. Interruption of normal sensory input may occur if the inferior alveolar nerve or mental nerve is damaged during osteotomy preparation or surgical flap management.

Typically, three branches of the mental nerve exit the mental foramen, providing sensory innervation to the chin, lower lip, labial mucosa in the region of the mandibular anterior dentition, and the skin overlying the body of the mandible, anterior temporal, and preauricular regions [4]. Although it is most common for one foramen to exit the mandible in this locale, accessory mental foramina may be present [5].

Radiographic assessment of the mental foramen location via periapical, vertical bitewing, and panoramic radiographs should be interpreted with caution as studies have shown that these conventional images may often not clearly or accurately reflect the true anatomic positioning of the foramen [6–8]. This difficulty in locating the mental foramen by conventional radiographic methods may be due to not capturing the foramen in the image because of its inferior position, a lack of contrast between the mental foramen and the underlying trabecular bone pattern, or the influence of the thick lingual cortical plate masking the ability of the imaging technique from detecting the decrease in bone density caused by the foramen [7, 8]. Recent utilisation of cone beam computed tomography (CBCT) scans have proven to be more accurate than conventional radiographs at determining the true anatomical location of the mental foramen (Figure 8.2) [9, 10].

The presence of an anterior loop, defined as 'an extension of the inferior alveolar nerve anterior to the mental foramen, prior to exiting the canal' [11] is subject to debate. Conventional radiographic methods detected the presence of an anterior loop very frequently [12], while surgical dissection of cadaveric mandibles exhibited a variety of results with some studies showing nearly all specimens having an anterior loop [13, 14], yet another showing the presence of such a loop far more infrequently [15]. Studies that have included dissection findings and radiographic findings of the same specimen have shown that radiographic determination of the presence of an anterior loop is of questionable value due to poor

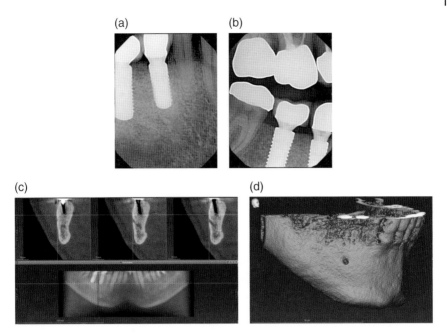

Figure 8.2 Comparison of imaging techniques on the same patient. The periapical image depicted in (a) captures the area where the mental foramen is anticipated, but cannot be discerned. The vertical bitewing (b) does not extend apically enough to capture the foramen. The cross-sectional view (c) and three-dimensional reconstruction (d) of the CBCT scan more clearly depict the correct anatomical relationships.

correlation between the data from radiographic and dissection assessment [16–18]. A more recent study comparing the dissection findings with CBCT scans has shown that these scans are both reliable and accurate means of detecting and measuring the anterior loop [19]. Similarly, studies on the size or magnitude of the anterior loop have been conflicting, with some radiographic studies showing broad ranges in size between 0 and 7.5 mm [12, 20], while cadaveric and CBCT studies show a range of 0–5.6 mm with an average closer to 1 mm [15, 21].

From the available evidence in the literature, it can be assumed that the anterior loop of the mental nerve may be present in some individuals is it has been identified by radiographic imaging, cadaveric dissection, and CBCT scan interpretation. The frequency with which the anterior loop is encountered and the size or length of the loop is more controversial at this time.

8.2.1 Importance in Oral Implantology

When considering implant surgery in the foraminal region it is of great importance to identify the location of the mental foramen and the magnitude of the anterior loop, if present, to avoid any damage to the neurovascular bundle during incision-making, flap reflection, or the creation of osteotomies. Other times pressure on the mental nerve can be caused by implant impingement, swelling or oedema, or trauma from dental anaesthetic injections in the vicinity. The nerve may become damaged, either by being severed completely or by being partially transected, compressed, or stretched [22].

Injuries to the mental nerve may result in paraesthesia (numbness), hypoaesthesia (reduced sensitivity), hyperaesthesia (increased sensitivity), dysaesthesia (painful sensation), or anaesthesia (complete absence of sensation) in the regions it typically provides sensory input. Nerve injuries may be described as follows [11]:

- *Neurotmesis*: This is complete transection or severing of the nerve, with a poor prognosis for resolution of altered sensation or paraesthesia.
- *Axontmesis*: In this nerve is damaged but not completely transected. Sensation often returns to normal within two to six months of injury.
- *Neurapraxia*: The nerve has been stretched or traumatised without losing its continuity. Typically sensation will return to normal in days to weeks.

To avoid injury to the mental nerve, consider obtaining a CBCT scan of the region to help determine the exact position of the foramen and neurovascular structures. If this information does not remove the uncertainty of the location of the mental foramen or presence of an anterior loop, consider careful surgical exposure and investigation of the structures for direct visualisation with a full thickness flap [3].

8.3 Mandibular Incisive Canal and Nerve

The mandibular incisive canal has been described as a continuation of the mandibular canal towards the incisor region, containing the relatively small mandibular incisive nerve and neurovascular bundle [4, 6, 23, 24]. The mandibular incisive canal is most frequently found in the middle third of the mandible, with respect to the superior and inferior borders. Although typically small in diameter, the width of the canal can range from being undetectable to nearly 3 mm [25]. The range of observed diameters may contribute to the conflicting data on the frequency of observation of the mandibular incisive canal. As detection methods and imaging capabilities have improved, it has been widely adopted that the mandibular incisive canal and nerve are normal anatomical structures [17, 26]. Functionally, the mandibular incisive nerve housed within the canal supplies innervation to the first premolar, canine, and lateral and central incisors.

8.3.1 Importance in Oral Implantology

Given that the mandibular incisive canal is comparatively difficult to detect using panoramic radiography versus CBCT scans, strong consideration should be given to CBCT imaging when planning implant placement interforaminally [6]. Most of the time implants can be planned and placed without too much consideration for the mandibular incisive canal. However, in the presence of a larger mandibular incisive canal, care should be taken to avoid encountering or damaging the structure during osteotomy preparation as patients may experience intraoperative or post-operative pain requiring implant removal [27, 28].

8.4   Genial Tubercles

The genial tubercles are relatively small paired bony elevations located on the lingual surface of the anterior mandible on either side of the midline. They are most often located in the inferior third of the mandible, but may appear level with or even superior to the residual mandibular ridge height in cases of severe mandibular resorption. Functionally, the genial tubercles serve as the insertion point for both the genioglossus and geniohyoid muscles [29], with the genioglossus inserting on the superior tubercle and the geniohyoid inserting on the inferior tubercle. The lingual foramen is located in between the tubercles at the midline.

8.4.1   Importance in Oral Implantology

The genial tubercles rarely interfere with implant planning or placement in dentate or partially edentulous patients, but may require more consideration in those individuals with severely resorbed mandibles. In these instances, accommodation for the space required for the tubercles, both surgically and restoratively, should be allowed. It is imperative to avoid obliteration of the tubercles when performing an osteoplasty to level the residual mandibular ridge or to completely reflect the genioglossus muscle from the superior tubercle during flap elevation as it might compromise the stability of the upper airway.

8.5   Lingual Foramen and Accessory Lingual Foramina

The lingual foramen contains a small artery formed by the anastomosis of the right and left sublingual arteries [30]. Additional smaller accessory foramina are often found accompanying the midline lingual foramen. The lingual foramen is typically less than 1 mm in diameter, while the accessory foramina are often even smaller, averaging around 0.5 mm [31].

8.5.1   Importance in Oral Implantology

Conventional periapical and panoramic radiographs do not consistently allow for detection of the lingual foramen, in part due to the small size, but also due to beam angulation challenges when imaging this region. Encountering either the lingual foramen and its contents or the neighbouring accessory foramina during osteotomy preparation is unlikely to cause complications. The lingual foramina can be clearly seen in the CBCT scan and 3D reconstruction depicted in Figure 8.3. However, if a larger canal is penetrated during osteotomy preparation, significant bleeding may result. In these instances where bleeding from the osteotomy is brisk the implant fixture can serve as a tamponade. The patient should be monitored for any development of a sublingual hematoma.

(a)

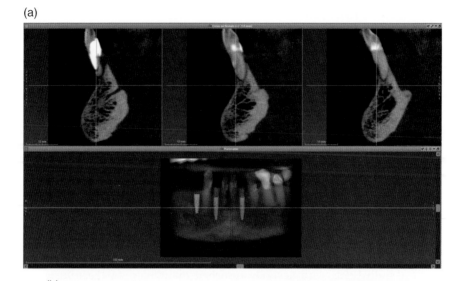

(b)

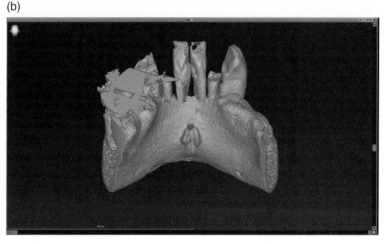

Figure 8.3 Imaging of the lingual foramen and proximity to the genial tubercle. Lying superior to the genial tubercle, the lingual foramen and associated vasculature may be encountered when placing implants in the anterior region of the mandible. (a) CBCT scan. (b) Three-dimensional reconstruction.

8.6 Sublingual Fossa

The sublingual fossa is a bilateral shallow depression often triangular in shape located on the medial surface of the mandible, occurring on both sides of the mental spine and resting above the anterior portion of the mylohyoid line. The sublingual salivary gland and duct, the lingual artery and vein, lingual nerve (branch of CN V), and branches of the glossopharyngeal (CN IX) and hypoglossal (CN XII) nerves are all contained in this fossa [32].

8.6.1 Importance in Oral Implantology

The sublingual fossa must be investigated via palpation or CBCT imaging prior to performing an osteotomy in the mandibular anterior region to avoid perforation of the lingual cortical plate and damage to the contents of the sublingual fossa. Consideration for the presence and depth of any undercut created by the fossa should be given to ensure osteotomy development and implant angulation are both safely contained within the cortical plates of the anterior mandible and suitable emergence angle for final prosthesis.

8.7 Submental and Sublingual Arteries

The submental artery is a branch of the facial artery approximately 2 mm in diameter that runs under the inferior border of the mylohyoid muscle in most instances, with some anatomical observations of the artery passing through the mylohyoid muscle [33]. The submental artery provides blood supply to both submandibular and sublingual salivary glands, the mylohyoid muscle, and the skin in the submental region.

   The sublingual artery is similar in size, also approximately 2 mm in diameter, and is located superior to the mylohyoid muscle. The sublingual artery is the major blood supply to the floor of the mouth [34].

8.7.1 Importance in Oral Implantology

The sublingual and submental arteries can be located in close proximity to the lingual cortical plate anteriorly, with some branches of these arteries entering the mandibular cortex via the lingual foramen and/or accessory foramina [35]. Although rare, serious complications can result if these arteries are injured or severed as submandibular or sublingual haematomas can develop and compromise the patency of the airway. Care should be taken both when performing osteotomies to avoid inadvertent penetration of the lingual cortical plate and when elevating a lingual flap to avoid severing vessels entering accessory foramina.

8.8 Inferior Alveolar Canal and Nerve

The inferior alveolar canal carries the inferior alveolar nerve (branch of the mandibular nerve), the inferior alveolar artery, vein, and lymphatic vessels as it courses anteriorly through the mandible from its entry point on the medial surface of the posterior mandible by the lingula [36]. The diameter of the inferior alveolar canal is approximately 3.4 mm, with the nerve being on average 2.2 mm in diameter [37]. The inferior alveolar nerve is a mixed sensory and motor branch of the posterior division of the mandibular division of the trigeminal nerve (CN V). The inferior alveolar nerve itself has three major branches: the nerve to the mylohyoid, the mental nerve, and the incisive nerve.

   The first branch, the nerve to the mylohyoid, occurs just before the inferior alveolar nerve enters the mandible and supplies the mylohyoid and anterior belly of the digastric muscle. As the canal passes anteriorly through the mandible from the lingula to the mental foramen a variety of anatomic configurations may be encountered. The inferior alveolar nerve and artery run parallel to one another within the canal; however, the relationship of one lying superior or inferior to the other varies [37]. The canal may move gently from a more superior to inferior position as it courses anteriorly, it may exhibit a steeper or more abrupt decline, or it may drape downward as if hanging between two points in a catenary fashion [38]. The inferior alveolar canal and its contents cross from its entry point on the lingual aspect of the posterior mandible to its buccal exit point at the mental foramen (Figure 8.4). The inferior alveolar canal is often centred between the buccal and lingual cortical plates in the region of the first molar [39]. During this

(a)

(b)

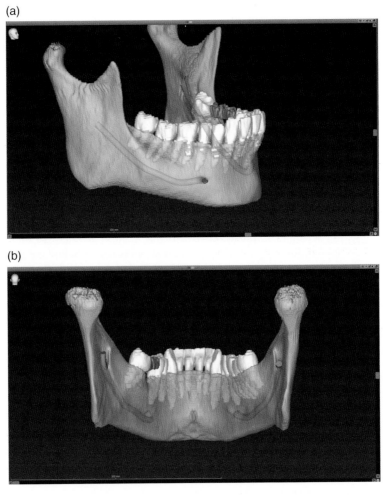

Figure 8.4 Tracing of inferior alveolar canal. The capture of CBCT imaging allows the course of the inferior alveolar canal to be traced from the buccal exit at mental foramen anteriorly to the lingual exit adjacent to the lingula posteriorly. This information can be invaluable in planning osteotomies and implant placement safely. (a) Buccal view; (b) lingual view.

progression anteriorly, small unnamed offshoots of the inferior alveolar nerve contribute to the inferior dental plexus which supplies sensory innervation to the three molars and two premolars. In the premolar region the inferior alveolar nerve again further divides, branching into the mental nerve which emerges from the mental foramen, supplying the skin and mucous membrane of the lower lip and buccal gingival tissue from the midline to second premolar, and the incisive nerve and canal which continue anterior to the mental foramen supplying sensory innervation to the canine and both central and lateral incisors [4].

8.8.1 Importance in Oral Implantology

Due in part to the variations between individual patients of the pathway of the inferior alveolar canal it is essential to definitively locate the inferior alveolar canal prior to surgery to avoid potential injury and adverse effects. Inferior alveolar nerve injury can occur during administration of local anaesthesia (via needle penetration), during flap reflection (by traction or improper manipulation), during incisions (by scalpel), during osteotomy preparation (via thermal insult or direct trauma), upon implant placement (direct compression), or due to surgery-induced swelling or hematoma formation (indirect compression). Although it is important to discuss potential injury to the neurovascular bundle during the informed consent process, injuries to the inferior alveolar nerve should be rare provided that the presurgical position of the canal space is clearly identified and avoided intraoperatively.

The drills used to prepare osteotomies for implant placement are typically 0.5–1.0 mm longer than the corresponding implant being placed. Surgeons must be familiar with the dimensions of the surgical instrumentation they are utilising in order to carry out osteotomy preparations safely and precisely. It is good practice to leave a zone of safety of 2 mm or more between the most apical end of the implant being placed and the most superior aspect of the inferior alveolar canal [40]. This concept of a zone of safety can also be applied to other vital structures to avoid unintentional complications.

8.9 Lingual and Mylohyoid Nerves

The lingual nerve stems from the mandibular branch of the trigeminal nerve (CN V). It travels inferiorly from a position slightly anterior and medial to the inferior alveolar nerve, descending to the area of the base of the tongue. The lingual nerve supplies sensory input to the anterior two-thirds of the tongue. Unlike the inferior alveolar nerve, which travels anteriorly in the relative safety of the inferior alveolar canal within the mandible itself, the lingual nerve typically travels medially in close proximity to the medial lingual cortical plate at a level below the crest of the ridge and posterior to the roots of the mandibular third molars [41]. In a smaller percentage of individuals, the lingual nerve is found at or above the crest of bone, lingual to the mandibular third molars [42].

The mylohyoid nerve is a branch of the inferior alveolar nerve, arising just before the inferior alveolar nerve enters the mandibular foramen posteriorly.

From the point it branches off the inferior alveolar nerve the mylohyoid nerve follows the mylohyoid groove towards the mylohyoid muscle, where it innervates the mylohyoid muscle and the anterior belly of the digastric muscle. Additionally, the mylohyoid muscle may provide accessory innervation to anterior and posterior mandibular teeth [43, 44].

8.9.1 Importance in Oral Implantology

Due to the frequent positioning of the lingual nerve at or near the alveolar crest, and frequent direct contact of the nerve with the lingual cortical plate, care should be taken when reflecting flaps in this region to avoid traction or compression injuries to the nerve. Lingual vertical releasing incisions are to be avoided in this area, with incisions made distal to the second mandibular molar made towards the buccal aspect of the ridge to avoid the lingual nerve. The mylohyoid nerve may require additional anaesthesia if a profound block is not achieved when anaesthetising the inferior alveolar nerve. In patients exhibiting objective signs of inferior alveolar anaesthesia, but who may be experiencing intraprocedural discomfort, an additional infiltration injection on the lingual aspect of the posterior mandible may provide added comfort and more profound anaesthesia.

8.10 Submandibular Fossa

The submandibular fossa is located on the medial surface of the mandible inferior to the mylohyoid line in the region of the mandibular molars. It contains the submandibular salivary gland and duct, branches of the facial and lingual arteries, and the nerve to the mylohyoid (Figure 8.5). The mild concavity formed by the fossa cannot be visualised accurately on a panoramic radiograph [45], nor can it be visualised intraorally due to the position of the mylohyoid being superior to

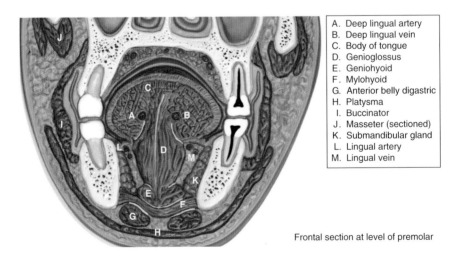

A. Deep lingual artery
B. Deep lingual vein
C. Body of tongue
D. Genioglossus
E. Geniohyoid
F. Mylohyoid
G. Anterior belly digastric
H. Platysma
I. Buccinator
J. Masseter (sectioned)
K. Submandibular gland
L. Lingual artery
M. Lingual vein

Frontal section at level of premolar

Figure 8.5 Contents of the submandibular fossa and closely related structures.

the fossa. Digital palpation via compression of the tissues can allow for interpretation of lingual anatomy, but a CBCT scan provides the most accurate assessment of lingual mandibular contour and anatomy.

8.10.1 Importance in Oral Implantology

There are two major limiting factors in determining the maximum dental implant length when performing surgery in the mandibular posterior region, namely the position of the inferior alveolar nerve and canal and the anatomy of the submandibular fossa [46]. Determining the true height and width of bone available for placement of a dental implant can help reduce the risk of lingual cortical plate penetration during osteotomy preparation or in placing the implant itself. Perforation in this region can cause arterial bleeding and haemorrhage either immediately or with some delay following injury. Haemorrhages occurring in the floor of the mouth may cause a rare but serious airway obstruction where the floor of the mouth is displaced superiorly and posteriorly and impinging on the airway space.

8.11 Mandibular Ramus

The mandibular ramus houses the lingual and mandibular foramen, where the inferior alveolar nerve enters the mandibular cortex as it courses anteriorly. The foramen is located approximately two-thirds from its leading or anterior border, with the entire antero-posterior dimension averaging about 30.5 mm [47]. The location of the buccal notch can be palpated along the inferior border of the mandible and locates the position of the facial artery, vein, and nerve.

8.11.1 Importance in Oral Implantology

Understanding the anatomy of the mandibular ramus is imperative in the consistent and effective delivery of local anaesthetic to the inferior alveolar nerve. Additionally, the ramus buccal shelf serves as a common osseous donor site for block grafts [48, 49].

References

1 Kieser, J., Kuzmanovic, D., Payne, A. et al. (2002). Patterns of emergence of the human mental nerve. *Arch. Oral Biol.* 47: 743–747.

2 Fishel, D., Buchner, A., Hershkowith, A., and Kaffe, I. (1976). Roentgenologic study of the mental foramen. *Oral Surg. Oral Med. Oral Pathol.* 41: 682–686.

3 Greenstein, G. and Tarnow, D. (2006). The mental foramen and nerve: clinical and anatomical factors related to dental implant placement: a literature review. *J. Periodontol.* 77: 1933–1943.

4 Mraiwa, N., Jacobs, R., Moerman, D., and Lambrichts, I. (2003). Presence and course of the incisive canal in the human mandibular interforaminal region: two dimensional imaging versus anatomical observations. *Surg. Radiol. Anat.* 25: 416–423.

5 Sawyer, D., Kiely, M., and Pyle, M. (1998). The frequency of accessory mental foramina in four ethnic groups. *Arch. Oral Biol.* 43: 417–420.

6 Jacobs, R., Mraiwa, N., Van Steenberghe, D. et al. (2004). Appearance of the mandibular incisive canal on panoramic radiographs. *Surg. Radiol. Anat.* 26: 329–333.

7 Yosue, T. and Brooks, S. (1989). The appearance of mental foramina on panoramic radiographs. I. Evaluation of patients. *Oral Surg. Oral Med. Oral Pathol.* 68: 360–364.

8 Yosue, T. and Brooks, S. (1989). The appearance of the mental foramina on panoramic and periapical radiographs. II. Experimental evaluation. *Oral Surg. Oral Med. Oral Pathol.* 68: 488–492.

9 Klinge, B., Petersson, A., and Maly, P. (1989). Location of the mandibular canal: comparison of macroscopic findings, conventional radiography, and computed tomography. *Int. J. Oral Maxillofac. Implants* 4: 327–332.

10 Sonick, M., Abrahams, J., and Faiella, R. (1994). A comparison of the accuracy of periapical, panoramic, and computerized tomographic radiographs in locating the mandibular canal. *Int. J. Oral Maxillofac. Implants* 9: 455–460.

11 Jalbout, Z. and Tabourian, G. (2004). Glossary of Implant Dentistry, 16e. Upper Montclair, NJ: International Congress of Oral Implantologists.

12 Arzouman, M., Otis, L., Kipnis, V., and Levine, D. (1993). Observations of the anterior loop of the inferior alveolar canal. *Int. J. Oral Maxillofac. Implants* 8: 295–300.

13 Nieva, R., Gapski, R., and Wang, H. (2004). Morphometric analysis of implant-related anatomy in Caucasian skulls. *J. Periodontol.* 75: 1061–1067.

14 Solar, P., Ulm, C., Frey, G., and Matejka, M. (1994). A classification of the intraosseous paths of the mental nerve. *Int. J. Oral Maxillofac. Implants* 9: 339–344.

15 Rosenquist, B. (1996). Is there an anterior loop of the inferior alveolar nerve? *Int. J. Periodontics Restorative Dent.* 16: 40–45.

16 Kuzmanovic, D., Payne, A., Kieser, J., and Dias, G. (2003). Anterior loop of the mental nerve: a morphological and radiographic study. *Clin. Oral Implants Res.* 14: 464–471.

17 Mardinger, O., Chaushu, G., Arensburg, B. et al. (2000a). Anatomic and radiologic course of the mandibular incisive canal. *Surg. Radiol. Anat.* 22 (3–4): 157–161.

18 Mardinger, O., Chaushu, G., Arensburg, B. et al. (2000b). Anterior loop of the mental canal: an anatomical radiologic study. *Implant Dent.* 9: 120–125.

19 Santana, R.R., Lozarda, J., Kleinman, A. et al. (2012). Accuracy of cone beam computerized tomography and a three-dimensional stereolithographic model in identifying the anterior loop of the mental nerve: a study on cadavers. *J. Oral Implantol.* 38 (6): 668–676.

20 Bavitz, J., Harn, S., Hansen, C., and Lang, M. (1993). An anatomical study of mental neurovascular bundle – implant relationships. *Int. J. Oral Maxillofac. Implants* 8: 563–567.

21 Filo, K., Schneider, T., and Locher, M.C. (2014). The inferior alveolar nerve's loop at the mental foramen and its implications for surgery. *J. Am. Dent. Assoc.* 145 (3): 260–269.

22 Bartling, R., Freeman, K., and Kraut, R. (1999). The incidence of altered sensation of the mental nerve after mandibular implant placement. *J. Oral Maxillofac. Surg.* 57: 1408–1412.

23 Mraiwa, N., Jacobs, R., Moerman, P. et al. (2003). Presence and course of the incisive canal in human mandibular interforaminal region: two-dimensional imaging versus anatomical observations. *Surg. Radiol. Anat.* 25 (5–6): 416–423.

24 Mraiwa, N., Jacobs, R., van Steenberghe, D., and Quirynen, M. (2003). Clinical assessment and surgical implications of anatomic challenges in the anterior mandible. *Clin. Implant Dent. Relat. Res.* 5: 219–225.

25 Obradovic, O., Todorovic, L., Pesic, V. et al. (1993). Morphometric analysis of mandibular canal: clinical aspects. *Sci. Stomatol. Odontol.* 36 (3–4): 109–113.

26 De Andrade, E., Otomo-Corgel, J., Pucher, K.A. et al. (2001). The intraosseous course of the mandibular incisive nerve in the mandibular symphysis. *Int. J. Periodontics Restorative Dent.* 21 (6): 591–597.

27 Kohavi, D. and Bar-Ziv, J. (1996). Atypical incisive nerve: a case report. *Implant Dent.* 5: 281–283.

28 Romanos, G. and Greenstein, G. (2009). The incisive canal: considerations during implant placement: case report and literature review. *Int. J. Oral Maxillofac. Implants* 24 (4): 740–745.

29 Norton, N. (2007). Netter's Head and Neck Anatomy for Dentistry. Philadelphia: Saunders.

30 Liang, H., Frederiksen, N., and Benson, B. (2004). Lingual vascular canals of the interforaminal region of the mandible: evaluation with conventional tomography. *Dentomaxillofac. Radiol.* 33: 340–341.

31 Galheitner, A., Hofschneider, U., and Tepper, G. (2001). Lingual vascular canals of the mandible: evaluation with dental CT. *Radiology* 220: 186–189.

32 Al-Faraje, L. (2013). Surgical and Radiologic Anatomy for Oral Implantology. Chicago: Quintessence Publishing Co.

33 Quirynen, M., Mraiwa, N., van Steenberghe, D., and Jacobs, R. (2003). Morphology and dimensions of the mandibular jaw bone in the interforaminal region in patients requiring implants in the distal areas. *Clin. Oral Implants Res.* 14 (3): 280–285.

34 Martin, D., Pascal, J., and Baudet, J. (1993). The submental island flap: a new donor site. Anatomy and clinical applications as a free or pedicled flap. *Plast. Reconstr. Surg.* 92: 867–873.

35 Hofschneider, U., Tepper, G., Gahleitner, A., and Ulm, C. (1999). Assessment of the blood supply to the mental region for reduction of bleeding complications during implant surgery in the interforaminal region. *Int. J. Oral Maxillofac. Implants* 14: 379–383.

36 Tammisalo, T., Happonen, R., and Tammisalo, E. (1992). Stereographic assessment of mandibular canal in relation to the roots of impacted lower third molar using multiprojection narrow beam radiography. *Int. J. Oral Maxillofac. Surg.* 21 (2): 85–89.

37 Ikeda, K., KC, H., Nowicki, B., and Haughton, V. (1996). Multiplanar MR and anatomic study of the mandibular canal. *AJNR Am. J. Neuroradiol.* 17: 579–584.

38 Anderson, L., Kosinski, T., and Mentag, P. (1991). A review of the intraosseous course of the nerves of the mandible. *J. Oral Implantol.* 17: 394–403.

39 Miller, C., Nummikoski, P., Barnett, D., and Langlais, R. (1990). Cross-sectional tomography. A diagnostic technique for determining buccolingual raltionship of impacted mandibular third molars and the inferior alveolar neurovascular bundle. *Oral Surg. Oral Med. Oral Pathol.* 70: 791–797.

40 Worthington, P. (2004). Injury to the inferior alveolar nerve during implant placement: a formula for protection of the patient and clinician. *Int. J. Maxillofac. Implants* 19: 731–734.

41 Behnia, H., Kheradvar, A., and Shahrokhi, M. (2000). An anatomic study of the lingul nerve in the third molar region. *J. Oral Maxillofac. Surg.* 58: 649–651.

42 Pogrel, M. and Goldman, K. (2004). Lingual flap retraction for third molar removal. *J. Oral Maxillofac. Surg.* 62: 1125–1130.

43 Bennet, S. and Townsend, G. (2001). Distribution of the mylohyoid nerve: anatomical variability and clinical implications. *Aust. Endod. J.* 27: 109–111.

44 Stein, P., Brueckner, J., and Milliner, M. (2007). Sensory innervation of mandibular teeth by the nerve to the mylohyoid: implications on local anaesthesia. *Clin. Anat.* 20: 591–595.

45 Thunthy, K., Yeadon, W., and Nasr, H. (2003). An illustrative study of the role of tomograms for the placement of dental implants. *J. Oral Implantol.* 29: 91–95.

46 Yildiz, S., Bayar, G.R., Guvenc, I. et al. (2015). Tomographic evaluation on bone morphology in posterior mandibular region for safe placement of dental implant. *Surg. Radiol. Anat.* 37: 167–173.

47 Misch, C. (2010). Distance between external cortical bone and mandibular canal for harvesting ramus graft: a human cadaver study. *J. Periodontol.* 81: 1103–1104.

48 Clavero, J. and Lundgren, S. (2003). Ramus or chin grafts for maxillary sinus and local onlay augmentation: comparison of donor site morbidity and complications. *Clin. Implant Dent. Relat. Res.* 5: 154–160.

49 Hwang, K., Shim, K., Yang, S., and Park, C. (2008). Partial-thickness cortical bone graft from the mandibular ramus: a non-invasive harvesting technique. *J. Periodontol.* 79: 941–944.

9

Extraction Ridge Management
Tino Mercado

9.1 Principles

Extraction and replacement of maxillary anterior teeth is one of the most challenging tasks in oral surgical rehabilitation. Healing of fresh extraction sockets involves physiological resorption and remodelling resulting in three-dimensional changes affecting alveolar ridge height and width and total volume [1–3]. The disruption of blood supply form the periodontal ligament after tooth extraction and increase in local osteoclastic activity in the area initiates the bone resorptive process [1, 2] resulting in an average of 1.5–3 mm vertical and 3–4.5 mm horizontal alveolar bone loss [1, 4, 5]. Most of these dimensional changes in the alveolar bone ridge morphology take place in the first three months following tooth extraction [1, 6, 7]. In the anterior maxillary cosmetic areas, these 3D changes represent the key causative factor for aesthetic implant complications and failures [8, 9].

In a systematic review that looked at dimensional changes after tooth extraction, it was found that the vertical dimensional reduction on the buccal side amounted to 11–22% (−1.24 to 0.11 mm) after six months, whereas the horizontal dimensional reduction on the buccal side was greater, reaching 29–63% (−3.79 to 0.23 mm) after six to seven months [10]. Alveolar ridge management procedures have been developed to improve the quantity and also quality of both hard and soft tissues on the alveolar ridge after extraction. To preserve the soft tissue profile, a variety of materials have been used, such as subepithelial connective tissue graft, free gingival graft (FGG) or a soft tissue substitute or a resorbable membrane that enhances closure of the soft tissue wound [11–14]. The majority of these procedures are performed as a flapless approach, particularly if the buccal bone has been preserved after tooth extraction. The primary purpose of using these soft tissues, apart from achieving complete closure of the socket, is to gain keratinized tissue. When it comes to the hard tissue filler of the extraction socket, materials such as autogenous bone, allografts, xenografts, and alloplasts have been used with varying degrees of success [12, 15, 16].

Practical Procedures in Implant Dentistry, First Edition. Edited by Christopher C.K. Ho.
© 2022 John Wiley & Sons Ltd. Published 2022 by John Wiley & Sons Ltd.
Companion website: www.wiley.com/go/ho/implant-dentistry

The consensus of the above studies is that alveolar ridge management can reduce the dimensional changes of the extraction socket when compared to an 'unpreserved' extraction socket.

9.2 Osteoconductive Materials for Ridge Management

Variable outcomes have been obtained in numerous ridge preservation studies using different osteoconductive particulate grafting materials to maintain post-extraction ridge dimensions in the anterior maxilla [15, 17]. In general, favourable outcomes have been obtained with slowly resorbing materials, such as deproteinised bovine bone mineral (DBBM) and DBBM stabilised with 10% collagen (DBBMC) [18–20]. A randomised clinical trial on ridge management compared (i) DBBMC covered with FGG, (ii) DBBMC covered with collagen xenograft, (iii) tricalcium phosphate (β-TCP), and (iv) spontaneous healing socket [12]. The study reported that sockets filled with DBBMC covered in free gingival graft or collagen xenograft resulted in less vertical changes of the alveolar ridge compared with sockets that had spontaneous healing and sockets filled with β-TCP [12]. The −0.3 to −1.4 mm reduction in the buccal bone height (BH) and palatal bone height (PH) in the DBBMC gingival graft group in the study by Jung et al. [12] is also within the range of −0.8 to −1.2 mm reported in a study where the socket was filled with DBBMC or DBBM then sealed with collagen membrane [21], which showed that DBBM and DBBMC demonstrated similar behaviour histologically and in terms of minimising ridge resorption after tooth extraction. The study by Jung et al. [12], however, did not consider the possible influence of buccal wall thickness on volume changes after ridge management procedures. Taken together, the findings of these two studies [12, 21] demonstrate the reproducibility of minimising the post-extraction buccal and palatal wall resorption to a range of 1–1.5 mm when utilising DBBMC.

9.3 Biologically Active Materials for Ridge Management

One of the perceived limitations of using xenografts on healing sockets is that these slowly resorbing materials can also interfere with new bone formation in the healing socket [22], which may compromise the osseointegration of implants subsequently placed in these sites. Because of this, biologically active materials, such as platelet-rich plasma [23, 24], platelet-rich fibrin [25], and recombinant bone morphogenic protein 2 [26] have been used to improve the performance of osteoconductive materials with mixed results. Enamel matrix derivative (EMD) is an insoluble matrix derived from an extract of naturally occurring enamel matrix proteins (EMPs), which are formed during amelogenesis by ameloblasts in Hertwig's epithelial root sheath (HERS) during tooth formation. HERS regulates the formation of the periodontal attachment apparatus, particularly the maturation of acellular extrinsic fibre cementum, producing cementoblasts from progenitor cells [27–29]. Emdogain®, a regenerative product introduced in the 1990s, is a gel product extracted from porcine tooth buds which contains mainly amelogenins and propylene glycol alginate (PGA) as carriers. Although the effectiveness of EMD in promoting periodontal regeneration is well documented [30, 31], the majority of the evidence that suggests EMD has osteogenic potential comes from *in vitro* studies [32–35]. A recent study explored for the first time the effect of incorporating EMD with DBBMC for ridge preservation in the anterior maxilla, reporting no beneficial effect on ridge dimensional outcomes [36], but the osteogenic effect of EMD or any other biologically active material was not explored.

Our group [37] conducted an anterior ridge management study comparing DBBMC alone versus DBBMC with EMD. We studied the radiographic difference in the ridge volume before and after extraction and also collected histological trephine biopsies four months after ridge preservation studies to assess bone quality with or without the adjunctive EMD. The aims of this prospective randomised controlled clinical study were: (i) to assess dimensional changes of grafted extraction sockets using either DBBMC alone or DBBMC with enamel matrix derivative (DBBMC-EMD) in preservation of the maxillary anterior ridge; and (ii) to assess the osteogenic potential of EMD by assessing histomorphometrically a tissue biopsy harvested from the treated alveolar ridge (Figure 9.1).

Our study [37] demonstrated that the application of DBBMC and DBBMC-EMD into extraction sockets covered with a FGG resulted in similar ridge dimensional reduction in volume four months after tooth extraction. Except for ridge width (RW), there were no significant dimensional changes in BH or PH in both test (DBBMC-EMD) and control (DBBMC only) groups four months after tooth extraction, confirming the relative effectiveness of this technique in minimising ridge reduction following tooth extraction (Figure 9.2). In other words, the use of EMD as an adjunct to DBBMC in this study did not help in minimising volumetric ridge reduction after tooth extraction. Although the percentage reduction in BH and PH is smaller in the test group where EMD was added with DBBMC, this did not reach statistical significance. This is consistent with a recently published study which also compared ridge preservation using DBBMC with and without EMD and similarly did not report a difference in ridge dimensional outcomes [36].

Although the use of biologically active materials (EMD) did not seem to improve the quantity of volume of the alveolar ridge after ridge management procedures, in terms of improving bone quality, the histomorphometric analysis of the study showed readily identifiable components of more new bone, less residual graft (RG) and less soft tissue matrix (STM) in sockets treated with DBBMC-EMD [37, 38] (Figure 9.3). The observation that most of the xenograft particles were surrounded by bone of varying maturity with no associated inflammatory reaction corroborates the excellent biocompatibility of DBBMC (Bio-Oss collagen®, Geistlich Pharma AG, Switzerland) that has been reported in the literature [40]. The histomorphometric analysis showed statistically significant differences in terms of percentage of new bone, RG, and soft tissue and marrow spaces between the test and control groups. The increased amount of new bone in the test group shows that the addition of EMD with DBBMC had

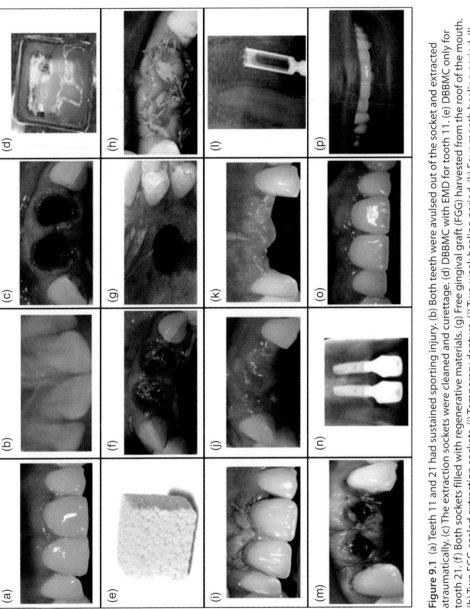

Figure 9.1 (a) Teeth 11 and 21 had sustained sporting injury. (b) Both teeth were avulsed out of the socket and extracted atraumatically. (c) The extraction sockets were cleaned and curettage. (d) DBBMC with EMD for tooth 11. (e) DBBMC only for tooth 21. (f) Both sockets filled with regenerative materials. (g) Free gingival graft (FGG) harvested from the roof of the mouth. (h) Two FGG-sealed extraction sockets. (i) Temporary denture. (j) Two-week healing period. (k) Four-month healing period. (l) Trephine used to harvest bone core biopsy. (m) Two implants placed four months after extraction. (n) The implants restored eight weeks after extraction. (o) The implants after final restoration. (p) Final patient profile.

(a)

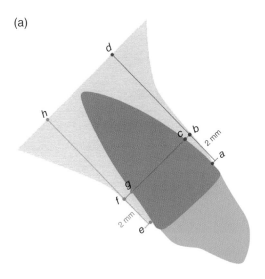

(b)

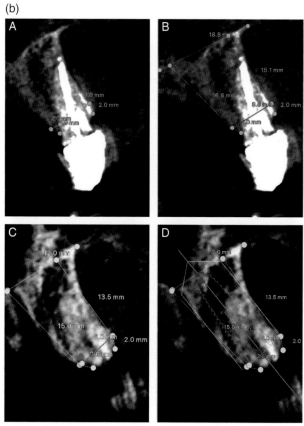

Figure 9.2 (a) CBCT measurement schematic. Points *a–d*: buccal bone height, *b–c*: buccal wall thickness (BT), *e–h*: palatal wall height (PH), *f–g*: palatal wall thickness (PT). (b) Representative CBCT scans. (A) and (B) Before extraction. (C) and (D) Four months after extraction [37–39].

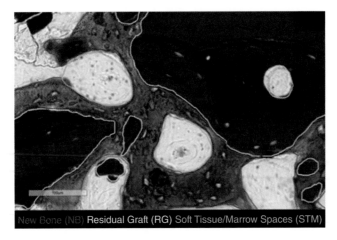

New Bone (NB) Residual Graft (RG) Soft Tissue/Marrow Spaces (STM)

Figure 9.3 Histological image (20× magnification) showing new bone, residual graft (yellow), and soft tissue/marrow (green) space within a biopsy core.

increased the osteogenic potential of this biomaterial. Evidence to support the increased osteogenic potential of EMD has been reported in *in vivo* studies showing that ameloblastin degradation products stimulated cementum formation, bone growth, and craniofacial bone formation [41, 42]. Furthermore, combining EMD with absorbable collagen sponge (ACS) influenced the activity of induced pluripotent stem cells (iPSCs) by upregulating the expression of bone sialoprotein and osteopontin and increasing the levels of osteoblastic differentiation and mineralisation, when compared to ACS alone [43]. Another possible effect of EMD in the present study is that it may promote resorption of the RG particles. This hypothesis is supported by studies that showed the ability of EMD to induce osteoclast formation in mouse bone marrow cells via the RANK-OPG-RANKL pathway *in vitro* [44], and *in vitro* evidence that a purified EMD fraction enhanced osteoclast activity and bone resorption in the monocytic cell line RAW 264.7 [45]. Whether EMD increased the formation of new bone or whether it increased the rate of resorption of the xenograft cannot be elucidated from the present study.

Because of the broad effects of EMD on various host cells and proteins, and not just exclusively on osteoblast and osteogenic activity, EMD has been described as osteopromotive rather than osteoinductive [41, 46, 47]. Indeed, the general pro-wound healing effects of EMD are reflected in its established clinical effectiveness in periodontal regeneration [48], root overage procedures [38, 39], and the management of peri-implantitis [49, 50].

To the best of our knowledge, ours is the first clinical study to demonstrate the osteogenic potential of EMD in fresh extraction sockets [37]. The clinical relevance of the present study, where more percentage new bone was noted four months after extraction in the test group, may translate clinically to earlier implant placement, enhanced implant osseointegration due to the presence of more bone, and better primary implant stability. This kind of study should be repeated in bigger randomised multi-centre clinical trials.

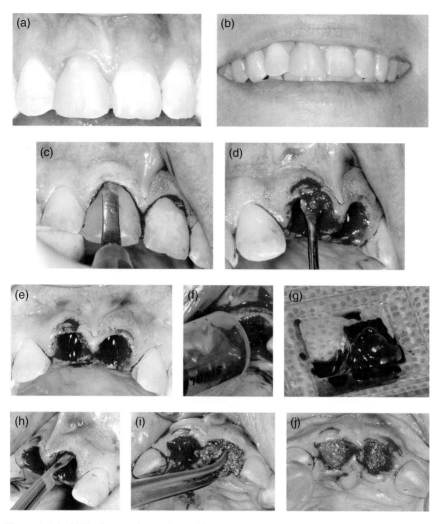

Figure 9.4 (a, b) Teeth 11 and 21 indicated for extraction. (c) Minimally traumatic extraction of tooth 11 using No.69 Swann-Morton® blade without any buccal and palatal movement (only rotary) to preserve buccal and palatal bone. (d) Extraction sockets thoroughly cleaned and curetted after minimally traumatic extraction of teeth. (e, f) Fresh autogenous blood harvested from thoroughly cleaned extraction socket (can use or mix other biologically active material such as Emdogain). (g) Deproteinised bovine bone mineral with 10% collagen (DBBMC, Bio-Oss Collagen™) mixed with the fresh autogenous blood harvested from the thoroughly cleaned socket (can use or mix other biologically active material such as Emdogain). (h) Gingival margin of the socket 'freshened-up' by de-epithelialising the extraction socket to ensure better vascularisation of the FGG or xenograft that will be adapted and sutured around the gingival margin. (i) DBBMC (Bio-Oss Collagen) densely packed into the socket. (j) DBBMC densely packed into the socket, leaving a 2 mm space below the gingiva for free gingival margin or xenograft (Mucograft™) closure. (k) Sterile paper template cut according to the size of the extraction sockets to assist in the free gingival graft stabilisation. (l) Palatal donor site, bleeding stopped by cellulose hemostatic fibre (Surgicel™) and stabilised by resorbable suture. (m) Two free gingival grafts stabilised by 5-0 monofilament suture (4–5 sutures around the circumference. (n) Temporary 'teeth-borne' denture during the first six to eight weeks of healing while the healing socket is filled with inflammatory and eventually 'non-load bearing' woven bone. A healing period of at least three to four months is needed prior to dental implant placements. (o) Two implants placed four months after 11 and 21 extraction and restored two to three months after implant placement.

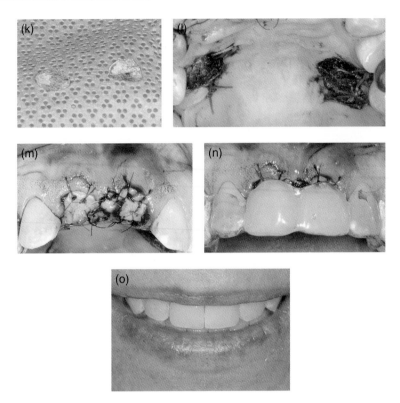

Figure 9.4 (Continued)

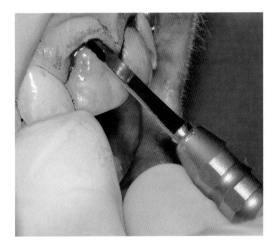

Figure 9.5 The No.69 Swann-Morton® mini-blade can act as a surgical blade and also as 'luxator' to 'loosen' the tooth and widen the periodontal ligmanent space without breaking the buccal and palatal wall.

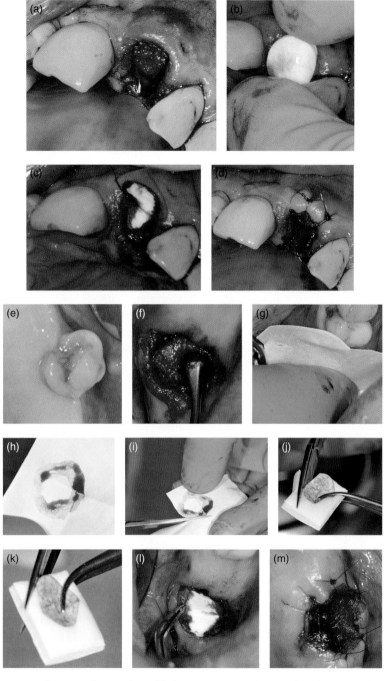

Figure 9.6 (a–d) For maxillary and mandibular anterior or single-rooted teeth (a), a circular Mucograft Seal™ (b) is available as substitute for free gingival graft to close the DBBMC-filled socket chamber (c). The minimum number of sutures to achieved maximum passive stabilisation is preferred (4–5 sutures) (d). (e–m) For maxillary or mandibular posterior teeth (e) where the extraction sockets are larger in circumference, the same protocol can be followed where DBBMC is plugged into each root up to the coronal area with 2 mm space below the gingival margin (f). A sterile paper template is adapted on top of the socket (g) to create an impression of the socket wound (h). This impression will give the clinician an idea on the size and shape of the extraction socket (i). The prepared paper template can be used or transferred into the Mucograft (j and k). This will create a tailor-made Mucograft firmly and passively adapted on the socket (l). Suture the tailor-made Mucograft with 4–5 circumferential monofilament sutures (m).

9.4   Influence of Buccal Wall Thickness on Ridge Management

After the analysis of ridge dimensional changes according to the treatment performed (Test DBBMC with EMD versus Control DBBMC only), the patients' radiographic data were grouped according to the thickness of the buccal wall (BT ≥1 mm versus BT <1 mm). Significant differences in the ridge dimensions were noted after the four-month healing period. Patients with <1 mm BT sustained ridge reductions of 1.0 to −1.5 mm (or −5.8 to −14%) (RW, BH, PH) compared to the minimal ridge reduction of 0.17 to −0.4 mm (or −2 to −5.4%) when the initial buccal wall thickness was ≥1 mm. It has been reported that the thickness of the buccal bone crest significantly influences the amount of vertical crestal resorption after tooth extraction [51–53]. In a study in which 93 subjects had extractions and implants immediately placed in the maxillary anterior area, it was demonstrated that patients with thin buccal walls (≤1 mm, 43% ridge reduction) sustained greater percentage ridge reduction than patients with thick buccal walls (>1 mm, 21% ridge reduction) 16 weeks after implant placement [52]. Therefore, although our study shows that the ridge preservation outcomes were improved in the presence of thicker buccal walls, when taken in the context of the increased resorption associated with thin buccal walls in the absence of ridge preservation [52], the results show that patients with a thin buccal wall (<1 mm) may benefit as much, if not more, from the socket management technique.

It has been reported that thin buccal walls (<1 mm) have a prevalence of 50–80% in the anterior maxilla, and are more common than thick buccal walls (>1 mm), which have a prevalence of 10–12% [51, 54]. Considering the large prevalence of patients susceptible to significant ridge resorption after extraction of maxillary anterior teeth, pre-extraction radiographic analysis of the buccal bone wall using cone beam computed tomography (CBCT) may be recommended prior to deciding on the ridge management approach.

The treatment planning for implant rehabilitation starts prior to the tooth extraction. Before tooth extraction (anterior or posterior) a radiographic examination (preferably CBCT scan) needs to be requested and the ridge dimension measured (Figure 9.2b). The dimension of buccal wall thickness (1.5–2.0 mm from the tip of the buccal crest and perpendicular to the root surface, Figure 9.2b) is a valuable parameter for predicting how much bone volume will be lost and how much the anterior ridge management procedure described in this chapter (Figures 9.4–9.6) will benefit the future implant site and result in possibly improved long-term implant outcomes. The use of biologically active materials as an adjunct to osteoconductive materials in preserving jawbone for future implant rehabilitation should be examined in larger multicentre clinical trials, whereby the long-term outcome of implant placement in these sites is also evaluated.

References

1 Araújo, M.G., Sukekava, F., Wennström, J.L. et al. (2005). Ridge alterations following implant placement in fresh extraction sockets: an experimental study in the dog. *J. Clin. Periodontol.* 32 (6): 645–652.

2 Cardaropoli, G., Araújo, M., and Lindhe, J. (2003). Dynamics of bone tissue formation in tooth extraction sites. *J. Clin. Periodontol.* 30 (9): 809–818.

3 van der Weijden, F., Dell'Acqua, F., and Slot, D.E. (2009). Alveolar bone dimensional changes of post-extraction sockets in humans: a systematic review. *J. Clin. Periodontol.* 36 (12): 1048–1058.

4 Iasella, J.M., Greenwell, H., Miller, R.L. et al. (2003). Ridge preservation with freeze-dried bone allograft and a collagen membrane compared to extraction alone for implant site development: a clinical and histologic study in humans. *J. Periodontol.* 74 (7): 990–999.

5 Lekovic, V., Camargo, P.M., Klokkevold, P.R. et al. (1998). Preservation of alveolar bone in extraction sockets using bioabsorbable membranes. *J. Periodontol.* 69 (9): 1044–1049.

6 Schropp, L., Wenzel, A., Kostopoulos, L., and Karring, T. (2003). Bone healing and soft tissue contour changes following single-tooth extraction: a clinical and radiographic 12-month prospective study. *Int. J. Periodont. Restorat. Dent.* 23 (4): 313–323.

7 Sun, D., Lim, H., and Lee, D. (2019). Alveolar ridge preservation using an open membrane approach for sockets with bone deficiency: a randomized controlled clinical trial. *Clin. Implant Dent. Relat. Res.* 21 (1): 175–182.

8 Belser, U.C., Grütter, L., Vailati, F. et al. (2009). Outcome evaluation of early placed maxillary anterior single-tooth implants using objective esthetic criteria: a cross-sectional, retrospective study in 45 patients with a 2- to 4-year follow-up using pink and white esthetic scores. *J. Periodontol.* 80 (1): 140–151.

9 Chen, S.T. and Buser, D. (2009). Clinical and esthetic outcomes of implants placed in postextraction sites. *Int. J. Oral Maxillofac. Implants* 24: 186–217.

10 Tan, W.L., Wong, T.L.T., Wong, M.C.M., and Lang, N.P. (2012). A systematic review of post-extractional alveolar hard and soft tissue dimensional changes in humans. *Clin. Oral Implants Res.* 23 (5): 1–21. https://doi.org/10.1111/j.1600-0501.2011.02375.x.

11 Barone, A., Aldini, N.N., Fini, M. et al. (2008). Xenograft versus extraction alone for ridge preservation after tooth removal: a clinical and histomorphometric study. *J. Periodontol.* 79 (8): 1370–1377.

12 Jung, R.E., Philipp, A., Annen, B.M. et al. (2013). Radiographic evaluation of different techniques for ridge preservation after tooth extraction: a randomized controlled clinical trial. *J. Clin. Periodontol.* 40 (1): 90–98.

13 Kassim, B., Ivanovski, S., and Mattheos, N. (2014). Current perspectives on the role of ridge (socket) preservation procedures in dental implant treatment in the aesthetic zone. *Aust. Dent. J.* 59 (1): 48–56.

14 Sisti, A., Canullo, L., Mottola, M.P. et al. (2012). Clinical evaluation of a ridge augmentation procedure for the severely resorbed alveolar socket: multicenter randomized controlled trial, preliminary results. *Clin. Oral Implants Res.* 23 (5): 526–535.

15 Avila-Ortiz, G., Chambrone, L., and Vignoletti, F. (2019). Effect of alveolar ridge preservation interventions following tooth extraction: a systematic review and meta-analysis. *J. Clin. Periodontol.* 46 (S21): 195–223.

16 Vignoletti, F., De Sanctis, M., Berglundh, T. et al. (2009). Early healing of implants placed into fresh extraction sockets: an experimental study in the beagle dog. II: ridge alterations. *J. Clin. Periodontol.* 36 (8): 688–697.

17 Darby, I., Darby, I., Chen, S.T. et al. (2009). Ridge preservation techniques for implant therapy. *Int. J. Oral Maxillofac. Implants* 24: 260–271.

18 Iorio-Siciliano, V., Blasi, A., Nicolo, M. et al. (2017). Clinical outcomes of socket preservation using bovine-derived xenograft collagen and collagen membrane post-tooth extraction: a 6-month randomized controlled clinical trial. *Int. J. Periodont. Restorat. Dent.* 37 (5): E290–E296.

19 Maiorana, C., Poli, P., Deflorian, M. et al. (2017). Alveolar socket preservation with demineralised bovine bone mineral and a collagen matrix. *J. Periodont. Implant Sci.* 47 (4): 194–210.

20 Manfro, R., Fonseca, F.S., Bortoluzzi, M.C., and Sendyk, W.R. (2014). Comparative, histological and histomorphometric analysis of three anorganic bovine xenogenous bone substitutes: bio-oss, bone-fill and gen-ox anorganic. *J. Maxillofac. Oral Surg.* 13 (4): 464–470.

21 Nart, J., Barallat, L., Jimenez, D. et al. (2017). Radiographic and histological evaluation of deproteinized bovine bone mineral vs. deproteinized bovine bone mineral with 10% collagen in ridge preservation. A randomized controlled clinical trial. *Clin. Oral Implants Res.* 28 (7): 840–848.

22 Araujo, M.G., Lindhe, J., and Institutionen för odontologi, Institute of Odontology, Sahlgrenska akademin, Göteborgs universitet, Sahlgrenska Academy (2009). Ridge alterations following tooth extraction with and without flap elevation: an experimental study in the dog. *Clin. Oral Implants Res.* 20 (6): 545–549.

23 Cheah, C.W., Vaithilingam, R.D., Siar, C.H. et al. (2014). Histologic, histomorphometric, and cone-beam computerized tomography analyses of calcium sulfate and platelet-rich plasma in socket preservation: a pilot study. *Implant Dent.* 23 (5): 593–601.

24 Strauss, F.J., Stähli, A., and Gruber, R. (2018). The use of platelet-rich fibrin to enhance the outcomes of implant therapy: a systematic review. *Clin. Oral Implants Res.* 29 (S18): 6–19.

25 Marenzi, G., Riccitiello, F., Tia, M. et al. (2015). Influence of leukocyte- and platelet-rich fibrin (L-PRF) in the healing of simple postextraction sockets: a split-mouth study. *Biomed. Res. Int.* 2015: 369273–369276.

26 Lim, H., Yoon, S., Cha, J. et al. (2018). Overaugmentation to compensate for postextraction ridge atrophy using a putty-type porcine bone substitute material with recombinant bone morphogenetic protein-2: 4 weeks of healing in a canine model. *Clin. Oral Investig.*: 1–10.

27 Gestrelius, S., Andersson, C., Johansson, A.C. et al. (1997). Formulation of enamel matrix derivative for surface coating. Kinetics and cell colonization. *J. Clin. Periodontol.* 24: 678–684.

28 Hammarström, L. (1997). Enamel matrix, cementum development and regeneration. *J. Clin. Periodontol.* 24 (9): 658–668.

29 Heijl, L. (1997). Periodontal regeneration with enamel matrix derivative in one human experimental defect a case report. *J. Clin. Periodontol.* 24 (9): 693–696.

30 Miron, R.J., Sculean, A., Cochran, D.L. et al. (2016). Twenty years of enamel matrix derivative: the past, the present and the future. *J. Clin. Periodontol.* 43 (8): 668–683.

31 Wu, Y., Lin, L., Song, C. et al. (2017). Comparisons of periodontal regenerative therapies: a meta-analysis on the long-term efficacy. *J. Clin. Periodontol.* 44 (5): 511–519.

32 Galli, C., Macaluso, G.M., Guizzardi, S. et al. (2006). Osteoprotegerin and receptor activator of nuclear factor-kappa B ligand modulation by enamel matrix derivative in human alveolar osteoblasts. *J. Periodontol.* 77 (7): 1223–1228.

33 Kappa, B. Ligand modulation by enamel matrix derivative in human alveolar osteoblasts. *J. Periodontol.* 77 (7): 1223–1228.

34 Klein, M., Reichert, C., Koch, D. et al. (2007). in vitro assessment of motility and proliferation of human osteogenic cells on different isolated extracellular matrix components compared with enamel matrix derivative by continuous single-cell observation. *Clin. Oral Implants Res.* 18 (1): 40–45.

35 Reichert, C., Al-Nawas, B., Smeets, R. et al. (2009). in vitro proliferation of human osteogenic cells in presence of different commercial bone substitute materials combined with enamel matrix derivatives. *Head Face Med.* 5 (1): 1–9.

36 Lee, J.H., Kim, D.H., and Jeong, S.N. (2020). Comparative assessment of anterior maxillary alveolar ridge preservation with and without adjunctive use of enamel matrix derivative: a randomized clinical trial. *Clin. Oral Implants Res.* 31 (1): 1–9.

37 Mercado, F., Vaquette, C., Hamlet, S., and Ivanovski, S. (2020). Enamel matrix derivative promotes new bone formation in xenograft assisted maxillary anterior ridge preservation – a randomized controlled clinical trial. *Clin. Oral Implant. Res.*, 5/2020: in press.

38 Mercado, F., Hamlet, S., and Ivanovski, S. (2020). A 3-year prospective clinical and patient-centered trial on subepithelial connective tissue graft with or without enamel matrix derivative in class I-II Miller recessions. *J. Periodontal Res.* 55 (2): 296–306.

39 Mercado, F., Hamlet, S., and Ivanovski, S. (2020). Subepithelial connective tissue graft with or without enamel matrix derivative for the treatment of multiple class III–IV recessions in lower anterior teeth: a 3-year randomized clinical trial. *J. Periodontol.* 91: 473–483.

40 Alayan, J., Vaquette, C., Saifzadeh, S. et al. (2016). A histomorphometric assessment of collagen-stabilized anorganic bovine bone mineral in maxillary sinus augmentation – a randomized controlled trial in sheep. *Clin. Oral Implants Res.* 27 (6): 734–743.

41 Grandin, H.M., Gemperli, A.C., and Dard, M. (2012). Enamel matrix derivative: a review of cellular effects in vitro and a model of molecular arrangement and functioning. *Tissue Eng. Part B Rev.* 18 (3): 181–202.

42 Tamburstuen, M.V., Reseland, J.E., Spahr, A. et al. (2010). Ameloblastin expression and putative autoregulation in mesenchymal cells suggest a role in early bone formation and repair. *Bone* 48 (2): 406–413.

43 Hisanaga, Y., Suzuki, E., Aoki, H. et al. (2018). Effect of the combined used of enamel matrix derivative and atelocollagen sponge scaffold on osteoblastic differentiation of mouse induced pluripotent stem cells in vitro. *J. Periodontal Res.* 53: 240–249.

44 Gruber, R., Roos, G., Caballe-Serrano, J. et al. (2014). TGF-[beta]RI kinase activity mediates emdogain-stimulated in vitro osteoclastogenesis. *Clin. Oral Investig.* 18 (6): 1639.

45 Itoh, N., Kasai, H., Ariyoshi, W. et al. (2006). Mechanisms involved in the enhancement of osteoclast formation by enamel matrix derivative. *J. Periodontal Res.* 41 (4): 273–279.

46 Bosshardt, D.D. (2008). Biological mediators and periodontal regeneration: a review of enamel matrix proteins at the cellular and molecular levels. *J. Clin. Periodontol.* 35 (8): 87–105.

47 Miron, R.J., Chandad, F., Buser, D. et al. (2016). Effect of enamel matrix derivative liquid on osteoblast and periodontal ligament cell proliferation and differentiation. *J. Periodontol.* 87 (1): 91–99.

48 Esposito, M., Grusovin, M., Papanikolaou, N. et al. (2009). Enamel matrix derivative (Emdogain) for periodontal tissue regeneration in intrabony defects. A Cochrane systematic review. *Eur. J. Oral Implantol.* 2 (4): 247–266.

49 Isehed, C., Svenson, B., Lundbergp et al. (2018). Surgical treatment of peri-implantitis using enamel matrix derivative, an RCT: 3 and 5 year follow-up. *J. Clin. Periodontol.* 45: 744–753.

50 Mercado, F., Hamlet, S., and Ivanovski, S. (2018). Regenerative surgical therapy for peri-implantitis using deproteinized bovine bone mineral with 10% collagen, enamel matrix derivative and doxycycline- a prospective cohort study. *Clin. Oral Implants Res.* 29: 583–591.

51 Braut, V., Braut, V., Bornstein, M.M. et al. (2011). Thickness of the anterior maxillary facial bone wall-a retrospective radiographic study using cone beam computed tomography. *Int. J. Periodontics Restorative Dent.* 31 (2): 125–131.

52 Ferrus, J., Cecchinato, D., Pjetursson, E.B. et al. (2010). Factors influencing ridge alterations following immediate implant placement into extraction sockets. *Clin. Oral Implants Res.* 21 (1): 22–29.

53 Nevins, M., Camelo, M., Paoli, S.D. et al. (2006). A study of the fate of the buccal wall of extraction sockets of teeth with prominent roots. *Int. J. Periodont. Restorat. Dent.* 26 (1): 19–29.

54 Januário, A.L., Duarte, W.R., Barriviera, M. et al. (2011). Dimension of the facial bone wall in the anterior maxilla: a cone-beam computed tomography study. *Clin. Oral Implants Res.* 22 (10): 1168–1171.

10

Implant Materials, Designs, and Surfaces
Jonathan Du Toit

10.1 Principles

Materials science can be overwhelming for many dentists. Implant dentistry is a significant industry, and understanding the materials science can be complex. The aim of this chapter is to demystify the main topics related to implants, including their materials, designs, and surfaces, and provide clinically relevant knowledge.

The main questions one should be able to answer after reading this chapter are:

- What are the types of implant designs available?
- What are the differences between implant connections?
- What are types of surfaces are available?
- What are the differences in thread design?
- What are the clinical effects of all these different features?

To comprehensively describe in this chapter every available design feature of every implant available is simply not possible. There are more than 2000 different dental implants [1], each claiming unique and superior designs. Thus, the information here will focus on the features a clinician will most often encounter.

10.2 Implant Bulk Materials

A dental implant and its crown may be made up of many different materials. The term 'implant bulk material' refers to the main material the bulk of the actual dental implant is manufactured from. The main materials are:

- Pure titanium
- Titanium alloys
- Zirconia
- Other.

Practical Procedures in Implant Dentistry, First Edition. Edited by Christopher C.K. Ho.
© 2022 John Wiley & Sons Ltd. Published 2022 by John Wiley & Sons Ltd.
Companion website: www.wiley.com/go/ho/implant-dentistry

10.2.1 Pure Titanium Used for Implant Bulk Material

As mentioned in earlier chapters, results from titanium as an implanted material in dentistry were published in the late 1960s, but the first experiments were as far back as the 1950s [2]. You may often hear the term 'commercially pure titanium'. That means, titanium metal that does not have other metals incorporated with it, and thus is not an alloy. Titanium is also graded. You may hear most often of grades 3, 4, and 5 titanium in implant dentistry. In fact, there are 37 grades of titanium available across many industries. Grades 1, 2, 3, 4, 7, and 11 are pure titanium. Grade 3 is no longer used; grade 4 titanium is possibly the most widely used [3].

This titanium is produced in long rods, and the individual dental implants are 'cut' from these rods (Figures 10.1–10.3). There are newer manufacturing processes, even three-dimensional printing of titanium, but these are too new and will not be discussed here. The cut implants may then be treated to alter its properties, such as strength, surface roughness, etc. (Figures 10.4–10.6).

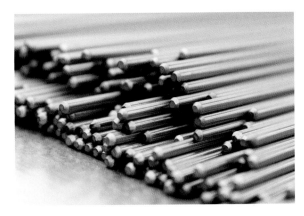

Figure 10.1 Titanium rods prior to dental implants being cut from these. *Source:* Image courtesy of MegaGen, South Korea.

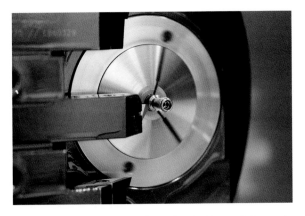

Figure 10.2 An individual dental implant cut from the titanium rod. *Source:* Image courtesy of MegaGen, South Korea.

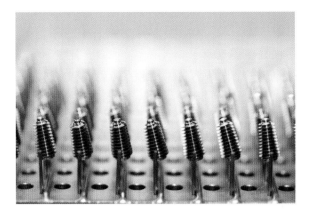

Figure 10.3 The cut implants prior to any surface treatments. *Source:* Image courtesy of MegaGen, South Korea.

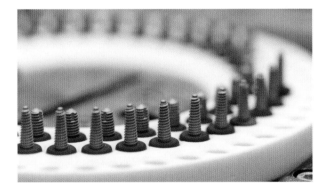

Figure 10.4 The implants after sandblasting. *Source:* Image courtesy of MegaGen, South Korea.

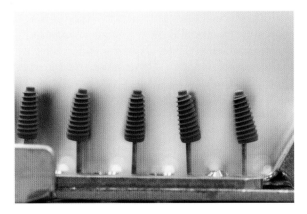

Figure 10.5 The implants are then acid etched to remove surface impurities and further create surface roughness. *Source:* Image courtesy of MegaGen, South Korea.

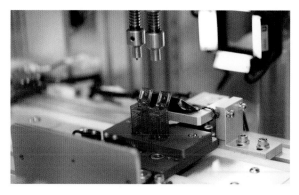

Figure 10.6 Finally, the implants are sterilised and packaged. *Source:* Image courtesy of MegaGen, South Korea.

There is no conclusive evidence that any one manufacturer's implant design, surface, material, or feature is superior over another [4]. There is, however, some data to support expert opinion and theory why a given feature is possibly better, or why another feature that may be undesirable. Also, no one feature ensures better outcomes, rather several factors combined may produce a better implant [5].

With regards to implant bulk materials, titanium and its alloys remain the gold standard in implant dentistry (Figures 10.7a–f). The survival rates are in the middle to upper 90% [6]. Survival means the implant has osseointegrated and remains osseointegrated, but does not explain about overall treatment success. The survival performance for titanium is higher than that for other bulk materials.

10.2.2 Titanium Alloys Used for Implant Bulk Material

Strong implants are going to be successful implants. Logically, we do not want implants to fracture. Because of their small size, the componentry they interact with, the forces in the mouth, and parafunction they are prone to fracture. Thus, many companies make an effort to improve implant strength. A common method is to 'cold work' the titanium. In this process the metal is squeezed or bent without heating, to produce a harder and less plastic metal [7]. Grade 4 pure titanium can be cold worked, but grade 5 titanium alloy cannot. Grade 5 combines titanium with 6% aluminium and 4% vanadium (Figure 10.7) (e.g. MIS Implants, Israel; Bicon implants, USA). Grade 23 is yet another alloy variation (e.g. Ditron Implants, Israel).

The 'mix' of metals are what give grade 5 titanium its supposed improved mechanical properties. Another common alloy for strength is Roxolid®, which is made of 85% titanium with 15% zirconia (Straumann Implants, Switzerland). That said, implant fracture is a very rare complication (less than 1% after five years in function) [8]. This should be remembered when considering manufacturers' claims of superior strength.

10.2.3 Zirconia Used for Implant Bulk Material

Zirconia is a complex material, and to fully describe it is outside the scope of this chapter. It is a metal oxide with other metals and additives, and when prepared as a dental implant is white in colour [9]. The main purpose of using zirconia

(a)

- Tapered implant
- Parallel neck
- Micro-threads at neck
- Progressive thread, both shallow and deep thread depth
- Aggressive thread
- Rectangular thread design
- Narrow thread pitch
- Internal connection
- Conical connection
- Platform switch

(b)

- Tissue level implant
- Parallel implant body
- Machined neck/collar
- Non-aggressive thread
- Reverse buttress thread design
- Shallow thread depth
- Wide thread pitch
- Internal conical

(c)

- Tapered implant body
- Machined bevel
- Aggressive thread
- V-shaped thread design
- Deep thread depth
- Narrow thread pitch
- Internal conical
- Morse-taper-like connection

(d)

- Tissue level implant
- 1-piece
- Tapered implant body
- Machined neck/collar
- Non-aggressive thread
- Rectangular thread design
- Shallow thread depth
- Narrow thread pitch
- External connection

(e)

- Bone level implant
- Mostly parallel implant body
- Short implant (6 mm length)
- Beveled neck/collar
- Non-aggressive thread
- Rectangular thread design
- Shallow thread depth
- Narrow thread pitch
- Internal conical "morse-taper-like" connection

(f)

- Bone level implant
- Both parallel and tapered implant body
- Machined neck/collar
- Non-aggressive thread
- Trapezoidal thread design
- Shallow thread depth
- Narrow thread pitch
- External hexagonal connection

(g)

- Zirconia implant
- Tissue level implant
- 1-piece / monotype
- Parallel implant body
- Non-aggressive thread
- Reverse buttress thread design
- Shallow thread depth
- Narrow thread pitch
- External connection

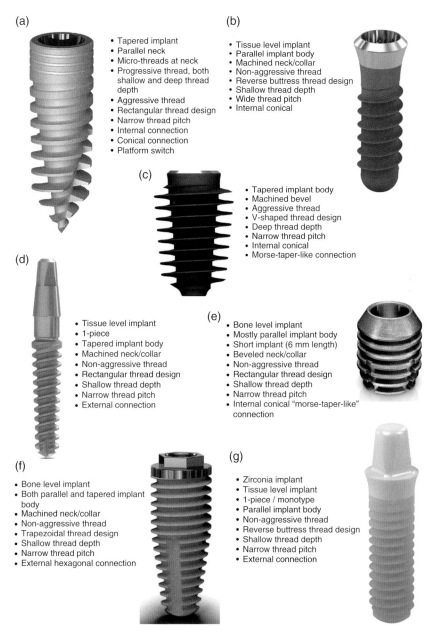

Figure 10.7 Examples of various implant designs. (a) Tapered implant with parallel neck. *Source:* Folkman, M., Becker, A., Meinster, I. et al. Comparison of bone-to-implant contact and bone volume around implants placed with or without site preparation: a histomorphometric study in rabbits. Sci. Rep. 2020;10:12446. https://doi.org/10.1038/s41598-020-69455-4. (b) Tissue level implant with parallel body. *Source:* By kind permission of the Straumann Group. (c) Tapered implant body. *Source:* MegaGen, South Korea. (d) One-piece tissue level implant. *Source:* MIS, Israel. (e) Bone level implant with mostly parallel body. *Source:* Bicon, USA. (f) Bone level implant with both parallel and tapered body. *Source:* Southern Implants, South Africa. (g) Zirconia tissue level implant. *Source:* By kind permission of the Straumann Group.

implants is to improve optics; a titanium implant is dark grey whereas a zirconia implant is white and does not discolour the tissue as much (Figure 10.7g). A second reason to use would be to avoid titanium allergy, which is said to affect 0.6% of patients [10]. Other patients (and dentists) may opt for 'metal-free' dentistry, which is, in fact, a misnomer.

Zirconia implants have a proven performance record lower than that of titanium implants. The survival rate for one-piece immediate zirconia implants is so low (85%) they are contraindicated [11]. Overall, zirconia implants are to be used in select cases only, where the above indications are implicit. These implants support a maximum of a three-unit fixed partial denture.

10.2.4 Other Materials as Bulk Implant Material

Tests on implants made of polyetheretherketone (PEEK) have been reported. The rationale for using this material is that it has properties close to those of bone and it is tooth-coloured. The osseointegration of this material is far poorer than that of titanium, and at this time it cannot be recommended [3].

10.3 Implant Surface Treatments

The process of osseointegration has been explained in earlier chapters. To summarise, initially the implant is inserted into a bony hole drilled into alveolar bone (an implant osteotomy). The initial friction between the bone tissue and the implant surface is called primary stability. As the surface of this bony wound is resorbed and remodelled, the implant slowly loses this primary stability, as it slowly gains secondary stability. That is, the wound heals and slowly new bone is formed around and onto the implant's surface, which is covered in a titanium oxide layer [7, 12]. The wound heals better if the cells function better. The functions of the blood clot cells are to achieve haemostasis, recruit inflammatory cells via mediator release, and provide a scaffold for fibroblasts and bone-forming cells to migrate into. Bone-forming cells (osteoblasts and pre-osteoblasts) produce a functional matrix. Ideally, these cells attach to and spread out on the implant surface and begin releasing chemical mediators, producing collagen and then mineralizing it. These cells and components function better and attach better if the implant surface has high wettability [13–15]. Consider, for example, a drop of blood applied to an implant made of Teflon (dense polytetrafluoroethylene, basically plumber's tape). What would you expect to see? Beading possibly. Beading looks like complete droplets on a surface. The drop of blood would not 'coat' the surface very well. All the steps mentioned above that ideally lead to bone forming on the surface then also would not occur. Teflon as a material has a very low wettability and low surface energy. In materials science, wettability is measured by the angle a droplet forms with a surface and the angle determines whether the material is hydrophilic or hydrophobic (Figure 10.8). If the blood and blood clot are to wet the surface of a dental implant well and the cells to adhere, the implant material should have good wetting, high surface energy, and thus be hydrophilic.

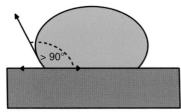

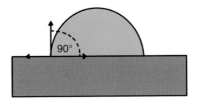

- Hydrophobic surface
- Low wettability
- Low surface energy

- Hydrophilic if contact angle < 90°

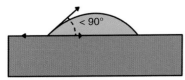

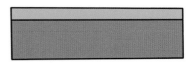

- Hydrophilic surface
- High wettability
- High surface energy

- Super-hydrophilic surface
- Contact angle zero

Figure 10.8 Measuring wettability by the sessile water droplet test.

Table 10.1 Classification of implant surface treatments.

Surface treatment	Type	Example
Additive	Anodised electrochemical oxidation	Xpeed surface, MegaGen implants
	Anodised electrochemical oxidation	TiUnite, Nobel Biocare implants
	Plasma-sprayed	No longer widely available
Subtractive	Sandblasted	
	Acid etched	
	Sandblasted and acid etched (SLA)	Most implants today
	Alumina blasting	Southern Implants, South Africa

The topic of wettability is complex. There is, however, some very practical information to apply. Remember that implant surfaces should ideally be hydrophilic to better achieve osseointegration. When a rod of titanium is 'cut' into an implant, the cut surface is referred to as 'machined'. Machined surfaces have no additional surface treatment (see Figure 10.3 for an image of implants prior to surface treatment). Early implants consisted only of this type of manufacture and had lower survival rates than the implants now available. Today, surfaces are treated to improve their hydrophilicity. The surface treatments are broadly classified into additive or subtractive (Table 10.1). A widely used surface treatment is sandblasting and acid etching (SLA) (Figure 10.9). This is a subtractive treatment. The surface is made micro-rough to improve its wettability. Most implant companies jostle for positioning as the 'best surface', and truly such a best surface does not exist. In fact, the majority of implant surfaces are SLA, and

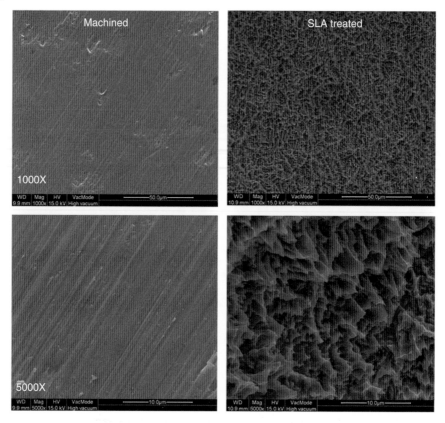

Figure 10.9 Scanning electron microscope (SEM) view of an untreated, machined titanium surface (left) compared to a sandblasting and acid etching (SLA)-treated titanium surface (right). Source: Kim et al. 2015. Cell Adhesion and in Vivo Osseointegration of Sandblasted/Acid Etched/Anodized Dental Implants. *Int. J. Mol. Sci.* 2015;16:10324–10336. https://doi.org/10.3390/ijms160510324. CC BY 4.0.

are classified as moderately rough (Figure 10.10). There is a theoretical concern that rough implants may become more rapidly colonised by peri-implant disease-causing bacteria if exposed to these pathogens. Review of the evidence does show that the roughest implants (plasma sprayed) are the most hydrophilic, but also have higher failure rates [14, 16].

If the choice of implant product becomes overwhelming, the decision-maker can rest assured that most surfaces are quite similar. There are minor differences promoted by manufacturers. For example, the Xpeed™ surface by the MegaGen company incorporates calcium in the surface after SLA treatment, and a different treatment is used to produce the SLActive™ surface from the Straumann company. When exposed to the air out of its packaging a sterile implant with surface treatment will become contaminated with hydrocarbons and will lose its hydrophilicity [15]. For this reason, SLActive implants (and some others) are stored in sterile saline to limit contamination.

To summarise, a moderately rough surface improves osseointegration and most implants today are moderately rough and SLA treated. There is histological

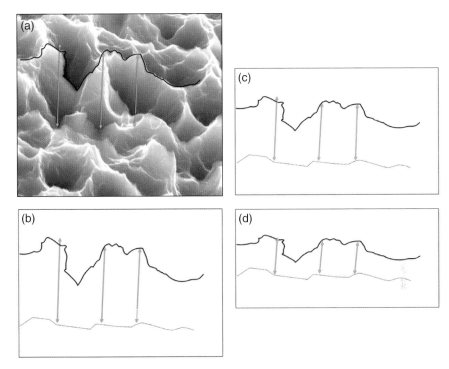

Figure 10.10 Classification of implant surface roughness: (a) treated implant surface; (b) rough: valley to hill >2 μm; (c) moderately rough: valley to hill 1–2 μm; (d) smooth: valley to hill <1 μm.

data of different stages of osseointegration in animals [17]. In the first few weeks there is slightly higher bone-to-implant contact (BIC) in the first two weeks, but in weeks four to six onward, BIC for most implants is the same [18]. Most implants will osseointegrate adequately. As mentioned earlier, no great differences in clinical performance have been proven between the various implant surfaces beyond what has been mentioned here.

10.4 Implant Design

This section provides a summary of the most important and clinically relevant knowledge on implant body shapes, and thread patterns, and implant connections.

10.4.1 Implant Body Shape Design

Broadly, implants are either tapered or parallel. A tapered implant is a 'root-form' implant – wider at its neck or platform and narrowest at its apex. The implant thus has a 'wedging' effect when turned into an osteotomy. These implants are especially suited for softer type bone (type D-4). In fact, most implants today are tapered. Some implants are a combination of both parallel and tapered. The disadvantage may be that a taper design exerts compression where the implant is widest and where bone can least tolerate it – at the cortex [19]. For this reason, older implant designs were commonly parallel, or straight, and thus exerted less pressure on bone (Figure 10.7b). The disadvantage with these implants is poorer primary stability. Arguably, a good implant design should exert compression in areas where cancellous bone can accommodate this for good primary stability, and have little or no compression where cortical bone cannot accommodate this and may resorb [3, 19].

Also note that some implants are placed at or just below the bone crest – referred to as 'bone level'. These implants allow for variability in treatment approach (whether to submerge and allow for healing first or to attach a transmucosal abutment the same day, or even to immediately load). Conversely, some implants have the transmucosal part built into the implant – referred to 'tissue level' (Figure 10.7b). Abutments attach to both these types, and thus these implants are two-piece. Another design is similar to the tissue level implant, but no other abutment attaches to it. Such one-piece implants have a rough bone level portion and a polished tissue level portion that continues to emerge in the mouth, typically for an overdenture to seat onto (Figures 10.7d and 10.7f).

10.4.2   Implant Thread Design

Biting force exerts substantial force, especially if a patient lacks proprioception from an absent peridontal ligament. When the forces are too great, the weakest link in the 'chain' will fail – either the implant and its components or the bone [3, 19]. Shear forces and excessive compressive forces on bone are also undesirable, as is occlusal overload that may cause microfractures of bone and thus bone loss. Implant threads have numerous shapes and designs to overcome this (Figures 10.11 and 10.12) [5]. The theoretical goal is to dissipate biting force through the bone and to limit shear force. Studies often state that 'most of the occlusal load is transferred to cortical bone'. Thus, modifying the implant design/ geometry affects this transfer of stress. However, this can only be investigated by software using finite element analyses that theoretically replicate these forces [5, 20]. In theory, the data from these experiments report the following:

- Threads closer to each other (lesser thread pitch) create less stress
- Longer threads create better load distribution
- Rectangular threads create less stress than trapezoidal
- Micro-threads at the implant neck may reduce stress to cortical bone
- Narrow implants transfer more stress to cortical bone.

It must be stressed that this data on the effect of thread design on bone is theoretical and the direct clinical application is challenging. No single implant features all these designs. A lesser thread pitch can also have deeper thread depth (Figure 10.7c). Deeper threads are typically also not rectangular, etc.

10.4.3   Implant Connection Designs

The different connection types are classified in Table 10.2. Historically, most implants had an external connection with a hexagonal anti-rotation feature (commonly termed external hex) (Figure 10.7f). This connection still exists today, but

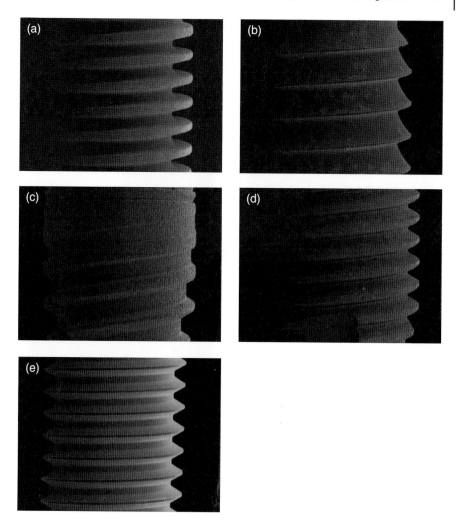

Figure 10.11 Differing thread designs: (a) plateau; (b) reverse buttress; (c) square; (d) trapezoidal; (e) V-shaped, narrower tip. *Source:* Images courtesy of Delgado-Ruiz, R.A., Calvo-Guirado, J.L., and Romanos, G.E. (2019). Effects of occlusal forces on the peri-implant-bone interface stability. *Periodontol 2000* 81: 179–193.

is less frequently available – and for good reasons. As stated, oral biting forces have significant magnitude that is transferred from the prosthesis/crown through the implant abutment, through the implant, and to the bone. Instability anywhere in that 'unit' will cause movement [21]. Movement can cause wear and tear on the components, which may then loosen, be damaged, and fracture. Certain connections already have inherent microgaps. They are greatest at external hexagon, internal hexagon, and internal tri-lobe connections. Movement creates gaps for oral fluids and endotoxin-producing bacteria to populate (Figure 10.13) [22]. Such unstable connections rely on the tension of a tightened screw to hold the prosthesis/crown to the implant (Table 10.2). Screw-loosening thus is the most common prosthetic complication in implant dentistry.

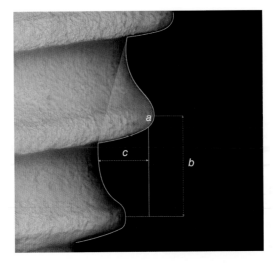

Figure 10.12 (*a*) Thread geometry, reverse buttress design. (*b*) Thread pitch, distance from the tip of one thread to the tip of the adjacent thread. (*c*) Thread depth, variable depth from a line connecting the tip of two adjacent threads to the implant wall.

Table 10.2 Classification of implant connections.

External	Internal	
	Non-conical	Conical
Hexagon	• Hexagon	• Taper-integrated screwed-in abutment
	• Tri-lobe	
		* Relies on a screw to retain the abutment
		• Purely tapered interference fit
		* Does not rely on a screw to retain

10.4.4 Which Implant Connections Are Better and Why?

When the abutment fits inside the implant, the platform of the implant is automatically wider than the abutment (Figures 10.13–10.16). The term for this is 'platform switch'. If there is a microgap (and worse, micromotion) between the implant and the abutment, the gap may fill with oral fluid and bacteria that causes inflammation of the adjacent tissues. Bone will resorb in an effort retreat from this zone of inflammation (Figures 10.13 and 10.15). At platform-switched implants, this gap (if any at all) is moved farther away from bone. Thus, bacteria and source of inflammation is also moved away from bone (Figure 10.16). At stable implant connections (with minimal or no microgap/micromotion) this narrower abutment also allows for more soft tissue in the area. Soft tissue thickness is often shown in the literature to be symbiotic for peri-implant bone health and stability [23]. At these stable implant connections, bone can be seen to remain above the platform, instead of being resorbed apically to the 1st/2nd/3rd threads. Such stable connections have a built-in platform switch. They do not rely on the screw to retain the prosthesis/crown. The friction between the coni-

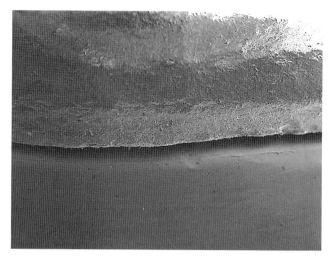

Figure 10.13 An external hexagonal connection. Note the visible gap between abutment and implant. (SEM view, unknown magnification.)

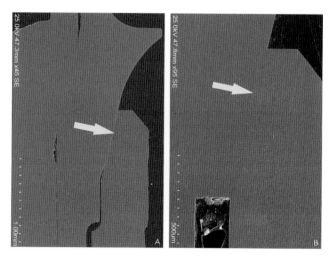

Figure 10.14 An internal conical connection. Note the intimate contact between abutment and implant (arrow). (SEM view, unknown magnification.) *Source:* Images courtesy of Fokas, G., Ma, L., Chronopoulos, V. et al. (2019). Differences in micromorphology of the implant–abutment junction for original and third-party abutments on a representative dental implant. J. Prosthet. Dent. 121(1): 143–150.

cal portion of the abutment inserted into the conical portion of the implant is what retains the crown. In other industries, this friction, which meets exact specifications, is referred to as Morse taper (connections). Morse taper in implant dentistry in fact does not exist. A Morse taper connection is determined by a formula that includes the material's coefficient of friction, the length of contact, and the angle of the conical connection [24]. It would be more accurate to refer to the most stable of conical connections rather as 'Morse-taper-like connections'.

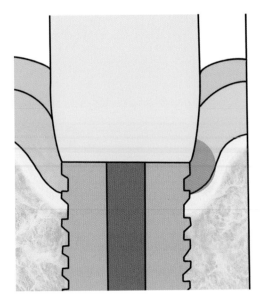

Figure 10.15 An external, 'flat-on-flat' connection. Abutment and implant are the same diameter. This unstable connection typically has a microgap filled with oral fluid and bacteria. Bone resorbs to retreat away from the zone of inflammation (arrow).

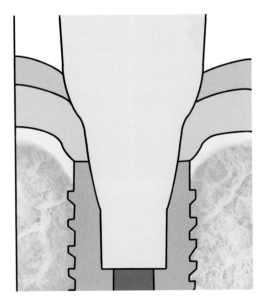

Figure 10.16 The internal conical connection moves a potential gap away from bone, called 'platform switch'. Also, the steeper the internal angle the more stable the connection, a 'morse-taper-like' connection. Less microgap and less micromovement.

There is no angle or other parameter to designate such a connection, other than connections that require a screw for retention, and connections that do not (Table 10.2).

10.5   Summary

There are a wide variety of implant designs, shapes, and sizes that may suit a particular application among a wide variety of situations. To answer 'which is better or the best?' is not entirely objective. Moreover, research does not always help. Thus, implant selection will likely be the clinician's preference. One should rather ask, 'what works best in my hands?' and 'what is best for this situation?'. That said, some general recommendations can be made: (i) A stable connection better ensures healthy peri-implant tissues, leading to smaller microgaps, less micromovement, and less screw-loosening. (ii) Tapered implants with an aggressive thread better ensure primary stability that leads to osseointegration. (iii) A platform switch implant probably allows for more peri-implant abutment tissues. (iv) All surfaces available today perform more or less equally in the end and almost all will osseointegrate adequately.

References

1 Jokstad, A. and Ganeles, J. (2018). Systematic review of clinical and patient-reported outcomes following oral rehabilitation on dental implants with a tapered compared to a non-tapered implant design. *Clin. Oral Implants Res.* 29 (Suppl 16): 41–54.

2 Branemark, P.I., Adell, R., Breine, U. et al. (1969). Intra-osseous anchorage of dental prostheses. I. Experimental studies. *Scand. J. Plast. Reconstr. Surg.* 3: 81–100.

3 Bonfante, E.A., Jimbo, R., Witek, L. et al. (2019). Biomaterial and biomechanical considerations to prevent risks in implant therapy. *Periodontol.* 81: 139–151.

4 Esposito, M., Ardebili, Y., and Worthington, H.V. (2014). Interventions for replacing missing teeth: different types of dental implants. *Cochrane Database Syst. Rev.* (7): CD003815.

5 Abuhussein, H., Pagni, G., Rebaudi, A., and Wang, H.L. (2010). The effect of thread pattern upon implant osseointegration. *Clin. Oral Implants Res.* 21: 129–136.

6 Roehling, S., Schlegel, K.A., Woelfler, H., and Gahlert, M. (2018). Performance and outcome of zirconia dental implants in clinical studies: a meta-analysis. *Clin. Oral Implants Res.* 29 (Suppl 16): 135–153.

7 Özcan, M. and Hämmerle, C. (2012). Titanium as a reconstruction and implant material in dentistry: advantages and pitfalls. *Materials (Basel).* 2012 Aug 24; 5 (9): 1528–1545. https://doi.org/10.3390/ma5091528. eCollection 2012 Sep.

8 Lee, D.W., Kim, N.H., Lee, Y. et al. (2019). Implant fracture failure rate and potential associated risk indicators: an up to 12-year retrospective study of implants in 5,124 patients. *Clin. Oral Implants Res.* 30: 206–217.

9 Burgess, J.O. (2018). Zirconia: the material, its evolution, and composition. *Compend. Contin. Educ. Dent.* 39: 4–8.

10 Sicilia, A., Cuesta, S., Coma, G. et al. (2008). Titanium allergy in dental implant patients: a clinical study on 1500 consecutive patients. *Clin. Oral Implants Res.* 19: 823–835.

11 Roehling, S., Astasov-Frauenhoffer, M., Hauser-Gerspach, I. et al. (2017). in vitro biofilm formation on titanium and zirconia implant surfaces. *J. Periodontol.* 88: 298–307.

12 Terheyden, H., Lang, N.P., Bierbaum, S., and Stadlinger, B. (2012). Osseointegration--communication of cells. *Clin. Oral Implants Res.* 23: 1127–1135.

13 Gittens, R.A., Scheideler, L., Rupp, F. et al. (2014). A review on the wettability of dental implant surfaces II: biological and clinical aspects. *Acta Biomater.* 10: 2907–2918.

14 Rupp, F., Gittens, R.A., Scheideler, L. et al. (2014). A review on the wettability of dental implant surfaces I: theoretical and experimental aspects. *Acta Biomater.* 10: 2894–2906.

15 Rupp, F., Liang, L., Geis-Gerstorfer, J. et al. (2018). Surface characteristics of dental implants: a review. *Dent. Mater.* 34: 40–57.

16 Wennerberg, A., Albrektsson, T., and Chrcanovic, B. (2018). Long-term clinical outcome of implants with different surface modifications. *Eur. J. Oral Implantol.* 11 (Suppl 1): S123–s136.

17 Berglundh, T., Abrahamsson, I., Lang, N.P., and Lindhe, J. (2003). De novo alveolar bone formation adjacent to endosseous implants. *Clin. Oral Implants Res.* 14: 251–262.

18 Schwarz, F., Ferrari, D., Herten, M. et al. (2007). Effects of surface hydrophilicity and microtopography on early stages of soft and hard tissue integration at non-submerged titanium implants: an immunohistochemical study in dogs. *J. Periodontol.* 78: 2171–2184.

19 Delgado-Ruiz, R.A., Calvo-Guirado, J.L., and Romanos, G.E. (2019). Effects of occlusal forces on the peri-implant-bone interface stability. *Periodontol.* 81: 179–193.

20 Calì, M., Zanetti, E.M., Oliveri, S.M. et al. (2018). Influence of thread shape and inclination on the biomechanical behaviour of plateau implant systems. *Dent. Mater.* 34: 460–469.

21 Zipprich, H., Weigl, P., Lange, B., and Lauer, H.-C. (2007). Micromovements at the implant–abutment interface: measurement, causes, and consequences. *Implantologie* 15: 31–46.

22 Sasada, Y. and Cochran, D.L. (2017). Implant-abutment connections: a review of biologic consequences and peri-implantitis implications. *Int. J. Oral Maxillofac. Implants* 32: 1296–1307.

23 Linkevicius, T., Puisys, A., Steigmann, M. et al. (2015). Influence of vertical soft tissue thickness on crestal bone changes around implants with platform switching: a comparative clinical study. *Clin. Implant. Dent. Relat. Res.* 17: 1228–1236.

24 Oberg, E. (2012). *Machinery's Handbook*, 29e. New York: Industrial Press.

11

Timing of Implant Placement
Christopher C.K. Ho

11.1   Principles

The placement of dental implants for the restoration of missing teeth is a well-established procedure with the original protocol requiring two to three months of alveolar bone remodelling following tooth extraction, and an additional six months of load-free healing to ensure implant stability during the early stages of bone healing. According to conventional protocol, implant placement was performed after the edentulous site had healed, which would resolve any infection and allow bony and soft tissue healing for implant placement. Such a long treatment period can be an obvious drawback to patient acceptance, and the conventional protocol has been challenged in recent decades by reducing the time between extracting a tooth to placing and loading of the implant. Placing implants immediately may minimise the number and time of surgical interventions the patient must undertake, however this should be carefully assessed to ensure predictability and success of procedures.

11.1.1   Classification for Timing of Implant Placement

There are varying descriptions on the timing of how implants are placed. For example, Esposito et al. in a Cochrane Review [1] described a classification as follows:

- Immediate implants – those that are placed in dental sockets after tooth extraction
- Immediate–delayed implants – those inserted after a couple of weeks up to a couple of months to allow for soft tissue healing
- Delayed implants – those placed thereafter in partially or completely healed bone.

An alternative descriptive classification introduced at the Third ITI Consensus Conference by Hämmerle and co-workers [2] is based on the clinical outcome of the wound-healing process, rather than rigid time frames (Table 11.1).

Practical Procedures in Implant Dentistry, First Edition. Edited by Christopher C.K. Ho.
© 2022 John Wiley & Sons Ltd. Published 2022 by John Wiley & Sons Ltd.
Companion website: www.wiley.com/go/ho/implant-dentistry

Table 11.1 Classification system for timing of implant placement [2].

Classification	Descriptive terminology	Period after extraction	Desired clinical scenario
Type 1	Immediate placement	0	Post-extraction site with no soft or hard tissue healing
Type 2	Early placement with soft-tissue healing	Typically 4–8 weeks	Post-extraction site with healed soft tissue but without significant bony healing
Type 3	Early placement with partial bone healing	Typically 12–16 weeks	Post-extraction site with healed soft tissue and significant bony healing
Type 4	Late placement	Typically 6 months +	Fully healed site

Source: Based on Chen, S.T., Wilson, T.G., and Hämmerle, C.H.F. (2004). Immediate or early placement of implants following tooth extraction: review of biologic basis, clinical procedures and outcomes. Int. J. Oral Maxillofac. Implants 19(Suppl): 12–25.

- **Type 1** – immediate implant placement occurring at time of tooth extraction within the same surgical procedure
- **Type 2** – placement after soft tissue healing, but before any significant bone fill of the socket. Typically, this would be around four to eight weeks
- **Type 3** – placement following bone fill of the socket. This would be around 12–16 weeks
- **Type 4** – placement in a fully healed site around six months or longer.

11.1.2 Immediate Placement

More recently, studies have reported promising high success rates and aesthetic outcomes for implants placed into extraction sockets (Figure 11.1–11.5). The potential advantages of immediate implants are that treatment time can be short-

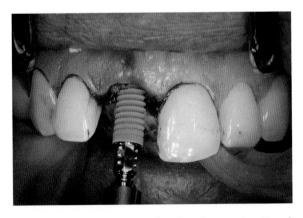

Figure 11.1 Immediate implant placement on day of tooth extraction. Use of a tapered threaded implant for maximum implant stability.

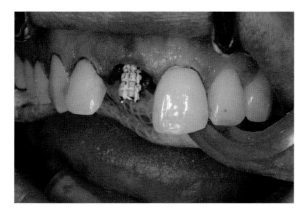

Figure 11.2 Temporary cylinder *in situ* opaqued with opaque tints to block metal show-through.

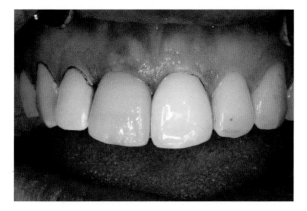

Figure 11.3 Denture tooth converted into immediate provisional crown.

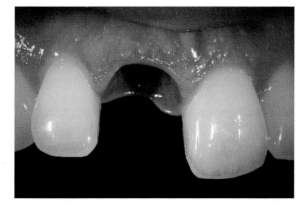

Figure 11.4 Prosthetically guided soft tissue healing with provisional crown recreates natural harmonious gingival contours.

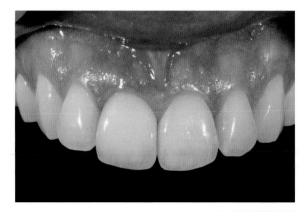

Figure 11.5 Final all-ceramic crown and abutment in place, recreating natural aesthetics.

ened, with fewer surgical procedures and that bone volumes might be partially maintained, thus possibly providing good aesthetic results. The potential disadvantages are an increased risk of infection and failures. After implant placement in post-extraction sites, gaps can be present between the implant and the bony walls. It is possible to fill these gaps and to augment bone simultaneously to implant placement. There are many techniques to achieve this but it is unclear when augmentation is needed and which could be the best augmentation technique.

Immediate implant placement has been proposed to:

- preserve soft tissue form and contour
- reduce the number of surgical appointments
- preserve bone dimensions (although this has been refuted)
- reduce treatment time, thereby improving patient satisfaction and comfort
- reduce costs for treatment due to fewer appointments
- optimise aesthetic results.

It has been suggested that an immediate approach may minimise remodelling of the alveolus, and consequently maintain the original shape of the ridge. Conversely, recent literature in dog and human studies by Araujo et al. [3] and Botticelli et al. [4] fail to support this. It has been shown that irrespective of immediate or delayed placement, extraction leads to bony remodelling with loss of ridge height and width. Botticelli et al. placed 21 implants in the fresh extraction sockets of 18 patients. They recorded a horizontal resorption of about 50% at the buccal aspect and 30% at the lingual side of the implant, corresponding to an overall width reduction of 2.8 mm. Covani et al. [5] analysed healing around 15 implants placed immediately and found the mean bucco-lingual distance reported at time of implant placement (10.5 mm) reduced to 6.8 mm at time of second-stage surgery. They observed that immediate implant placement could not prevent resorption in the bucco-lingual direction of the alveolar process.

It is likely that immediate implant placement does not prevent resorption of the bony alveolus after extraction. The more pronounced bone loss seen from the buccal aspect may be because the buccal bone crest is composed of bundle bone, whereas the palatal plate is mainly cortical bone. This may be the cause of the mid-facial gingival recession often seen with remodelling of the alveolus after extraction.

Ideal positioning of dental implants is required for aesthetic and functional success. This requires correct three-dimensional positioning of the implant with maintenance of adequate buccal bone over the implant buccal surface. The positioning is made more difficult for immediate placement due to the need to negotiate the extraction socket and the remaining alveolus and to manage soft tissues. The buccal–lingual position should be positioned 1–2 mm lingual to the emergence of the adjacent teeth. Implants with shoulder position at or buccal to the line drawn between the cervical margins of adjacent teeth demonstrate three times more recession than those with shoulder position palatal to this line (1.8 mm compared to 0.6 mm) [6]. Alignment of the implant with immediate placement in this correct manner may be complicated due to the thinner cortical plate evident in extraction sockets, with the tendency for the osteotomy preparation to drift buccally. Complexity may also arise due to the clinician's attempt to obliterate sockets with the implant, leading to a buccal/labial alignment of the fixture.

The use of a threaded tapered implant with a moderately rough surface is recommended. Recent work on the surface activity of implants, such as UV treatment and the use of nitrogen atmosphere with rinsing of implants, has enhanced the free surface energy and hydrophilicity of implants. This promotes faster osseointegration and leads to quicker secondary stability.

Potential risk factors involved with an immediate placement approach include the possibility of infection, discrepancy between socket size and implant leading to gap formation and possible fibrous tissue formation, as well as implant micromovement during wound healing if it is immediately loaded or a healing abutment is placed [7, 8]. There are also aesthetic concerns with recession of gingival margins, especially in thin gingival biotype patients. To improve aesthetic outcomes and compensate for horizontal resorption of the ridge following tooth extraction, the use of adjunctive soft tissue grafts have been suggested to assist in contour augmentation and increasing the tissue thickness as well as keratinisation. These grafts are normally taken from the palatal mucosa or tuberosity region.

Prospective studies by Cornelini et al. [9], Fugazzotto [10], Covani et al. [5], and Kan et al. [11] as well as retrospective studies [12, 13] have reported high survival rates of over 95% for immediate implants. In a recent systematic review and meta-analysis by Cosyn et al. [14], significantly lower implant survival rates were noted for immediate implant placement (94.9%) compared to delayed implant placement (98.9%), and it was found that all were early implant failures.

11.1.3 Delayed Implant Placement

11.1.3.1 Resolution of Local Infection

Teeth often require extraction because of acute infection with purulent discharge or chronic infection that has led to major alveolar destruction. In these situations delaying implant placement for four weeks or more (types 2–4 implant placement) allows local infection to resolve. Implants should never be placed into infected sites as this may lead to complications or implant loss.

11.1.3.2 Dimensional Changes of the Alveolar Ridge

The extraction of a tooth results in dimensional changes in the socket due to resorption and remodelling of the facial bone. The crestal portion of the labial buccal plate is often thin and made up almost entirely of bundle bone. The vascular supply to bundle bone is derived from the periodontal ligament, and when teeth are extracted this interrupts the blood supply and the facial bone rapidly resorbs [15].

In a systematic review looking at post-extraction alveolar hard and soft tissue dimensional changes in humans, Tan et al. [16] found that six months after tooth extraction horizontal bone loss ranging from 29 to 63% had occurred and vertical bone loss of 11–22%. There was a rapid reduction in the first three to six months, followed by gradual reduction.

Early implant placement (type 2), in which insertion is within four to eight weeks of tooth extraction, allows soft tissue healing with minimal dimensional changes. Implants can be placed into favourable morphology with three or more bone walls with bony augmentation procedures often carried out simultaneously.

Early implant placement with partial bone healing (type 3) allows at least 12 weeks of healing, although the horizontal ridge resorption will be more advanced. This may lead to increased risk of insufficient bone width after healing.

In late placement (type 4) with over six months of healing after tooth extraction, the facial ridge contour may suffer further flattening of ridge contour from ridge resorption. This may require a staged approach, where the augmentation procedures are performed initially followed by several months of healing prior to implant placement. This is often seen in children or adolescents with traumatic loss of teeth because time must be allowed for skeletal maturation before placement of implants. In type 3 and 4 placements this might also occur when there are larger defects such as cysts or infections that may compromise implant stability. Ridge preservation procedures have also been recommended in these situations to minimise bone loss using low substitution bone fillers.

11.2 Procedures

Undertaking a comprehensive examination with careful assessment to assess the risk factors may influence placement approach, with a more conservative delayed placement approach indicated for a higher risk patient with local or systemic risk factors.

11.2.1 Systemic Risk Factors

Systemic risk factors include all medical conditions, medications, smoking, or diseases which may compromise wound healing and osseointegration. This has been discussed in details in Chapter 2: Patient Assessment and History Taking.

11.2.2 Local Risk Factors

There may be dental, aesthetic, and anatomic risk factors that need to be addressed prior to the implant placement procedure. These may include the following:

- *Bone quantity and quality*: Immediate implant placement requires adequate bone apical to the root for implants to engage in order to attain primary stability at placement (Figure 11.6).

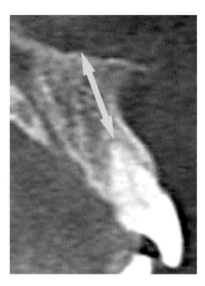

Figure 11.6 Assessment of the cone beam computed tomography (CBCT) radiograph reveals bone apical to the tooth for sufficient primary stability with an immediate implant.

- *Location of anatomical features*: Features such as maxillary sinus, incisive foramen, mental foramen, and inferior alveolar canal must be located and avoided.
- *Buccal plate thickness*: It has been demonstrated that the thickness of the buccal bone crest influences the amount of bony fill within a socket gap with immediate implant placement (Figure 11.7). After four months, in a thick buccal plate of 1 mm or more, the amount of horizontal bone fill is 100% compared to about 75% if less than 1 mm thick. The vertical resorption in a thick >1 mm site was −0.4 mm while in the <1 mm buccal plate there was loss of −1.2 mm [17]. With a thick buccal bone plate there is evidence of minimal bone resorption; however, a buccal bone thickness of >1 mm occurs only 13% of the time in the anterior maxilla and 41% of the time in the maxillary premolar region.
- *Keratinised tissue*: Immediate implants may be contraindicated with minimal keratinised tissue, as it may be simpler to plan for delayed placement with increased keranisation as tissue heals after tooth extraction.
- *Aesthetic risks*: There are certain anatomic risk factors that may influence the aesthetic outcome. These include the expectations of the patient, tissue biotype, contact points, lip line, shape of teeth as well as the bone crest height and thickness.

11.2.3 Biomaterials

The use of autogenous bone and other bone substitutes may be used to fill any socket gap to expedite bony healing. If the 'jumping distance' is less than 1.5 mm there may be no need to place any augmentation material into the gap as bone will form against the implant surface. If the gap is larger than 1.5 mm it has been recommended to use bone substitutes with low substitution rate (resorption) so that this enhances volume stability, combined with the use of autogenous which

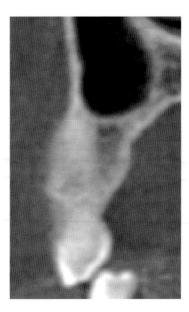

Figure 11.7 Assessment of the CBCT reveals a large root anatomy with minimal buccal plate thickness. This tooth may not be indicated for immediate implant placement because there is not enough bone apical to the root, along with the large root encompassing most of the bone volume. It may be difficult to attain sufficient primary stability with implant placement. Furthermore, this site has minimal buccal plate thickness, which will resorb after tooth extraction. In this situation it may be better to proceed with early implant placement and augmentation.

provides increased osteogenic potential. The graft materials act as a scaffold to maintain hard and soft tissue volume as well as the blood clot for healing.

Araujo et al. [18] found that placement of deproteinised bovine bone mineral with collagen (Bi-Oss® Collagen, Geistlich) in the buccal gap at immediate implants in dogs modified the process of hard tissue healing and provided additional amounts of hard tissue at entrance of the previous socket with improved level of bone–implant contact.

11.2.4 Socket Morphology

Understanding the morphology of a socket after tooth extraction may allow optimal placement as well as stability of an implant. The number of roots, configuration, and positioning in the alveolus may influence the complexity of the procedure.

- *Anterior teeth*: In the anterior maxilla there is often a concavity in the facial bone apically around the root apex region, so placement needs to avoid perforating the facial bone in this region. The osteotomy in the anterior maxilla often necessitates the osteotomy to be prepared into the palatal wall of the socket (Figure 11.8). Due to the palatal bone being dense, the osteotomy drills have a tendency to drift facially, which may result in malposition of the implant. Additionally, the clinician needs to assess whether there is bone apical to the root so that it is possible to attain sufficient primary stability for the implant.

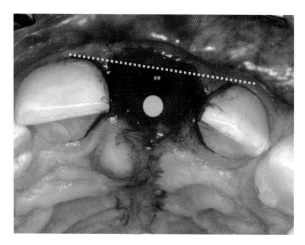

Figure 11.8 The initial osteotomy in the anterior maxilla needs to be initiated in the palatal wall and not the root apex. This first drill entry is placed half to two-thirds along the palatal wall and care should be taken to not allow the implant platform to be labial to the line taken from the emergence profile of the adjacent teeth, as implants placed facial to this line may experience gingival recession.

In the mandibular anterior region the dimensional spacing is often limited and the bone walls are thin with risk of facial or lingual perforation.

- *Premolar region*: The morphology of premolar sockets often will allow immediate placement with little difficulty. However, careful radiographic assessment is required to assess whether the maxillary sinus or mental foramen is in close proximity as often immediate placement will need to engage bone apical to the root apex while having sufficient clearance from neurovascular bundle and other critical anatomical structures.
- *Molar region*: The ideal prosthetic position is often in the centre of an extraction socket and is often placed into the inter-radicular septum. It can be difficult to attain initial entry due to the sloped bony ridge, and the use of a round bur or sharp needle/Lindemann bur may assist. The maxillary sinus should be avoided unless performing internal sinus lift procedures. It is not advisable to place implant into the root sockets of molars as the implant would not be located in the appropriate prosthetic position.

11.2.5 Flapless Protocol

A flapless approach may be made where a tooth has been atraumatically extracted and implants are placed immediately. It has been suggested that aesthetic outcomes may be improved by not raising a muco-periosteal flap and not compromising the blood supply derived from the periosteum. Flapless placement may be associated with less recession of the mid-facial mucosa and may have less morbidity. However, this is a more complex procedure as implant preparation is into the sloping anatomy of the palatal bone structure or septa within multi-root teeth. The visual access is impaired as this is a 'blind' technique with no visualisation of the alveolar ridge, and hence requires considerable clinical experience. It is indicated where there is sufficient bone volume in a thick alveolar ridge. Guided surgery may facilitate this technique with safe and predictable placement with less risk of complications. It must be remembered that these systems may still entail some deviation from what is planned and hence where bone quantity is limited these techniques should be used with caution.

11.2.6 Clinician Experience

The immediate placement of implant into an extraction socket involves significantly higher complexity, making it more difficult to place than in a healed site. It is critical to be able to remove the tooth atraumatically without damaging the bone. There may be advantages to doing this procedure without flap elevation to minimise vascular interruption with a flap, however this compromises visual access. Additionally, the need to achieve primary stability requires implants to be placed into bone that is often only found apically, and hence there is the need to underprepare/osseo-densify the osteotomy site to increase insertion stability.

11.2.7 Adjunctive Procedures with Implant Placement

11.2.7.1 Simultaneous Bone Augmentation with Implant Placement

It is a common protocol to simultaneously graft the post-extraction socket or marginal defects to reduce the extent of horizontal bone resorption performed with immediate type 1, early (type 2 and 3), and late placement (type 4) protocols. However, studies have shown that the loss of horizontal ridge dimensions cannot be prevented even with the placement of an immediate implant. It is advisable to place immediate implants in the anterior maxilla towards the palatal of the socket, allowing 2 mm or more space labially for augmentation with low substitution bone fillers. Grafting of the external surface of an intact socket with immediate implants can be a difficult challenge for accessibility, while early placement type 2 and 3 procedures result in an often-concave crater-like defect topography which may allow contour augmentation with appropriate soft tissue closure. A clinician must assess each patient to determine whether it is possible to undertake simultaneous bone augmentation or to use a staged approach where bony augmentation is performed followed by five to six months of healing.

11.2.7.2 Adjunctive Soft Tissue Grafting

In the anterior region the use of connective tissue grafts harvested from the palate can be used on the facial surface of the implant for contour augmentation and/or primary closure over the socket. The procedure involves releasing the periosteum at the base of the flap to advance the flap over the graft, and care must be taken to not over-graft as it may be difficult to close the flap correctly or the site may result in being over-contoured. The adjunctive use of soft tissue grafting may also assist when the tissue biotype is thin. Grunder et al. [19] reported on 24 patients treated consecutively with implants placed on the maxillary anterior region with one group (12) receiving immediate implants performed flaplessly, while the second group of 12 had a subepithelial connective

Table 11.2 Indications for different treatment approaches.

Treatment approach	Indications
Immediate placement (type 1)	Extraction socket with intact bony walls
	Appropriate socket morphology
	No infection
	Low aesthetic risks such as thick biotype, thick buccal bone wall, low lip line
	Sufficient bony quantity and quality for primary stability
Early placement with soft tissue healing (type 2)	Single-rooted teeth
	Minimal keratinised and tissue thickness. Allowing the ridge to heal may allow for keratinisation and tissue thickness
	Local infection
	Sufficient bone after extraction for primary stability
	In the aesthetic zone with low to moderate aesthetic risk
Early placement with partial bone healing (type 3)	Local infection
	Multi-rooted teeth
	Large apical bone defects where stability might not be possible with type 1 or 2 protocols
Late placement (type 4)	Skeletally immature patient – growing patient
	Where there has been significant infection or large cystic area
	Medical risk factors

tissue graft placed using a tunnel technique in the labial area. The labial volume was measured before treatment and after six months. The results showed an average loss of volume of 1.063 mm in the non-grafted group and in the grafted group a slight gain of 0.34 mm.

11.2.8 Selecting the Appropriate Treatment Protocol

The selection of the different treatment approaches post-extraction is based on the advantages and disadvantages of each and the desired treatment outcome (Table 11.2).

Current surgical and restorative treatment philosophies must strike an appropriate balance between expediency and predictability, with an individualised approach developed that is site-specific. There is insufficient evidence to determine possible advantages or disadvantages of immediate, immediate-delayed, or delayed implants, therefore preliminary conclusions are based on few underpowered trials often judged to be at high risk of bias. There is a suggestion that immediate implants may be at higher risks of implant failures and complications than delayed implants; on the other hand the aesthetic outcome might be better when placing implants just after teeth extraction. There is not enough reliable evidence supporting or refuting the need for augmentation procedures at immediate implants placed in fresh extraction sockets or whether any of the augmentation techniques is superior to the others.

11.3 Tips

- For immediate placement procedures ensure that care is taken in the implant alignment as it is easy for the osteotomy to drift. The handpiece must be held steady, especially in cases involving the anterior maxilla, where it is recommended to maintain a palatal force to the drill to prevent it drifting labially.
- Historically, there was a tendency to use large oversized implants in immediate implant in an extraction socket to achieve enhanced stability and to reduce the marginal gap between the implant and the socket walls. A prospective study by Small et al. [20] found that mucosal recession was observed around 88.7% of wide-diameter implant sites, compared with 48.6% for standard diameter implant sites. Implants with a wide diameter also require abutments which are large which may thin the marginal mucosa increasing risk of recession and poor aesthetics.
- In immediate implants, the author recommends packing the socket with bone substitutes with the final drill in place before then inserting the implant. This ensures that bone is packed into the socket, rather than placing an implant and then having to add the graft between the socket wall and implant.
- The placement of immediate implants may also involve placement to engage the cortical floor of the nose/sinus to attain better primary stability and engage bi-cortical stabilisation.

References

1 Esposito, M., Grusovin, M.G., Polyzos, I.P. et al. (2010). Timing of implant placement after tooth extraction: immediate, immediate-delayed or delayed implants? A Cochrane systematic review. *Eur. J. Oral Implantol.* 3 (3): 189–205.

2 Hämmerle, C.H., Chen, S.T., and Wilson Jr, T.G. (2004). Consensus statements and recommended clinical procedures regarding the placement of implants in extraction sockets. *Int. J. Oral Maxillofac. Implants* 1;19(Suppl): 26–28.

3 Araujo, M.G., Sukekava, F., Wennstrom, J.L., and Lindhe, J. (2005). Ridge alterations following implant placement in fresh extraction sockets: an experimental study in the dog. *J. Clin. Periodontol.* 32: 645–652.

4 Botticelli, D., Berglundh, T., and Lindhe, J. (2004). Hard-tissue alterations following immediate implant placement in extraction sites. *J. Clin. Periodontol.* 31: 820–828.

5 Covani, U., Bortolaia, C., Barone, A., and Sbordone, L. (2004). Bucco-lingual crestal bone changes after immediate implant placement in extraction sites. *J. Clin. Periodontol.* 75: 1605–1612.

6 Evans, C. and Chen, S.T. (2008). Esthetic outcomes of immediate implant placements. *Clin. Oral Implants Res.* 19: 73–80.

7 Brunski, J.B. (1999). in vivo; bone response to biomechanical loading at the bone/dental-implant interface. *Adv. Dent. Res.* 13: 99–119.

8 Gapski, R., Wang, H.L., Mascarenhas, P., and Lang, N.P. (2003). Critical review of immediate implant loading. *Clin. Oral Implants Res.* 14: 515–527.

9 Cornelini, R., Cangini, F., Covani, U., and Wilson, T.G. Jr. (2005). Immediate restoration of implants placed into fresh extraction sockets for single-tooth replacement: a prospective clinical study. *Int. J. Periodontics Restorative Dent.* 25 (5): 439–447.

10 Fugazzotto, P.A. (2006). Implant placement at the time of maxillary molar extraction: technique and report of preliminary results of 83 sites. *J. Periodontol.* 77 (2): 302–309.

11 Kan, J.Y., Rungcharassaeng, K., and Lozada, J. (2003). Immediate placement and provisionalization of maxillary anterior single implants: 1-year prospective study. *Int. J. Oral Maxillofac. Implants* 18: 31–39.

12 De Kok, I.J., Chang, S.S., Moriarty, J.D., and Cooper, L.F. (2006). A retrospective analysis of peri-implant tissue responses at immediate load/provisionalized microthreaded implants. *Int. J. Oral Maxillofac. Implants* 21 (3): 405-412.

13 Wagenberg, B. and Froum, S.J. (2006). A retrospective study of 1925 consecutively placed immediate implants from 1988 to 2004. *Int. J. Oral Maxillofac. Implants* 21 (1): 71–80.

14 Cosyn, J., De Lat, L., Seyssens, L. et al. (2019 Jun). The effectiveness of immediate implant placement for single tooth replacement compared to delayed implant placement: a systematic review and meta-analysis. *J. Clin. Periodontol.* 46: 224–241.

15 Araújo, M.G. and Lindhe, J. (2005). Dimensional ridge alterations following tooth extraction. An experimental study in the dog. *J. Clin. Periodontol.* 32 (2): 212–218.

16 Tan, W.L., Wong, T.L.T., Wong, M.C.M., and Lang, N.P. (2012). A systematic review of post-extractional alveolar hard and soft tissue dimensional changes in humans. *Clin. Oral Implants Res.* 23 (Suppl. 5): 1–21.

17 Ferrus, J., Cecchinato, D., Pjetursson, E.B. et al. (2010). Factors influencing ridge alterations following immediate implant placement into extraction sockets. *Clin. Oral Implants Res.* 21: 22–29.

18 Araújo, M.G., Linder, E., and Lindhe, J. (2011). Bio-Oss® Collagen in the buccal gap at immediate implants: a 6-month study in the dog. *Clin. Oral Implants Res.* 22 (1): 1–8.

19 Grunder, U. (2011 Feb 1). Crestal ridge width changes when placing implants at the time of tooth extraction with and without soft tissue augmentation after a healing period of 6 months: report of 24 consecutive cases. *Int. J. Periodontics Restorative Dent.* 31 (1): 9.

20 Small, P.N., Tarnow, D.P., and Cho, S.C. (2001). Gingival recession around wide-diameter versus standard-diameter implants: a 3-to 5-year longitudinal prospective study. *Pract. Procedures Aesthet. Dent.* 13 (2): 143.

12

Implant Site Preparation

Tom Giblin

12.1 Principles

An important decision to be made after a decision is taken to remove a tooth, is what you are going to do to replace the tooth.

There are four options for patients in replacing their missing teeth:

- *Do nothing – leave a gap*: This is always an option, but restoring the tooth is usually why the patient presents for treatment.
- *A removable prosthesis*: Although this is the most cost-effective method to restore multiple missing teeth, it is not usually the patient's first choice. It is, however, often necessary as a transitional measure and should not be dismissed in cases where implants may not be a suitable choice.
- *Fixed dental prosthesis*: Because this involves the preparation of adjacent teeth, this may not be a viable or preferred option. Having long-span bridges or other biomechanically questionable restorations may also make this an unsuitable choice, as will the absence of suitable abutments.
- *Dental implants*: Many would say this is the standard of care, but treatment can be lengthy and may not be suitable in some medically compromised patients. Implants can support either a fixed or removable prosthesis.

Before deciding on an implant, it is important to assess the site for suitability. This involves assessment not only of bone and soft tissue, but also restorative space, aesthetics, and the condition, position, and gingival levels of adjacent teeth. Critical assessment of the patient's overall situation not only avoids complications and disappointment in the future, but also allows the dentist to deliver more comprehensive care. If a dentist is restoring a central incisor with an implant-retained crown, but does not address issues with the surrounding teeth, such as periodontal health, crooked teeth, broken, chipped or worn teeth, and other more cosmetic issues, such as gingival levels and tooth colour, are they ever really going to deliver an optimal aesthetic and functional result?

Practical Procedures in Implant Dentistry, First Edition. Edited by Christopher C.K. Ho.
© 2022 John Wiley & Sons Ltd. Published 2022 by John Wiley & Sons Ltd.
Companion website: www.wiley.com/go/ho/implant-dentistry

12.2   Assessing Implant Sites and Adjacent Teeth

When assessing an implant site, the critical areas are the bone volume and soft tissues. There are many ways to assess these, and it is important to gather as much information as possible about a site before you formulate a treatment plan.

12.2.1   Periodontal Charting

It is important to know the periodontal status of the patient and also the nature and amount of attachment on the surrounding teeth. Bleeding on probing or mobile teeth may indicate active periodontal disease or occlusal/parafunctional issues. A phase of periodontal therapy may be required before commencing implant therapy to ensure a predictable result and ensure patient compliance with maintenance protocols. Occlusal assessment and the use of splints, occlusal equilibration, or selective tooth build-ups to optimise occlusion may be necessary for a stable long-term periodontal result.

12.2.2   Assessment of Gingival Biotype and Attached Mucosa

A thick biotype and 3–5 mm of attached mucosa are optimal for long-term implant health. If these conditions are not present, consider including soft tissue augmentation procedures either before commencing implant therapy or during implant placement or second-stage surgery.

12.2.3   Photography

Photography should be considered essential in modern implant placement, both from a planning and diagnosis perspective and from a medico-legal point of view. It is useful in showing the clinical situation to the patient as a teaching tool and is invaluable in discussing the case with other clinicians who may be involved in the procedure. Minimal photos recommended would be a 'nose to chin' shot in rest and at the patient's highest smile to assess aesthetics (Figure 12.1), a full

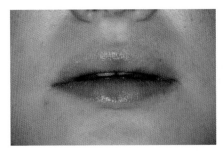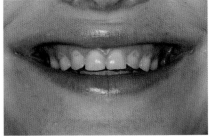

Figure 12.1 'Nose to chin' photos of the lips at rest and at high smile are essential for aesthetic evaluation. These are vital in determining where the correct incisal edge position needs to be. They also show tooth size, proportion, and colour and are important for assessing gingival contours and position, as well as lip position and mobility.

arch retracted shot, and close-up photos of the site from the buccal and occlusal. Full arch occlusal and lateral bite shots can also be useful in more complex cases.

12.2.4   Aesthetic Assessment

A missing tooth can be a major aesthetic issue. Assessment of the patient's aesthetic demands should be known at the start of treatment. Just because a patient has dark, stained, chipped, or worn teeth does not mean they want to keep them that way. One of the first questions when planning an implant case is to enquire whether the patient is happy with their current smile and if they are interested in improving it. Often, with a missing tooth in the aesthetic zone, a patient's mindset may only be how to eliminate the gap (out of embarrassment), not how to make their overall smile better. From a treatment planning point of view, knowing if the patient wants to make changes may affect the implant placement, tooth size, shape, and shade of the final result. There is nothing worse than placing an implant and restoring it, only to then have your patient say they are so happy with the result they now want tooth whitening, veneers, orthodontics, or gingival surgery and you cannot fully accommodate them without redoing your new crown or being compromised by the implant placement.

12.2.5   Radiography

A cone beam computed tomography (CBCT) scan can determine the bucco-lingual, vertical, and mesio-distal bone volume of an implant site, along with identifying structures such as adjacent teeth and their root angulations, bone levels, and apical pathologies. This should be done in conjunction with periapical radiographs (Figure 12.2) as cross-reference and to more accurately determine bone levels on adjacent teeth. Imaging is vital to determine the positions of nerves, vascular bundles, sinuses, anatomical abnormalities, and pathologies. A

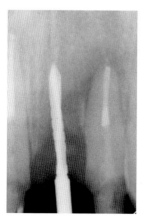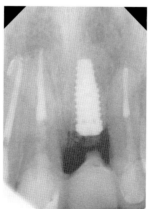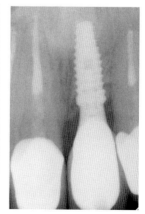

Figure 12.2 Periapical radiographs are essential in implant planning as they indicate where the levels of bone are on the adjacent teeth. This determines both implant depth, but also helps prosthetic planning in developing papilla.

CBCT scan can be taken in maximum intensity projection (MIP) to also adequately determine the 'crown height space', which is important in prosthetic planning. In conjunction with planning software, implants, abutments, crowns, and even grafts can be placed virtually to better plan the case and aid with informed consent and patient case acceptance.

12.2.6 Occlusal Analysis

Occlusal analysis is essential to assess and record prior to the planning process. Often the tooth that is being replaced was the result of occlusal trauma (cracked teeth, wear, bone loss, etc.). It is important to identify that and take that into account in the design of the restoration or plan to overcome the issue in other ways (occlusal splints, occlusal equilibration, restorative work, or orthodontics) in order to prevent the same problem recurring with your implant restoration.

12.2.7 Endodontic Status of Adjacent Teeth

An often-overlooked assessment is to check the status of adjacent root-filled teeth. The pathogenic flora associated with endodontic lesions can be very detrimental to implant placement and can result in implant failure and bone loss if an infection spreads to the adjacent implant site (Figure 12.3).

12.3 Site Preparation

If an implant site is assessed as not ideal for implant placement because of a lack of bone volume (height, width, or between two adjacent teeth), it is important to optimise the site through various means.

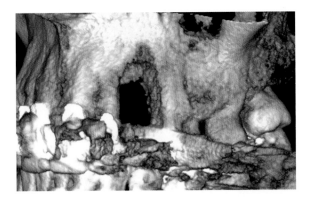

Figure 12.3 This image shows a large defect left when an implant became infected from an adjacent tooth with a leaking root canal treatment. The tooth was asymptomatic, showed only slight periodontal widening on pre-op X-rays, and was even cleared by an endodontist prior to treatment.

12.3.1   Grafting – Sinus, Buccal, Soft Tissue

Grafting will be covered in other chapters, but often the timing of this procedure is important in the planning of the whole case. Some grafts need time to mature prior to implant placement, others can be done concurrently. With soft tissue grafting, it is always less predictable to graft around implants, so best to have the soft tissue procedures done early on in the sequence so as to give them time to mature and ensure a predictable result.

12.3.2   Occlusion

Often, when a tooth fails, the occlusal component of the failure is overlooked, only to surface after the new restoration has been placed. There may be certain situations such as a plunger cusp that needs to be adjusted, or an out-of-position lower incisor to be moved orthodontically or reduced prior to the final restoration. These issues are best addressed with the patient during the planning phase.

12.3.3   Adjacent and Opposing Teeth

Assessment of the adjacent teeth is important as it may affect how successful the final crown, emergence profile, and soft tissue results are. The crown shapes of the adjacent teeth determine where the contact points of the teeth are and, according to papers by both Tarnow et al. [1] and Funato et al. [2], these are the primary determinants of papilla fill in the gingival embrasure spaces (Table 12.1). Even the best peri-implant tissues can be let down by incorrect crown shape and cause black triangles. One solution is to reshape the tooth and embrasure form restoratively to move the contact point closer to the crest of bone. This is another reason why a periapical X-ray determining the interproximal height of bone is vital in planning.

The chart shown in Table 12.1 is essential in planning soft tissue around restorations. It gives a guide as to where you have to place the contact point of your

Table 12.1 The Salama et al. classification of predicted height of interdental papilla [2].

Class	Restorative environment	Proximity limitations (mm)	Vertical soft tissue limitations (mm)
1	Tooth–tooth	1.0	5.0
2	Tooth–pontic	N/A	6.5
3	Pontic–pontic	N/A	6.0
4	Tooth–implant	1.5	4.5
5	Implant–pontic	N/A	5.5
6	Implant–implant	3.0	3.5

Source: Redrawn from Funato, A., Salama, M.A., Ishikawa, T. et al. (2007). Timing, positioning, and sequential staging in esthetic implant therapy: a four-dimensional perspective. *Int. J. Periodontics Restorative Dent.* 27(4): 313–323.

restoration in relation to the crest of the interproximal bone in order to get predictable papilla fill. An interesting observation is that the most predictable way to get papilla is with a pontic site, which is useful in determining temporisation and final restorations in aesthetic cases.

There is a need to assess the opposing teeth and their condition, as there may be little point in doing an implant if the opposing teeth are missing or of a poor or hopeless prognosis. Often if an implant is replacing a tooth in a space that has been edentulous for a long period, the opposing tooth must be checked to ensure that it has not over-erupted, making the implant difficult to restore without significantly reducing or removing the opposing tooth. This is something that occurs with surprising frequency.

12.3.4   Crown Lengthening and Gingivectomy

When determining how deep we need to place an implant, we usually use the proposed gingival margin as a guide, placing the implant 3–4 mm below that to ensure an optimal emergence profile. This is usually based on the adjacent teeth. However, if these adjacent gingival levels are uneven or in an unaesthetic position, this may need to be addressed in the early stages of planning. In a gummy smile patient, for example, the excessive gingival display may be due to altered passive eruption, which may be treated with a gingivectomy. Alternatively, it may be caused by vertical maxillary excess due to maxillary overgrowth, which may need surgical correction, or it may be a short or hyperactive upper lip. The gingival complex might also be classified as a high or low crest patient as described by Kois [3, 4], requiring aesthetic crown lengthening or gingivectomy to normalise and stabilise the gingival position prior to surgery. All of these conditions may determine where and how deep implants are placed and need to be taken into account to ensure a stable long-term result, as illustrated in Figure 12.4.

12.3.5   Orthodontics and Site Preparation

Orthodontics is a discipline often overlooked in the planning of dental implants. Orthodontics may be used effectively to create the ideal implant site and final aesthetic result by not only creating the ideal mesio-distal spacing between the adjacent teeth, but also correct root angulation. We know from Tarnow's work that we need at least 1.5 mm of space between an implant and adjacent natural tooth to provide for adequate soft tissue/papilla growth. If the smallest implant we have is 3 mm, that means we need a minimum of 6 mm between the adjacent teeth to achieve an acceptable soft tissue result. The ideal spacing aesthetically may be more, depending on the proportion of the adjacent teeth; larger teeth need more spacing to remain in proportion. A hazard of orthodontically moving teeth for site preparation is that the teeth are merely tipped and adequate space is not made between the roots for implant placement, as in Figure 12.5. This must be monitored and checked prior to the conclusion of orthodontic treatment. It must also be said that in the case of a missing lateral, it is very difficult to get canine substitution

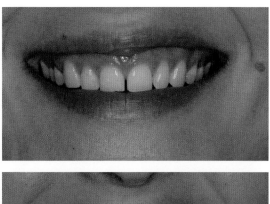

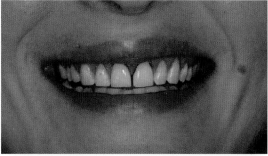

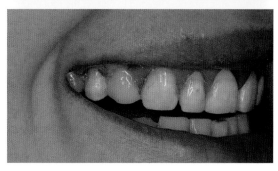

Figure 12.4 This patient presented with a failing first premolar. In planning for the case, the patient was not happy with her gummy smile and there was a diagnosis of altered passive eruption. Gingivectomies were performed at the time of implant placement. The new gingival levels then determined the depth of implant placement.

looking truly aesthetic because of the difference in size, especially at the neck, as well as the darker shade of a canine tooth. Functionally, occlusally, and aesthetically, it is often better to leave the canine in its correct position and to restore the missing lateral.

Another useful technique is to use orthodontics to create bone. In the case of a hopeless tooth or root stump, particularly where there is a soft tissue deficiency, orthodontically extruding a tooth out of the socket will enable the dentist to bring down bone and soft tissue at the implant site without having to do secondary bone or soft tissue grafting procedures, as in Figure 12.6. This can be done either rapidly (one to two weeks extrusion then three months of retention)

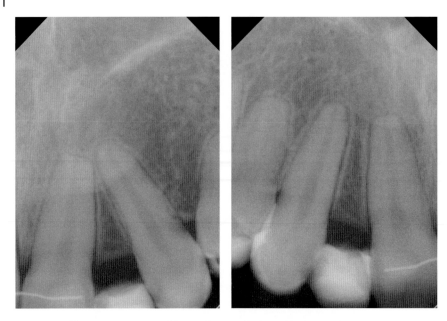

Figure 12.5 This patient presented for implants in the lateral incisor positions post orthodontics. More orthodontics are now needed to correct the root angulation.

or slowly over a few months. At the end of extrusion, there should only be a root stump to remove, and an immediate implant can often be placed into the site. An advantage of this technique is that there is an excess of soft tissue that can be manipulated later on. It should be noted that the tooth should have no periodontal or apical pathology and it will work most effectively if the buccal plate is present.

Orthodontics can also be used to create an implant site where there is a narrow ridge (Figure 12.7). By moving a tooth into a narrow site, a wider ridge will be created in the 'wake' of the tooth. This may be useful in substitution cases or in moving posterior teeth around in an arch.

Implants may also be used to facilitate more predicable orthodontic movement by providing rigid anchorage. This must be done with caution, however, as you need to plan exactly where the final tooth positions will be post ortho to enable you to accurately place the implant in the correct final position at the start. This traditionally has been achieved via the use of a Kessling setup to predict the final outcome.

12.3.6 Provisional Phase

Another overlooked part of the implant site preparation is the provisional phase. We must plan our provisionals to optimise the implant healing and the soft tissue result. If we again refer to Salama's table in Table 12.1 we can see that the most predictable restoration for soft tissue is a pontic–papilla fill, which is

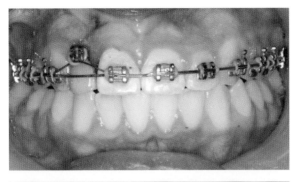

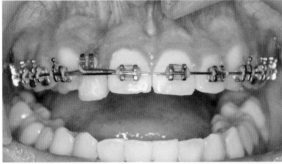

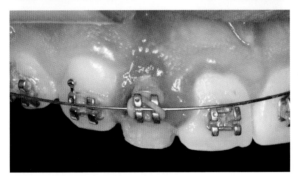

Figure 12.6 Orthodontic site preparation. In this case, an internally resorbed tooth was temporarily restored and then rapidly extruded over two weeks before being held in place for three months prior to extraction. This not only developed the bone and soft tissue, but also allowed for an easy extraction and immediate implant placement. As the tooth extruded, the incisal edge was regularly adjusted to remain out of occlusion.

better around a pontic than even two natural teeth together, and also better than an immediately loaded one-stage implant. A temporary partial denture can be detrimental to an implant site as it can load a healing site unpredictably, and cause bone loss and implant failure if not managed correctly. Removable solutions are also not as predicable for the maintenance of papilla as other methods, and in fact can load the implant sites and cause complications with implant healing.

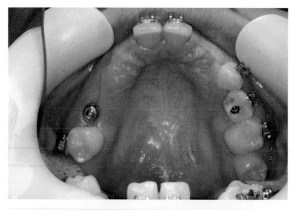

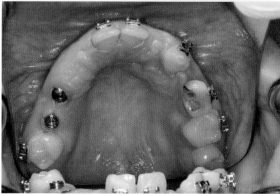

Figure 12.7 The ectopically erupted canine was moved not only to bring it back into its correct position, but also to develop the atrophic ridge surrounding it ready for implant placement.

References

1 Tarnow, D.P., Magner, A.W., and Fletcher, P. (1992). The effect of the distance from the contact point to the crest of bone on the presence or absence of the interproximal dental papilla. *J Periodontol* 63: 995–996.
2 Funato, A., Salama, M.A., Ishikawa, T. et al. (2007 Aug). Timing, positioning, and sequential staging in esthetic implant therapy: a four-dimensional perspective. *Int. J. Periodontics Restorative Dent.* 27 (4): 313–323.
3 Kois, J. (1994). Altering gingival levels: The restorative connection, Part 1: Biologic variables. *J Esthet Dent.* 6: 3–9.
4 Kois, J.C. (1996). The restorative-periodontal interface: Biological parameters. *Periodontol 2000* 11: 29–38.

Further Reading

Celenza, F. (2012). Implant interactions with orthodontics. *J. Evid. Based Dent. Pract. SI*: 192–201.

Hochman, M., Mark, N., Hochman Chu, S., and Tarnow, D. (September 2014). Orthodontic extrusion for implant site development revisited: a new classification determined by anatomy and clinical outcomes. *Semin. Orthod.* 20 (3): 208–227.

Kokich, V., Kinzer, G., and Janakievskic, J. (April 2011). Congenitally missing maxillary lateral incisors: restorative replacement. *Am. J. Orthod. Dentofac. Orthop.* 139 (4): 435.

Korayem, M., Flores-Mir, C., Nassar, U., and Olfert, K. (2008). Implant site development by orthodontic extrusion. *Angle Orthod.* 78: 752–760.

Kurth, J. and Kokich, V. (2001 Aug). Open gingival embrasures after orthodontic treatment in adults: prevalence and etiology. *Am. J. Orthod. Dentofac. Orthop.* 120 (2): 116–112.

Odman, J., Lekholm, U., Jemt, T., and Thilander, B. (1994). Osseointegrated implants as orthodontic anchorage in the treatment of partially edentulous adult patients. *Eur. J. Orthod.* 16: 187–201.

Roberts, W.E., Marshall, K.J., and Mozsary, P.G. (1990). Rigid endosseous implant utilized as anchorage to protract molars and close an atrophic extraction site. *Angle Orthod.* 60: 135–152.

Spear, F., Kokich, V., and Mathews, D. (1997 Mar). Interdisciplinary management of single-tooth implants. *Semin. Orthod.* 3 (1): 45–72.

Spear, F., Kokich, V., and Mathews, D. (2006 Feb). Interdisciplinary management of anterior dental esthetics. *J. Am. Dent. Assoc.* 137 (2): 160–169.

Thilander, B. (2008). Orthodontic space closure versus implant placement in subjects with missing teeth. *J. Oral Rehabil.* 35 (Suppl 1): 64–71.

13

Loading Protocols in Implantology

Christopher C.K. Ho

13.1 Principles

An osseointegrated implant is anchored directly to bone; however, in the presence of any movement during the healing phase a soft tissue interface may encapsulate the implant, causing failure [1]. To minimise the risk of fibrous encapsulation, it has been recommended to delay loading a prosthesis for three to four months in mandibles and six to eight months in maxillae [2].

Immediate loading of dental implants has gained popularity due to several factors, including reduction in treatment time and trauma, as well as aesthetic and psychological benefits to the patient. This may lead to higher patient acceptance and decreased patient anxiety. Much research has been undertaken to achieve shorter or immediate loading without jeopardising the success of this therapy.

13.1.1 Definitions

The following definitions of different implant loading protocols (Figure 13.1) have been described [3]:

- *Conventional (delayed) loading*: Implants are loaded after two months of healing.
- *Immediate loading*: Implants are placed into function within one week of placement. A further category within immediate loaded implants are 'occlusally' and 'non-occlusally' loaded implants. Non-occlusally loaded implants are those implants provisionally rehabilitated with restorations not in direct occlusion in static or dynamic lateral movements with the antagonistic dentition. Conversely, occlusally loaded implants are placed in function with the antagonist dentition.
- *Early loading*: Implants are put into function between one week and two months after placement.
- *Progressive loading*: The load of the implants is obtained by gradually increasing the height of the occlusal table in increments from a state of infra-occlusion to full occlusion.

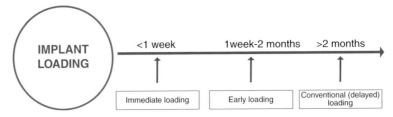

Figure 13.1 Implant loading timeline.

13.1.2 Conventional Loading

Traditionally, following implant insertion, delayed loading takes place anywhere from two to six months after placement. During this time a provisional is worn and care taken to ensure that it does not cause any micromovement on the healing implant; for example, the denture would be relieved and not allowed to impinge on the implant *in situ*. The majority of implant procedures are still performed in this manner, allowing undisturbed healing with no loading. It is particularly important to not load the implant in cases where there may be a need for bone or soft tissue augmentation, or cases where primary stability cannot be achieved, nor where this is no adequate control of occlusal forces.

13.1.3 Early Loading

There has been continual development of implant surfaces, including roughening by sandblasting, acid etching, and electrochemical modifying of surfaces to enhance hydrophilicity and surface energy, leading to accelerated bone healing. Early loading is defined as placing implants in function from one week to two months after insertion and certain implants are now being recommended to be loaded at six weeks. Further research in these areas is being conducted to reduce the length of time needed for osseointegration.

13.1.4 Progressive Loading

Appleton et al. [4] performed a controlled clinical trial with radiographic assessment of progressive loading on bone around single implants in the posterior maxilla. In the test group, acrylic implant crowns were placed in infra-occlusion, and then brought into occlusion, then a metal ceramic crown was fabricated. Digital image analysis and digital subtraction radiography at 12 months found less bone loss and higher density gain in the crestal area with progressively loaded implants.

Misch [5] described progressive loading protocols that generally controlled the load on a dental implant by controlling the size of the occlusal table, the direction and location of occlusal contact, an absence of cantilevers, and firmness of diet.

13.1.5 Immediate Loading

Schnitman et al. [6] performed the first longitudinal clinical trial suggesting implants could be loaded immediately or early in the mandibles of selected patients. The development of moderately rough implant surfaces has allowed improved integration times with better bone-to-implant contact. Implant

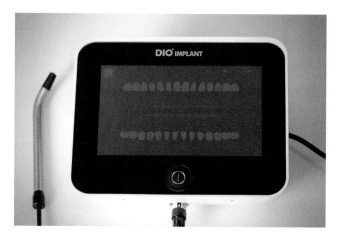

Figure 13.2 The Ostell IDX unit utilises resonance frequency analysis to measure implant stability quotient (ISQ).

macrostructure and microstructure developments have enabled enhanced primary stability, allowing early and immediate loading.

- *Single implant therapy*: Benic et al. [7] in a systematic review and meta-analysis on loading protocols for single implant crowns found immediately loaded and conventionally loaded single implant crowns are equally successful with regard to survival and marginal bone loss. This is supported by literature where implants were inserted with torque ≥30–45 Ncm or an implant stability quotient (ISQ) ≥60–65 with no need for simultaneous bone augmentation (Figure 13.2). There did not seem to be differences in papilla height after the first year of loading; however, there were difficulties in drawing clear conclusions about recession of the buccal mucosa.
- *Partially edentulous sites with extended edentulous sites*: Immediate loading in healed posterior extended edentulous sites results in survival rates similar to those of early or conventional loading. There is insufficient evidence to support immediate implant loading in anterior maxillary or mandibular extended edentulous sites [8].
- *Fully edentulous jaws*: High-level evidence exists for immediate loading of moderately rough implants with prostheses in both the edentulous maxilla and mandible being as predictable as early and conventional loading [8, 9]. The majority of studies have used criteria such as insertion torque ≥30 Ncm, ISQ ≥60 and minimal length of ≥10 mm for immediate loading.

13.2 Procedures

13.2.1 Selecting a Loading Protocol

In the majority of cases, clinicians prefer to perform conventional (delayed) loading, ensuring any provisional device does not lead to micromotion of the underlying implant disturbing osseointegration. Although the success of immediate loading (Figures 13.3–13.5) is evidenced in the literature, this is considered to be

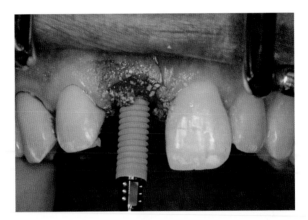

Figure 13.3 Immediate implant placement into socket after tooth extraction.

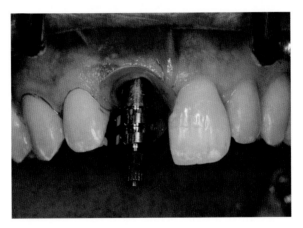

Figure 13.4 Impression of implant at time of placement. Note the protection of the socket from inadvertent contamination with small square of rubber dam to prevent ingress of foreign material into the surgical site.

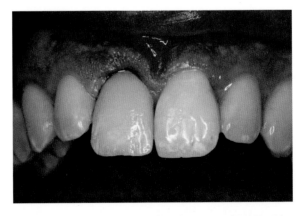

Figure 13.5 Immediate loading with provisional implant crown (PMMA with temporary engaging cylinder) issued at time of placement.

Table 13.1 Methods to improve primary stability.

Under-preparation and bone condensation techniques

Tapered moderately rough surface implant with threads

Bi-cortical stabilisation of implants

Splinting of adjacent implants

a more complex and technical procedure with the possibility of an impaired or failure of implant integration if patient compliance is poor with mastication or parafunction.

Immediate loading may lead to reduction of overall treatment times and less post-operative discomfort with removable prosthesis; however, careful patient selection and treatment planning are required. Some criteria are listed as follows:

- *High primary stability*: During implant healing, micromotion between 50 and 150 μm may negatively influence osseointegration and bone remodelling by forming fibrous tissues at the bone-to-implant interface, thereby inducing bone resorption [10]. The use of tapered implants with aggressive threads has enabled improved stability (Table 13.1). It is important to use sufficient length and diameter of implant. The correct length is necessary as the crown:implant ratio may be unfavourable for immediate loading. The use of amended surgical protocols such as under-preparation techniques, bi-cortical stabilisation, and bone condensation/densification procedures may be utilised to achieve improved stability. Poor bone quality may be a contraindication to immediate loading.
- *Implant design*: The screw or 'threaded' design minimises implant micromotion during function, thereby maintaining primary stability. Furthermore, threaded designs increase the implant surface area, offering a higher percentage of bone-to-implant contacts. The surface topography and roughness positively influence the healing process by promoting favourable cellular responses and cell surface interactions, enabling faster osteogenesis.
- *Medical and social history*: Patients with compromised medical status or history of tobacco use/alcohol abuse may be contraindications to early or immediate loading.
- *Numbers of implants*: In partially edentulous and fully edentulous cases sufficient numbers of implants must be used to support the prosthesis and are splinted (cross-arch in fully edentulous and partial splinting in partially edentulous arches) together for biomechanical advantage.
- *Control of occlusal forces*: In the single tooth implant it may be preferable to use a 'non-occlusal' immediate loaded approach where the restoration is not in occlusion in both static and dynamic occlusion. In cases of fixed dental prosthesis, where a prosthesis is 'occlusally loaded' the patient may be informed that they should consume a soft diet, and not to attempt to masticate hard foods on the prosthesis for the first six weeks to allow osseointegration. In patients with parafunction, immediate loading is contraindicated.

- *Clinician expertise*: Clinicians must have adequate knowledge, experience, and technical skills.
- *Patient compliance*: The patient needs to ensure that they do not masticate on a hard diet during the initial stages of osseointegration.
- *Need for augmentation*: The need for sinus or bone augmentation is a contraindication.

13.2.2 Methods of Evaluation of the Primary Stability for Immediate Loading

- *Periotest*: This instrument comprises a metallic tapping rod in a handpiece, and is electromagnetically driven and electronically controlled. Signals produced by tapping are converted to unique values called 'periotest' values.
- *Resonance frequency analysis (RFA)*: This can be used to monitor the changes in stiffness and stability at the implant–tissue interface and to discriminate between successful implants and clinical failures. However, presently no clinical data are available giving the necessary minimum RFA threshold required for immediate loading.
- *Cutting torque resistance analysis*: This is the energy required for an electric motor to cut bone during implant surgery. It has been shown to be significantly associated with bone density, which influences primary stability.
- *Insertion torque value*: This is the amount of torque applied to insert an implant into the prepared alveolar bone. It is normally expressed as the amount of rotational force require in Ncm, with much of the literature suggesting an insertion torque value of 30 Ncm or greater is needed for immediate loading.

13.3 Tips

- Immediate loading for single tooth implants may allow the opportunity to prosthetically guide soft tissue healing, and should be supportive of the soft tissue profile.
- It is good practice to inform the patient about the requirement for a soft diet protocol when using immediate loading to minimise the possibility of micromotion and disruption of the osseointegration process.
- With single-tooth implant treatment, ensure occlusal forces are kept to a minimum. Adjust occlusal contacts out of all centric and eccentric movements in immediate loading. For fixed dental prostheses, control of occlusion becomes more critical with careful adjustment in eccentric movements so that the prosthesis is free from destructive shear forces. Splinting of multiple implants (cross-arch or partial splinting) for fixed dental prostheses will improve the biomechanical stability of implants for immediate loading.
- If there is insufficient primary stability then delayed loading should be undertaken; a back-up plan for provisionalisation should be readily available.

References

1 Brunski, J.B., Moccia, A.F. Jr., Pollack, S.R. et al. (1979). The influence of functional use of endosseous dental implants on the tissue-implant interface. I. Histological aspects. *Journal of Dental Research* 58 (10): 1953–1969.
2 Brånemark, P.-I., Hansson, B.O., Adell, R. et al. (1977). *Osseointegrated Implants in the Treatment of the Edentulous Jaw. Experience from a 10-Year Period.* Stockholm: Almqvist & Wiksell International.
3 Esposito, M., Grusovin, M.G., Maghaireh, H., and Worthington, H.V. (2013). Interventions for replacing missing teeth: different times for loading dental implants. *Cochrane Database Syst. Rev.* (3): CD003878.
4 Appleton, R.S., Nummikoski, P.V., Pigno, M.A. et al. (2005). A radiographic assessment of progressive loading on bone around single osseointegrated implants in the posterior maxilla. *Clinical Oral Implants Research* 16 (2): 161–167.
5 Misch, C.E. (1999). *Contemporary Implant Dentistry.* St. Louis: Mosby.
6 Schnitman, P.A., Wohrle, P.S., and Rubenstein, J.E. (1990). Immediate fixed interim prostheses supported by two-stage threaded implants: methodology and results. *The Journal of Oral Implantology* 16 (2): 96–105.
7 Benic, G.I., Mir-Mari, J., and Hammerle, C.H. (2014). Loading protocols for single-implant crowns: a systematic review and meta-analysis. *The International Journal of Oral & Maxillofacial Implants* 29 (Suppl): 222–238.
8 Gallucci, G.O., Benic, G.I., Eckert, S.E. et al. (2014). Consensus statements and clinical recommendations for implant loading protocols. *The International Journal of Oral & Maxillofacial Implants* 29 (Suppl): 287–290.
9 Papaspyridakos, P., Chen, C.J., Chuang, S.K., and Weber, H.P. (2014). Implant loading protocols for edentulous patients with fixed prostheses: a systematic review and meta-analysis. *The International Journal of Oral & Maxillofacial Implants* 29 (Suppl): 256–270.
10 Brunski, J.B. (1993). Avoid pitfalls of overloading and micromotion of intraosseous implants (interview). *Dental Implantology Update* 4: 77–81.

14

Surgical Instrumentation
Christopher C.K. Ho

14.1   Principles

The skills and knowledge attained in the practice of implant dentistry are paramount to ensuring predictability. Furthermore, selection of the correct instrument
armamentarium is an important adjunct in performing precise surgical procedures. The instruments utilised should allow improved ergonomics, safety, and
efficiency in implant practice. The mouth can be a hostile environment, with
patient's oral musculature, tissues, saliva, and bleeding requiring the treating clinician's undivided attention when performing surgery. It is a worthwhile investment to acquire good-quality stainless steel instrumentation as these will provide
many years of service if looked after properly.

There are many different types of instruments designed for implantology
(Figure 14.1) and this chapter will outline the main instruments required for surgical placement, hard and soft tissue augmentation, and uncovering of submerged dental implants.

14.1.1   Mirror, Probe, and Tweezers

Every pack should possess a front surface mirror, periodontal probe, and college
tweezers. Front surface mirrors are preferred as they provide better visual acuity;
the use of a double-sided mirror can often be quite useful in that the mirror can
also help in retraction yet still illuminate the area of surgery as well as provide
further indirect vision. The surfaces of good-quality mirrors are often coated
with rhodium, which resists scratching.

14.1.2   Scalpel Handles

Although typical scalpel handles are flat, a round handle is recommended to
perform precise surgery because it allows improved tactile control, enabling
the clinician to perform minute rotation of the handles with fingers to enhance
control of the blade when incising intra-orally.

Practical Procedures in Implant Dentistry, First Edition. Edited by Christopher C.K. Ho.
© 2022 John Wiley & Sons Ltd. Published 2022 by John Wiley & Sons Ltd.
Companion website: www.wiley.com/go/ho/implant-dentistry

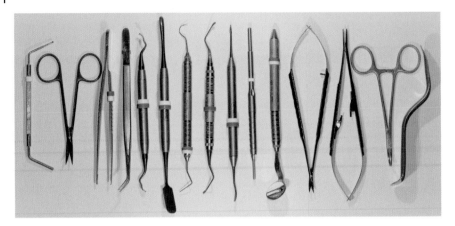

Figure 14.1 Surgical instrumentation. From left to right: Depth probe, Lagrange super-cut scissors, Debakey Permasharp tissue pliers, college tweezers, Buser modified bone scraper, Prichard periosteal, probe/periodontal probe, surgical curette, Buser periosteal, round scalpel handle, mirror with double-sided front surface mouth mirror, Castroviejo microsurgical scissors, Castroviejo needle holders, haemostat, Minnesota retractor.

14.1.3 Scalpel Blades

The typical blades used are No.15, No.15C, and No.12 blades, as well as micro-blades for perio-plastic procedures. No.15C blades, which have a narrower cutting edge, are often used in anterior regions, while No.15 blades can be used for anterior or posterior regions. No.12 blades may be useful in tipped teeth scenarios or cases where patients may have difficulty opening. The use of periodontal knives may also assist in situations where the angle of incision is awkward, allowing access in different regions.

14.1.4 Curettes

A spoon curette is used to ensure the ridge is free of any soft tissue, granulation or infected tissue from extraction sockets, alveolar ridge, and defects. It may be handy to also use periodontal curettes to debride root surface calculus present adjacent to implant sites.

14.1.5 Needle Holders

Selection of needle holders is dependent on individual surgeon preference and consists of either standard (conventional) style needle holders, such as, for example Mayo Hegar and Matthieu, or Castroviejo needle holders. The author recommends the use of Castroviejo needle holders because they allow an ergonomic pen-grip technique when suturing tissues, without having to move the whole wrist like conventional needle holders. This allows for very fine motor control with delicate handling of the soft tissues.

14.1.6   Periosteal Elevators

Periosteal elevators are designed for raising mucoperiosteal flaps. After full-thickness incision of the gingival tissues a periosteal elevator may assist in reflecting and retracting the mucoperiosteum. The sharp edge is held against the bone and the mucoperiosteum is carefully elevated from the bony ridge. Once the flap is reflected, often the elevator may be used to retract the flap from inadvertent damage during osteotomy procedures. It must be emphasised that full-thickness flap elevation requires inserting the elevator firmly against the bone to keep the mucoperiosteum intact, and care should be taken to ensure the elevator does not slip and injure any important anatomy or soft tissues. The most common periosteal elevators used in oral surgical procedures are Pritchard, Buser, Molt, and Papilla elevators.

14.1.7   Retractors

A variety of different retractors are available designed to retract lips, cheeks, tongues, and surgical flaps safely from the operative site. This provides protection of tissues from injury and allows direct visual access and better illumination of the surgical site. One commonly used universal retractor is the Minnesota retractor, which is used to retract the circumoral tissues and tongue and is also small enough to assist in retracting the surgical flaps. Another useful retractor is the Branemark lip retractor (Figure 14.2). This is a broad lip retractor providing a wide area of retraction allowing excellent access and visibility to the anterior maxilla and mandible. The Weider retractor can be used both as a cheek retractor and as a tongue retractor and is particularly useful in cases where the tongue is extremely uncooperative.

14.1.8   Depth Probe

It is useful to have a depth probe to assess the osteotomy. This consists of a rounded end probe which is used to check depth as well as to ensure that the osteotomy is fully contained within the alveolar ridge with no fenestration or perforation out of the bone. It can also be used to assess in sinus elevation procedures to check whether there has been perforation into sinus and whether the Schneiderian membrane is intact.

14.1.9   Tissue Forceps/Pliers

Tissue forceps are used to grasp and stabilise soft tissue upon reflection of the flap and while suturing. These can be standard or microsurgical in size, allowing for different size flaps. Due to the small size of microsurgical tissue forceps these

(a)
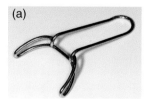
(b)
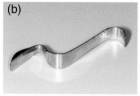
(c)
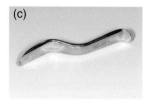

Figure 14.2 (a) Anterior (Branemark) retractor, (b) Bishop retractor, (c) Minnesota retractor.

can be gentler to soft tissues, minimising trauma. The tissue forceps are held in the non-dominant hand with a pencil grip; care is taken to apply minimal pressure to maintain soft tissue integrity and allow optimal wound healing. The tissue forceps can be either toothed or non-toothed. Toothed forceps are preferred by the majority of surgeons because the teeth penetrate the tissue to hold, rather than crushing the tissue. Additionally, with non-toothed forceps, more pressure may need to be applied to securely hold the tissues. Common examples of tissue forceps include Adson, DeBakey, Semkin-Taylor, and microsurgical tissue forceps.

14.1.10   Mouth Props/Bite Blocks

Mouth props are used to maintain mouth opening during dental procedures. They are particularly useful in implantology because of the longer procedures. In addition, they may be useful for patients with temporo-mandibular disorders or for cases involving conscious or intravenous sedation, where patients' jaws are relaxed. Examples are bite blocks and Molt mouth props.

14.1.11   Scissors

Scissors are used to cut sutures, as well as regenerative membranes and are available in different designs with curved or straight blades as well as in conventional or Castroviejo style for more ergonomic pen-style grip.

14.1.12   Extraction Forceps, Periotomes and Elevators

Clinicians should possess a selection of extraction forceps, including periotomes and elevators to extract teeth in an atraumatic manner. The objective is to remove teeth/roots with minimal trauma, preserving the alveolar ridge as intact as possible. There may be a need to section teeth to allow atraumatic extraction. The surgeon should be prepared to section teeth to remove multi-rooted teeth as well as in cases where the root remains within the ridge, when the offending sections of the root can often be sectioned and removed gently.

14.1.13   Kidney Dish

It is helpful to have a large kidney dish in which the scalpel, sutures or other sharps can be placed to minimise any chance of sharps injury. The sharps can be safely housed in the kidney dish separate from other instruments, preventing any harm to surgeon or staff.

14.1.14   Surgical Kit, Electric Motor, 20:1 Handpiece, and Consumables

Each implant manufacturer designs a specific surgical kit which effectively stores the drills, screw taps, directional indicators, implant torque wrench, etc. for their particular implants. The electric motor and a speed-reducing 20 : 1 handpiece are required for drilling protocols for each manufacturer's specific instructions. Other consumables include sutures, sterile drapes, drill sleeves, suction devices, and light covers.

14.1.15   Grafting Well

These are used to store biomaterials, and materials can be dispensed into them and hydrated prior to use. They are normally made of glass or ceramic, allowing them to be autoclaved.

14.2   Optional Instrumentation

14.2.1   Rongeurs

Rongeurs are used to trim and recontour bone and allow for gross tissue removal. This is particularly useful after tooth extraction to remove any sharp spurs as well as to perform osteoplasty or alveolectomy if required. These instruments can also be useful to harvest bone. Examples are Beyer and Friedman rongeurs.

14.2.2   Benex

The Benex® Extraction System is a specialised device for atraumatic removal of tooth roots (Figure 14.3). An extraction screw is inserted like a post down the root, and a pulley-like action is utilised with the other teeth as anchorage. An exertion force along the long axis of the root is applied, allowing for extraction in a minimally invasive manner without any compression or injury to the soft or hard tissues surrounding the root. Due to the innovative construction of the extractor, the root can be removed very easily and in an extremely controlled

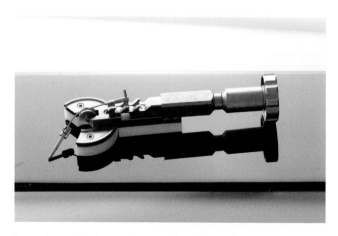

Figure 14.3 Benex® Extraction System is a specialised device for atraumatic removal of tooth roots.

manner. There are situations in which this may not be successful; if the root is fractured and the post has no anchor a conventional technique of root elevation or sectioning may be needed to perform complete removal.

14.2.3 Bone Harvesters

The use of bone scrapers is a minimally invasive option for obtaining autogenous bone (Figure 14.4). The manual harvesting of bone by scraping the blade against the bony ridge preserves the cortical bone tissue's cell vitality, thereby maximising the osteogenic potential of the graft. Harvesters are normally disposable cortical bone collectors with semicircular blades, and a curved tip. They allow clinicians to harvest autogenous bone from any intra-oral site, including near the defect in particulate form.

14.2.4 Anthogyr Torq Control

The Anthogyr Torq Control is a manual dynamometric declutching torque wrench fitted with an adjusting knob, allowing control of the tightening torque (Figure 14.5). It has a 100-degree angulated micro-head that provides an

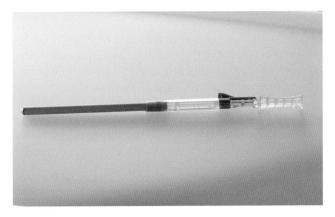

Figure 14.4 Micross (Meta) bone scraper. *Source:* Micross (Meta).

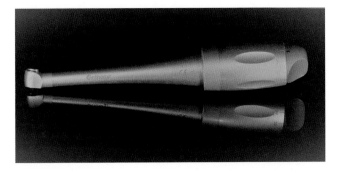

Figure 14.5 Anthogyr Torq Control.

improved access to tighten and loosen prosthetic screws. This is especially helpful in the posterior region where access is limited, as well as being safer to use
intra-orally than small screwdrivers, which may be ingested or aspirated.

14.2.5 Piezosurgery

Piezosurgery is a technique for osteotomy and osteoplasty that uses ultrasonic
vibration with modulated frequency and a controlled tip vibration range. The
ultrasonic frequency is modulated from 10, 30, and 60 cycles/s (Hz) to 29 kHz.
When it comes to cutting bone, you can use traditional burs and saw, but these do
not differentiate, so soft tissue getting in their way will also be lacerated. In piezosurgery the cut is safe because the ultrasonic frequency used does not cut soft tissue. The cutting action is also less invasive, producing less collateral tissue damage,
which results in better healing. Because of its cavitation effect on physiological
solutions (for example, blood), piezosurgery creates a virtually bloodless surgical
site that makes visibility in the working area much clearer than with conventional
bone cutting instruments. Unlike conventional burs and saws, piezosurgery inserts
do not become hot, which again reduces the risk of post-operative necrosis.

Kits are available with different tips and popular tips include the following:

- A periotome-type extraction tip can be used to separate the tooth root from
the bone, with care taken to prevent loss of the thin but intact labial bone. The
tooth root can then be elevated and removed with forceps.
- Sinus preparation tip can be used to safely open a lateral window to the sinus
with membrane elevation safely performed and minimal risk of damage to the
sinus cavity.
- Saws and bone harvesting tips. There may the need for osseous block augmentation, and piezosurgery excels as very fine cuts can be made within the bone
to allow removal. Other tips can be utilised to allow capture of bone for use in
augmentation procedures.

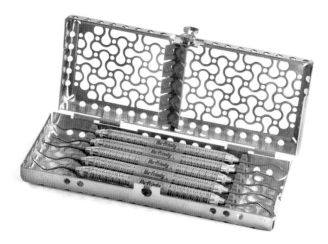

Figure 14.6 Surgical cassette housing instruments preventing damage and optimising safety.
Source: Hu Friedy.

14.3 Tips

- A good-quality surgical cassette is able to house instruments safely, protecting them from being damaged and reducing the risk of sharps injury to the dental team (Figure 14.6). It helps to organise the instruments so that they are always located in the same positions to allow efficient use.
- It is best to clean instruments soon after use to minimise blood clots and other debris sticking and drying onto them.
- It is recommended to have the instruments sharpened regularly to maximise their efficiency. They should be sharpened by approved technicians.

15

Flap Design and Management for Implant Placement

Christopher C.K. Ho, David Attia, and Jess Liu

15.1 Principles

15.1.1 Neurovascular Supply to Implant Site

It is essential for implant surgeons to develop a comprehensive knowledge and understanding of surgical head and neck anatomy to avoid inadvertent implant placement, or incision in areas that may compromise neurovascular bundles. This may lead to surgical complications including, but not limited to, paraesthesia or dysaesthesia, injuries to blood vessels that may result in haematomas, or in severe cases, compromise the airway leading to severe trauma or death. Furthermore, a poor understanding of vascular supply may also lead to compromised healing as a result of flap necrosis, which can lead to exposure of the surgical site and potential complications. The clinician should be aware of the anatomical variations that exist, especially after alveolar ridge remodelling that often occurs following tooth removal.

The key anatomical structures for dental implantology are as follows:

- Infraorbital foramen and nerve
- Maxillary sinus
- Nasal floor
- Anterior nasal spine
- Incisive canal and nerve
- Greater palatine foramen and artery
- Pterygomaxillary fissure
- External oblique ridge
- Inferior alveolar canal, nerve, and artery
- Mental foramen and nerve
- Lingual nerve and artery
- Genial tubercles
- Sublingual fossa
- Mylohyoid muscle.

Extreme caution should be exercised when carrying out incisions. For instance, around the mental foramen or when performing periosteal release in this region,

Practical Procedures in Implant Dentistry, First Edition. Edited by Christopher C.K. Ho.
© 2022 John Wiley & Sons Ltd. Published 2022 by John Wiley & Sons Ltd.
Companion website: www.wiley.com/go/ho/implant-dentistry

as sensory innervation may be disturbed. Placement of implants in the posterior mandible require cross-sectional imaging to determine the anatomy of the mandible, as two-dimensional imaging may not reveal concavities in the sublingual or submandibular fossa and encroachment of this area may lead to damage of lingual artery, which if uncontrolled can lead to airway obstruction. The drilling protocol for implants should allow a 2 mm safety zone. This allows for drills which are often 1 mm longer than labelled, as well as giving an additional 1 mm for a safety error. Hence if the vertical height of bone measured is 10 mm, the length of implant selected should be only 8 mm.

15.1.2 Flap Design and Management

There are a variety of flap designs available when performing implant surgery. It is important to thoroughly assess the clinical situation to determine the ideal flap design in order to achieve the goals of each case. Some factors to be considered in the design of the flap include the identification of anatomical structures, implant site location (e.g. aesthetic/non-aesthetic zone), number of implants being placed, need for soft or hard tissue grafting, and access for instrumentation. In cases where there is sufficient keratinised tissue and ridge dimensions, a flapless or more conservative flap design may be utilised. Cases that present with extensive horizontal and/or vertical ridge deficiencies may require more extensive flap reflection in order to facilitate hard and/or soft tissue ridge augmentation. In order to improve access and provide tension-free closure in these cases, vertical releasing incisions are commonly incorporated.

15.1.3 Types of Flap Reflection

When planning implant surgery, it is important to have a clear understanding of the procedure being performed in order to decide on the type of flap reflection required. In implant surgery, often, two common types of flap reflection are performed: full-thickness mucoperiosteal flap reflection and partial-thickness mucosal flap reflection (Figure 15.1a).

In clinical situations where there is sufficient hard and soft tissue volume, a full-thickness mucoperiosteal flap is routinely reflected, exposing the underlying bone to gain access and visibility of the underlying bony structure (Figure 15.1b). On the other hand, in clinical situations requiring simultaneous hard and or soft tissue augmentation, a combination of full-thickness and split-thickness flap reflection is often utilised (Figure 15.1c).

In full-thickness mucoperiosteal flap reflection, incisions are made through to the underlying bone. The epithelium, connective tissue, and periosteum are all reflected within the flap to expose the underlying bone. Although great visibility is achieved in full-thickness mucoperiosteal flap reflection, the blood supply to the underlying bony structure is reduced. In partial-thickness mucosal flap reflection, incisions are made within the epithelium and connective tissue. The epithelium and connective tissue are reflected within the mucosal flap, while the periosteum remains attached to the bone (Figure 15.1c). This type of flap reflection maintains blood supply to the underlying bone while allowing effective

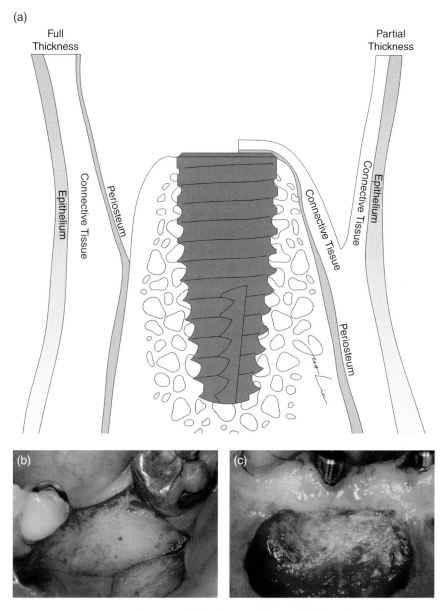

Figure 15.1 (a) Comparison between full-thickness and partial-thickness flaps. (b) Full-thickness flap reflection. (c) Partial-thickness flap reflection. *Source:* (b, c) Case by Dr. Jess Liu.

mobilisation of the mucosa. It is commonly used during implant surgery carried out with simultaneous hard and/or soft tissue augmentation procedures.

When planning full- or partial-thickness flap reflection, one factor to take into consideration is the gingival phenotype of the patient. A patient with a thick gingival phenotype is suitable for both full- and partial-thickness flap reflection. A thick gingival phenotype allows predictable flap dissection without risk of flap perforation or necrosis. Conversely, a patient with a thin gingival phenotype is often only suitable for full-thickness mucoperiosteal flap reflection because thin tissues are more technique-sensitive and have a higher risk of flap perforation. Thin partial-thickness flaps also have a compromised blood supply and this increases the risk of flap necrosis.

Clinicians can easily and predictably differentiate thin and thick gingival phenotype using a simple test with a standard periodontal probe as described by De Rouck et al. [1].

15.2 Procedures

15.2.1 Tissue Punch

Soft tissue punch techniques offer clinicians a flapless approach to implant therapy and are often used in conjunction with guided implant surgery (Figure 15.2). This has many advantages, including reduced surgical trauma, improved wound stability, and therefore minimised bone resorption. However, there is limited visibility of the surgical site and limited access for implant placement and ridge augmentation procedures. When considering the tissue punch technique, it is important to assess the presence or absence of keratinised tissue. After excision of a tissue punch, a minimum 2 mm of circumferential keratinised gingivae should be present. This provides an adequate band of keratinised gingivae to optimise peri-implant health. If there is insufficient keratinised gingivae to meet the minimum requirements, other techniques should be considered.

15.2.2 Envelope Flap

Envelope flaps are the most commonly used flap design in implant surgery. An envelope flap consists of a crestal incision and sulcular incisions around the adjacent teeth (Figure 15.3a). When increased flap mobility is required, the sulcular incision can be extended further away from the edentulous site. The envelope

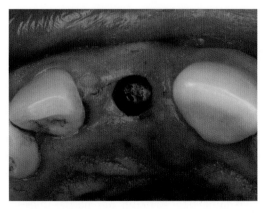

Figure 15.2 Soft tissue punch. *Source:* Case by Dr. Jess Liu.

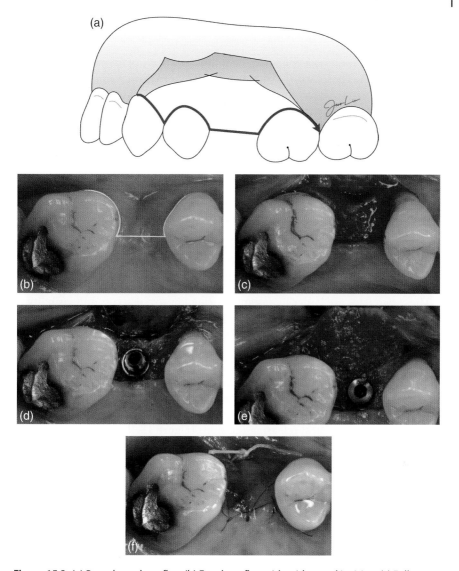

Figure 15.3 (a) Buccal envelope flap. (b) Envelope flap with mid-crestal incision. (c) Full-thickness envelope flap reflection. (d) Implant placement. (e) Biomaterial placed for buccal contour graft. (f) Double-layer closure with apical horizontal mattress suture and single interrupted sutures. *Source:* Case by Dr. David Attia.

flap can be modified by altering the position of the crestal incision. In cases where there is sufficient keratinised gingivae, a mid-crestal incision is commonly used (Figure 15.3b). On the other hand, the crestal incision is made 1–2 mm palatal/lingual to the middle of the crest in cases with a reduced amount of buccal keratinised gingivae. This modification allows the clinician to manipulate the keratinised tissue on the crest, moving it buccally to correct the pre-existing deficiency.

15.2.3 Triangular (Two-Sided) and Trapezoidal (Three-Sided) Flap

Triangular and trapezoidal flaps are often used in cases of reduced ridge volume where augmentation procedures are required prior to, or in conjunction with implant surgery. These two-flap designs are similar to the envelope flap, with the addition of one or two apically divergent vertical releasing incisions. The number of vertical releasing incisions to be incorporated is dependent upon access and visibility to the underlying bone or defect, as well as the amount of flap release required to gain tension-free primary closure. After the envelope flap incision has been outlined, the vertical releasing incisions are placed at the mesial or distal line angle of the teeth adjacent to the edentulous space (Figure 15.4a). The releasing incision should be made at 90 degrees to the gingival margin, allowing accurate flap approximation. When placing the vertical releasing incisions, it is important to avoid placing the vertical releasing incision:

- over any bony exostosis or prominent roots (e.g. maxillary canines) (Figure 15.4c)
- in the mid-facial aspect of the adjacent tooth (Figure 15.4c)
- to prevent bisecting of the interdental papilla.

These two flaps are larger in design, offering improved access and visibility to the surgical site. Having a wider base, the flap also carries an improved blood supply. When extensive ridge augmentation procedures are required, or the surgical site is in the aesthetic zone, some factors need to be taken into consideration. Large ridge augmentation procedures require increased flap mobility to achieve tension-free primary closure. Clinicians have the option of either extending the envelope aspect of the flap intrasulcularly further away from the bony defect, or alternatively, a trapezoidal flap may be used which combines an envelope flap with two vertical releasing incisions (Figure 15.4b). Additional scoring of the periosteum may be required to aid in flap advancement. Vertical releasing

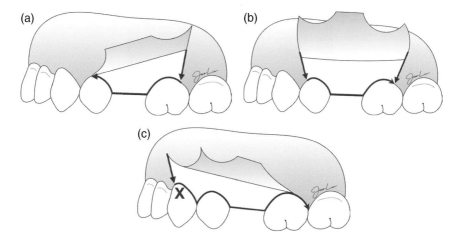

Figure 15.4 (a) Two-sided flap with distal vertical releasing incision at the first molar site. (b) Trapezoidal flap with mesial and distal vertical releasing incisions. (c) Vertical releasing incision incorrectly placed in the aesthetic zone, over the mid-facial aspect of a prominent maxillary canine root.

incisions should be avoided in the aesthetic zone as this can result in visible residual scarring that may compromise the final aesthetic outcome (Figure 15.4c). In these cases, one (or two) vertical releasing incisions can be placed distal to the aesthetic zone. Alternatively, the vertical releasing incisions can be placed within the buccal frenums, hiding any resulting scarring that may result.

15.2.4 Papilla-Sparing Flap

The papilla-sparing flap technique is often used in aesthetic cases where there is a need to preserve and avoid collapse of the interdental papilla. A papilla-sparing flap consists of a crestal incision that extends 1–2 mm away from the sulcus of the adjacent teeth (Figure 15.5a). Two vertical releasing incisions are made at each end of the crestal incision, preserving the entire papilla complex and reducing any crestal bone remodelling (Figure 15.5a). It is commonly used in cases where there is existing adjacent crown and bridge or implant supported restorations in order to prevent iatrogenic post-operative recession, exposing the existing restoration margins. It is also performed in cases of thin gingival phenotype and triangular-shaped teeth to minimise the loss of the interdental papilla.

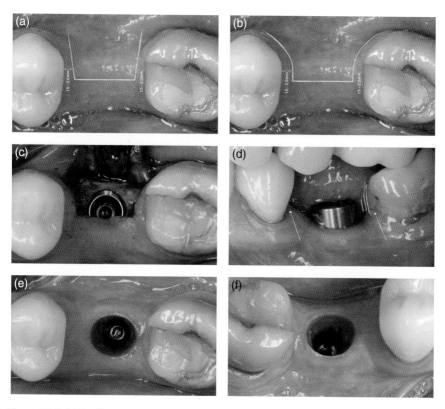

Figure 15.5 (a) Papilla-sparing incision. (b) Modified papilla-sparing incision incorporating semi-lunar vertical releasing incision. (c) Implant placement. (d) Preserved papilla height following implant osseointegration. (e) Healed peri-implant emergence profile (occlusal view). (f) Healed peri-implant emergence profile (buccal view). *Source:* Case by Dr. David Attia.

However, as it is a smaller flap, it can limit access and visibility to the surgical site and may result in a limited bloody supply. This flap design can be modified by replacing the two vertical releasing incisions with two semi-lunar incisions (Figure 15.5b). This results in a wider base of the flap, increasing the blood supply and also improving flap mobility.

15.2.5 Buccal Roll

The buccal roll flap technique is often used to correct a morphological soft tissue defect when there is sufficient bone volume to accommodate an implant for the edentulous site. The technique consists of an envelope flap design with a palatally/lingually placed crestal incision. After outlining the crestal incision with a No.15 blade, the crestal surface epithelial layer is removed using a high-speed diamond bur or the No.15 blade. A full-thickness pedicled mucoperiosteal flap is then reflected to expose the underlying bone in readiness for implant placement. Following implant placement, a buccal split-thickness dissection is performed. This creates a space to roll the de-epithelialised crestal soft tissue and restore the buccal morphological defect. One advantage of this technique is that it allows soft tissue augmentation of the ridge, without requiring a second donor site, therefore reducing patient morbidity. See Chapter 19 for a case example.

15.2.6 Palacci Flap

The Palacci flap is indicated in cases where papilla regeneration is required [2]. The flap consists of an envelope flap design with a palatally/lingually placed crestal incision (Figure 15.6a, c). A full-thickness mucoperiosteal flap is reflected and the underlying bone exposed. Following implant placement, the healing abutments are installed into the implants (if the desired primary stability is achieved). A semi-lunar incision is then made within the reflected buccal flap creating a pedicle (Figure 15.6b, d). The pedicle is then rotated 90 degrees to fill the interproximal space between the implant and adjacent tooth, or adjacent implants (Figure 15.6e, f).

15.3 Tips

- Incisions should be made with a sharp blade. When a blade touches bone, it becomes blunt. Dull blades should be replaced frequently during the surgical procedure to minimise trauma.
- Incisions should be perpendicular to the surface of the tissues to maximise thickness and blood supply at the flap margin, reducing the risk of necrosis and wound dehiscence.
- The technique to be used is case dependent. An appropriately sized flap should be used, allowing access and visibility and eliminating tension from the flap.
- The use of correct surgical instrumentation is key to minimising trauma to tissues. When handling flaps, microsurgical tissue forceps should be used to avoid flap perforation.

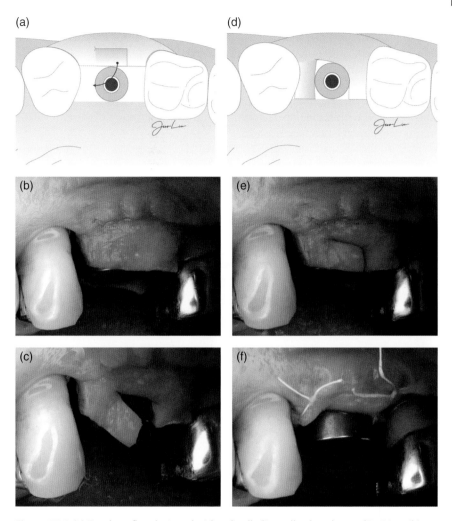

Figure 15.6 (a) Envelope flap designed with palatally/lingually placed crestal incision. (b) Semi-lunar incision made within the buccal flap to create a pedicle. (c) Full-thickness buccal flap following installation of healing abutment. (d) Semi-lunar incision made within the buccal flap to create a pedicle. (e) Pedicle is rotated towards the deficient mesial papilla. (f) Flap is adapted around healing abutment using sutures. *Source:* Case by Dr. Jess Liu.

- When raising full-thickness mucoperiosteal flaps, periosteal elevators should maintain contact with the underlying bone allowing atraumatic flap reflection by ensuring the flap is raised in its entirety – epithelium, connective tissue, and periosteum.
- Surgical sites must remain well hydrated throughout the entire surgical procedure. This will prevent tissue shrinkage and maintain flap elasticity, allowing atraumatic handling of the tissues at all times.
- Two- or three-sided flaps should have a wider base to ensure adequate blood supply to the surgical site.

- Vertical releasing incisions should be made at 90 degrees to the free gingival margin and should not be placed over prominent root eminences or at the gingival zenith, or bisect the interdental papilla.
- Vertical releasing incisions must extend beyond the mucogingival line, reaching the alveolar mucosa to allow for adequate release of the flap.
- In cases requiring ridge augmentation, periosteal releasing incisions should be incorporated within the flap design. This allows mobilisation of the flap, facilitating tension-free primary closure.

References

1 De Rouck, T., Eghbali, R., Collys, K. et al. (2009). The gingival biotype revisited: transparency of the periodontal probe through the gingival margin as a method to discriminate thin from thick gingiva. *J. Clin. Periodontol.* 36: 428–433.
2 Palacci, P. (1995). Papilla regeneration technique. In: *Optimal Implant Positioning & Soft Tissue Management for the Branemark System* (eds. P. Palacci, I. Ericsson, P. Engstrand and B. Rangert), 59–70. Chicago: Quintessence Pub. Co.

16

Suturing Techniques

Christopher C.K. Ho, David Attia, and Jess Liu

16.1 Principles

The primary objective of suturing is to secure surgical flaps by re-approximating the wound margins. This allows haemostasis to promote optimal healing and improve patient comfort. Following full-thickness mucoperiosteal flap reflection, healing by primary intention is intended. However, prolonged exposure of the alveolar bone due to incomplete wound closure may result in pain, bone loss, and delayed healing by secondary intention. On the other hand, in partial-thickness flap reflection, the periosteum and overlying connective tissue remains attached to the bone, serving as a protective barrier to minimise pain, bone loss, and delayed healing in cases of incomplete wound closure.

Correct suturing techniques ensure accurate and effective closure of the surgical site, allowing direct apposition of the tissues to provide an environment for favourable healing. Having a good understanding of the various suturing techniques and materials available allows the clinician to recognise when and where each technique should be utilised in order to achieve ideal healing and the desired outcomes.

Ineffective application of suturing techniques and materials, especially in cases involving ridge augmentation, may result in compromised healing or early wound dehiscence. This is often accompanied by exposure of the surgical site, hard and soft tissue grafts, and dental implants which can lead to post-operative infection and possible failure of the procedure.

16.1.1 Types of Sutures

Surgical sutures are commonly classified based on material (absorbable or non-absorbable), structure (monofilament or multifilament), coating (coated or non-coated), and source (natural or synthetic). Selecting the correct suture material in dental implantology is often dependent upon the nature of the procedures being performed, with both absorbable and non-absorbable sutures commonly incorporated. In cases where longer tension is desired, non-absorbable sutures

Practical Procedures in Implant Dentistry, First Edition. Edited by Christopher C.K. Ho.
© 2022 John Wiley & Sons Ltd. Published 2022 by John Wiley & Sons Ltd.
Companion website: www.wiley.com/go/ho/implant-dentistry

or sutures with a slow absorption time are used, whereas in cases where prolonged tension is not required, absorbable sutures are preferred. Because of this, sutures in this chapter will be classified based on absorption time.

16.1.1.1 Absorbable Sutures

Natural Absorbable Sutures

- Multifilament sutures are composed of purified collagen that is derived from bovine or sheep intestines and are broken down by the body's enzymes. Because they can be absorbed, post-operative appointments for suture removal may not be required, which reduces chair time.
- The absorption rate of these sutures is influenced by the body's pH. Patients who present with xerostomia, Sjögren's syndrome, gastric reflux, or eating disorders may experience quicker absorption of these sutures.
- Types:
  - Plain gut – lose approximately 50% of tensile strength within one day and are absorbed within five days following surgery.
  - Chromic gut – are plain gut sutures treated in a chromium salt solution, extending the absorption time. The chromic salt acts as a cross-linking agent and increases the tensile strength and resistance to absorption time to 10–15 days.

Synthetic Absorbable Sutures

- Synthetic absorbable sutures can be classified as braided multifilament or non-braided monofilament:
  - Braided multifilament sutures are composed of polyglycolic acid (PGA), manufactured from a polymer of glycolide and lactide which renders the thread extremely smooth, soft, and knot safe (e.g. Vicryl, Ethicon Inc.). This suture material has an absorption time of approximately three weeks.
  - Non-braided monofilament sutures include Resorba® Glycolon™, and Monocryl (Ethicon Inc.). Glycolon is composed of PGA and polycaprolactone. These sutures have an absorption time of 11–13 days. Monocryl is composed of poliglecaprone 25 and has an absorption time of 7 days.
  - Synthetic absorbable sutures are primarily resorbed by the process of hydrolysis.

16.1.1.2 Non-absorbable Sutures

- Silk sutures are braided multifilament sutures constructed from silk filaments with good handling properties and visibility. These sutures have a 'wick-effect' which results in accumulation of bacteria.
- Nylon sutures are made of a synthetic non-absorbable material (e.g. prolene). They are available in multifilament and monofilament variations. They are inert, with minimal tissue reaction. The advantage of these sutures is that they can stretch, accommodating any swelling that occurs post-operatively.
- Polypropylene (Ethicon Inc.) is a synthetic, non-absorbable, monofilament suture exhibiting good tensile strength and minimal tissue reaction. One

disadvantage of polypropylene is its shape-memory effect, which results in more technique-sensitive handling properties.

• Polytetrafluoroethylene (PTFE) sutures are soft, monofilament sutures that do not exhibit bacterial wicking into the surgical site. They are inert and biocompatible, offering excellent soft tissue response, while maintaining the flexibility and patient comfort usually associated with braided sutures. Additionally, they retain a high tensile strength and are easily visible in the mouth (e.g. Cytoplast™).

16.1.2 Suture Adjuncts

Tissue adhesive (e.g. GluStich Periacryl®) is a cyanoacrylate tissue adhesive that adheres to moist tissues with no toxic or foreign body reaction. It is violet in colour for visibility and sets quickly. It acts as a securing agent for free gingival grafts and as a liquid dressing for donor sites and biopsies, and for securing other types of dental dressings. It is haemostatic and bacteriostatic, and does not need to be removed during the post-operative follow-up.

16.1.3 Suture Size

Sutures are sized according to the diameter of the suture material (Figure 16.1), measured from sizes 1-0 (largest) to 10-0 (smallest). In dental implantology, suture sizes range from 3-0 to 7-0, with 4-0/5-0 commonly used for macro-surgery, while 6-0/7-0 are often utilised in microsurgical procedures.

16.1.4 Needle

A surgical needle has three parts (Figure 16.2):

1) Point
2) Needle body
3) Swaged (press fit) end.

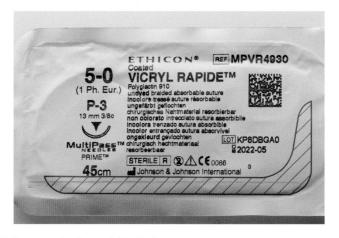

Figure 16.1 Suture packaging and descriptions.

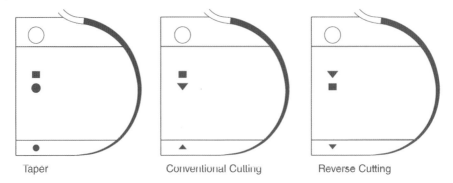

Taper   Conventional Cutting   Reverse Cutting

Figure 16.2 Suture needles.

The most commonly used needles in dentistry are 3/8 and ½ circle needles with a round, reverse cutting, or cutting point. Round needles are less traumatic, requiring more force to enter the tissue, while reverse cutting has a sharp tip downwards and is safer in more delicate tissue.

16.2 Procedures

16.2.1 Simple/Interrupted Sutures

The simple interrupted suture technique is the most commonly used technique (Figure 16.3). The individual sutures are not connected. It is simple to perform, and the effectiveness of each suture is independent. It is indicated for re-approximation of flap margins at specific points. This is usually in the

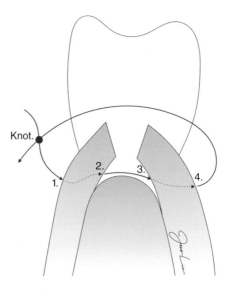

Figure 16.3 Simple interrupted sutures.

interproximal tissue or in the meeting point between a vertical and a sulcular incision, termed a 'key suture'.

16.2.2 Continuous/Uninterrupted Suture

A continuous or uninterrupted suture uses a single strand of suture material to close crestal incisions that are placed on a long edentulous span (Figure 16.4). Unlike single interrupted sutures, which are independent of one another, each possessing their own knot, a continuous or uninterrupted suture only uses one knot. The technique begins with a simple interrupted suture. The tail end of this suture is cut, leaving the needle end of the suture material to complete the remaining part of the suture. The needle end of the suture begins to engage the flap in a buccal-lingual/palatal direction until the entire span of the flap margins have been approximated. In the last pass of the suture needle, the suture material is not pulled completely through the flap, leaving a small loop which is then used as the 'tail-end' of the suture material and the knot is tied. One advantage of this suturing technique is that it saves time; only two knots need to be tied in order to complete the suture. On the other hand, if the buccal and palatal bites are not evenly spaced along the span of the flap, excessive tissue may accumulate towards the end of the incision line, leading to an overlap of flap margins called a 'dog-ear'. This also results in uneven tension within the suture. Furthermore, if one of the two knots become loose, the entire suture may be compromised and may even unravel completely.

16.2.3 Mattress Sutures

Mattress sutures can be either horizontal or vertical, offering a means of providing flap security. They are categorised as either internal or external mattress sutures (Figure 16.5). The horizontal mattress suturing technique is used to provide a resistance to muscle pull by relieving the tension from the flap, and approximating the wound margins. Horizontal mattress sutures are commonly used in combination with simple interrupted or continuous sutures,

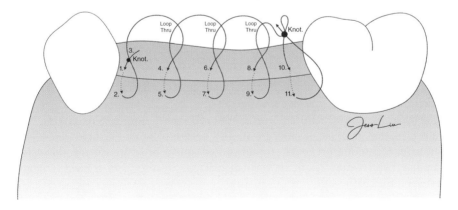

Figure 16.4 Continuous/uninterrupted sutures.

(a)

(b)

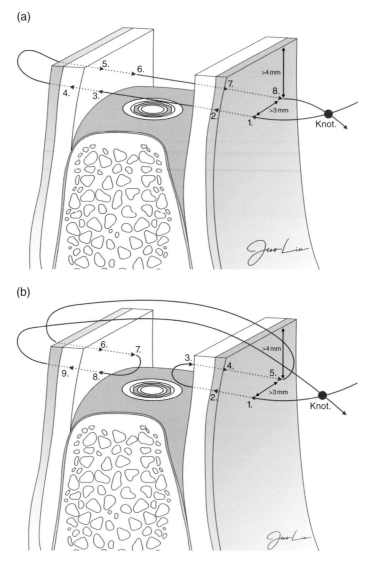

Figure 16.5 (a) Internal horizontal mattress suture continuous. (b) External horizontal mattress suture continuous.

especially in guided bone regeneration procedures where tension-free primary closure is required.

Vertical mattress sutures are commonly used for approximating the interproximal papillae, especially in the aesthetic zone (Figure 16.6). This suturing technique prevents any unwanted apical pressure on the tip of the papillae, which may result in vertical collapse, resulting in a black triangle between the teeth.

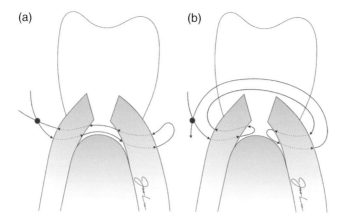

Figure 16.6 (a) Internal vertical mattress suture continuous. (b) External vertical mattress suture continuous.

16.2.3.1 Horizontal Mattress

1) Suturing starts from the vestibular aspect of the buccal flap, 4–5 mm from the flap margin.
2) The needle passes through to the internal aspect of the palatal/lingual flap at the same vertical position as the buccal counterpart.
3) The needle is then passed back through from outer surface on the palatal/lingual flap at a minimum of 3 mm from the initial palatal/lingual exit point.
4) The suture is completed with the needle passing through the internal aspect of the buccal flap at the same horizontal and vertical position as the palatal/lingual counterpart.
5) A surgeon's knot is tied to complete the suture.

16.2.3.2 Vertical Mattress

1) Suturing starts from the vestibular aspect of the buccal flap, 4–5 mm from the flap margin.
2) The needle passes through to the internal aspect of the palatal/lingual flap at the same vertical position as the buccal counterpart.
3) The needle is then passed back through from outer surface on the palatal/lingual flap in a more coronal position from the initial palatal/lingual exit point, maintaining a minimum of 1 mm from the wound margin/tip of the papilla.
4) The suture is completed with the needle passing through the internal aspect of the buccal flap/tip of the papillae at the same vertical position as the palatal/lingual counterpart.
5) A surgeon's knot is tied to complete the suture.

16.2.4 Suture Removal

Suture removal should take place once the wound has attained sufficient healing, which normally occurs around 7–10 days post-operatively. The use of diluted peroxide or chlorhexidine may be used to clean the wound and sutures prior to removal. The knot is elevated with diamond-coated tissue pliers and the suture loop is cut close to the tissue surface in order to minimise the amount of suture material (which can often accumulate plaque) passing through the tissue.

16.3 Tips

- Multifilament sutures should be avoided in contaminated wounds because bacteria can accumulate, which can lead to infection.
- Do not grasp the needle at the tip or the swage of the needle. The needle should be grasped approximately 1/3 to ½ the distance from the swage end.
- The needle should enter the tissue perpendicular to the surface and the knot should not be placed over the incision line.
- Do not tighten sutures excessively as this may cause ischaemia and necrosis of the flap at the margins.
- Adequate flap release may often be required in order to achieve tension-free primary closure of the surgical flaps, especially in guided bone regeneration procedures. This will ensure optimal healing without early wound dehiscence.
- Commonly used suture materials in implant therapy include PTFE, nylon, and polypropylene. These monofilament suture materials often result in less plaque accumulation at the surgical site during the healing period.

17

Pre-surgical Tissue Evaluation and Considerations in Aesthetic Implant Dentistry
Sherif Said

17.1   Principles

When considering implant therapy in the aesthetic zone, replicating the natural soft tissue frame may present challenges for the treating clinician. A harmonious gingival form and architecture are fundamental not only for adequate peri-implant pink aesthetics but also for simulating a natural emergence for the future restoration. When dealing with clinical situations in which adequate tissue architecture and volume are present, preserving or further enhancement of the available support may provide an improved aesthetic outcome with less associated morbidity and treatment duration. Nevertheless, reconstruction of atrophic sites due to lost hard and soft tissue volume is often inevitable in the anterior zone, which may necessitate more complex grafting procedures with varying degrees of predictability in achieving ideal peri-implant soft tissues. This chapter will highlight clinical scenarios and evidence-based treatment of cases in which the lack of hard and soft tissue volume poses difficulty in achieving optimal peri-implant aesthetics. Contemporary clinical strategies and minimally invasive techniques will also be discussed, to allow clinicians to better manage hard and soft tissue deficiencies when dealing with implant therapy in the aesthetic zone.

17.2   The Influence of Tissue Volume on Peri-implant 'Pink' Aesthetics

Aesthetics and patient-centred outcomes have evolved to become integral components of daily practice, especially in the aesthetic zone (Figure 17.1). The clinician must consider that aesthetics are also highly subjective and should be directed towards providing treatment tailored to each individual patient depending on their situation.

Implant aesthetics can be classified into pink and white aesthetics. The 'pink' refers to the soft tissue form, contour, colour, and texture surrounding the implant, while the 'white' focuses on the implant-supported restoration.

Practical Procedures in Implant Dentistry, First Edition. Edited by Christopher C.K. Ho.
© 2022 John Wiley & Sons Ltd. Published 2022 by John Wiley & Sons Ltd.
Companion website: www.wiley.com/go/ho/implant-dentistry

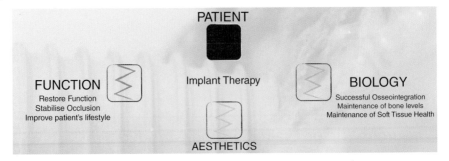

Figure 17.1 Triad of contemporary implant dentistry. *Sources:* Buser, D., Chappuis, V., Belser, U.C., and Chen, S. (2017). Implant placement post extraction in esthetic single tooth sites: when immediate, when early, when late? Periodontology 2000 73(1): 84–102; Linkevicius, T., Apse, P., Grybauskas, S., and Puisys, A. (2009). The influence of soft tissue thickness on crestal bone changes around implants: a 1-year prospective controlled clinical trial. Int. J. Oral Maxillofac. Implants 24(4): 11–17 [1–3].

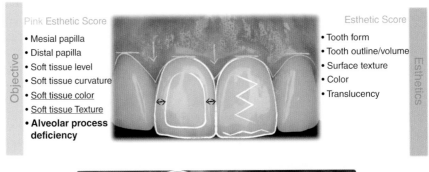

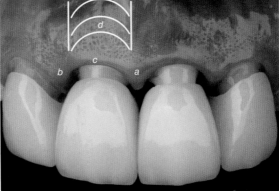

Figure 17.2 Pink Esthetic Score criteria include: mesial papilla (*a*), distal papilla height (*b*), soft tissue level (*c*), and soft tissue colour, texture and curvature (*d*). White Esthetic Score criteria include: tooth form, tooth outline, surface texture, colour, and translucency [5].

Objective assessment criteria have been introduced in the literature, such as the Pink Esthetic Score (PES) and White Esthetic Score (WES) [4] to standardise how clinicians and researchers evaluate the aesthetics of implant-supported restorations (Figure 17.2). For anterior implant therapy, evaluation of both the pink and white aesthetics is imperative, and consequently surgical therapy should be geared towards optimising functional and biological outcomes without neglecting the aesthetic component.

17.3 Tissue Volume Availability and Requirements

Preservation of the existing architecture of the soft tissues prior to tooth extraction offers clinicians an ideal method of obtaining a more 'natural' appearance of the final implant restoration. The soft tissue 'curtain' surrounding implant-supported restorations requires sufficient, three-dimensional hard and soft tissue volume to attain a long-term stable result. Unfortunately, the tissue volume requirements for dental implants is often more than what is needed for maintenance of the natural dentition. Consequently, preservation of the tissue architecture alone following tooth extraction may not be adequate to maintain tissue stability around the future implant and thus additional soft and hard tissue augmentation is often required.

17.3.1 Hard Tissue Requirements (Figure 17.3 and 17.4)

Hard tissue requirements include the following:

- Buccal bone to the implant:
  - Minimum of 2 mm [6]
  - Recommended 2–4 mm [3]

(a)   (b)   (c)   (d)

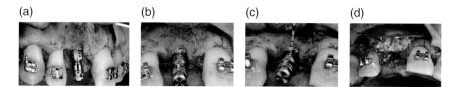

Figure 17.3 (a) Implant placement in an upper central incisor area. (b) Note the grey shadow of the implant fixture apparent through the thin buccal bone. (c) Buccal bone thickness less than 1 mm will possess minimal vascularity and is highly susceptible to further resorption following implant placement or loading. (d) Buccal veneer grafting to compensate for the remodelling of the thin buccal plate.

(a)   (b)   (c)

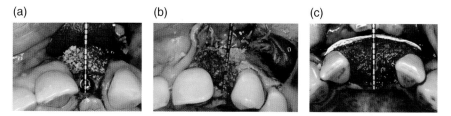

Figure 17.4 (a) Buccal veneer grafting performed at the time of implant placement with a xenograft material to further augment the buccal contour. (b) Grafting of more than 4 mm buccal to the anticipated implant position to compensate for remodelling of the bone graft material. (c) Utilising a non-resorbable membrane to shape the bone graft to the desired ridge shape.

(a)   (b)

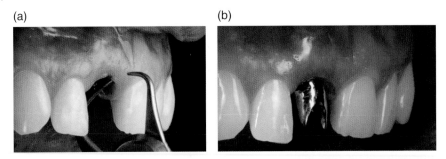

Figure 17.5 (a, b) Robust buccal volume augmentation following combined connective tissue grafting and dual zone protocols to simulate a natural emergence of the final restoration and mask any show-through of the abutment material.

Significance:

- Sufficient buccal bone thickness is required for long-term stability of the marginal bone over time.
- Decrease the incidence of marginal tissue recession long term.

17.3.2   Soft Tissue Requirements (Figure 17.5)

Soft tissue requirements include the following:

- 2–3 mm of facial peri-implant soft tissue thickness [7, 8].

Significance:

- Protective function to maintain the underlying bone integrity.
- Avoid soft tissue show through of the underlying implant restorative components.

Teeth with intact periodontium may require minimal augmentation. However, in cases where the integrity of the socket is compromised or in cases with severe tissue deficiencies more extensive augmentation may be required to achieve the desired outcomes.

17.4   Pre-operative Implant Site Assessment (Figures 17.6 and 17.7)

Because of the inherent anatomy of the alveolar topography in the anterior zone, post-extraction ridge dimension alterations are more common than in posterior sites. Tomographic studies have demonstrated that the average buccal bone thickness is less than 1 mm in 90% of anterior teeth [9].

This is compounded by the fact that the buccal plate (bundle bone) stems from the periodontal ligament of the tooth and inevitably undergoes remodelling/ resorption once the tooth is removed. Araújo et al. [10, 11] demonstrated a 40% reduction in ridge width following tooth extractions in dogs. Such dimensional changes often require more invasive procedures to restore sufficient ridge volume to satisfy the biologic, functional, and aesthetic demands. Subsequently, efforts to maximise the remaining ridge topography and tissue volume should be

(a)   (b)   (c)

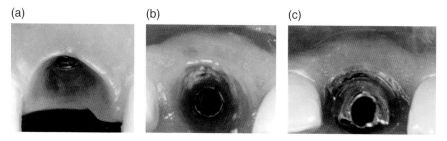

Figure 17.6 (a) Clinical situation following bone and soft tissue augmentation at the time of implant placement. (b) Note the bone graft particles encapsulated within the soft tissue. (c) Occlusal view of the final abutment in place.

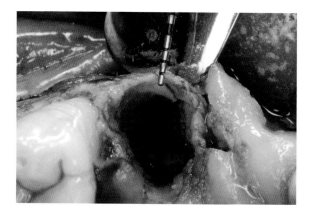

Figure 17.7 Close-up view of the buccal plate of a canine socket following extraction. Flap reflection was performed revealing a greenstick fracture of the bone that was not noted at the time of tooth removal.

made at the time of tooth extraction. If residual deficiencies are still present, further augmentation may be required at the time of implant placement and/or second stage uncovering.

Clinical decision-making requires appropriate timing of implant placement, and augmentation procedures can be performed at the following phases of treatment [12].

1) At the time of tooth extraction
2) At the time of implant placement
3) At the time of second stage uncovering or post implant provisionalization.

17.5   Key Factors in Diagnosis of the Surrounding Tooth Support Prior to Extraction

Accurate diagnosis of the periodontal integrity of both the tooth to be extracted and neighbouring teeth must be attained in order to determine the need for prior corrective procedures and/or plan for the augmentations required prior to tooth extraction. Furthermore, analysis of the clinical situation becomes a critical determinant in the viability of proceeding with immediate implant placement upon tooth extraction [13].

17.5.1 Integrity of the Interproximal Height of Bone

It has been well established in the literature that the height of the peri-implant papilla is not dictated by the level of bone surrounding the implant but by the presence of the supra-crestal periodontal fibres on the adjacent teeth. It has been further shown in recent literature that the papillary height in sites of multiple adjacent missing teeth is significantly less than when the tooth is present. Therefore, the periodontal integrity and height of bone on the adjacent teeth become a key determinant in the final aesthetics of the implant-supported restoration. In the presence of periodontal pathology or interproximal attachment loss on the adjacent teeth, interdisciplinary techniques such as orthodontic extrusion or changes to the tooth shape by restorative means may be required to compensate for the deficiencies in the interproximal papilla (Figure 17.8).

17.5.2 Essential Criteria Evaluation Prior to Extraction

Evaluation prior to extraction should include:

- Comprehensive periodontal evaluation
- Radiographic analysis
- Bone sounding of the interproximal and buccal bone.

The buccal bone and interproximal bone height integrity are essential diagnostic factors prior to tooth extraction in order to anticipate the final outcome and diagnose any deficiencies that may be present. Furthermore, the

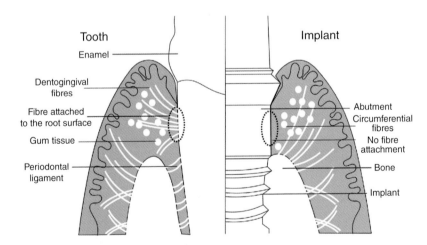

Figure 17.8 Schematic illustrating the differences between the peri-implant and periodontal attachment. Note the perpendicular orientation of the periodontal attachment which creates a protective barrier from physical and bacterial insults in addition to support of the supra-crestal tissue. The difference in fibre orientation histologically contributes to the difference in the macro-anatomy of the peri-implant papilla and gingiva.

clinician must be cognisant of any mesio-distal tooth malpositioning and/or root proximity that may render the interdental bone more susceptible to resorption. The choice of flap reflection and design may also modified in attempt to avoid stripping of the periosteum and blood supply overlying thin (<1.5 mm) or compromised inter-radicular bone [14, 15]. Therefore, radiographic evaluation of the neighbouring teeth and bone sounding of the dentition to be extracted should be performed prior to deciding to extract the tooth. Furthermore, a clinician should be cautious when reflecting soft tissue flaps in the maxillary anterior region. Should there be any signs of interproximal bone loss evident on the radiographs or bone-sounding measurements exceeding 5 mm, flap designs should be modified to involve papillary sparing techniques to avoid soft tissue collapse of the interproximal papilla.

17.5.3 Integrity of the Buccal Plate of Bone

Cone beam computed tomography scan, clinical periodontal evaluation, and bone sounding are combined to ascertain the integrity and level of the buccal plate prior to extraction. Compromise in the buccal plate integrity can ultimately lead to collapse of the tissue in the bucco-lingual aspect, giving an unaesthetic implant-supported restoration and facial tissue recession exposing the underlying restorative components (Figure 17.9.). If the level of the gingival margin in relation to the adjacent teeth and in relation to the final implant-supported restoration is located in an apical position, it may be prudent for the clinician to consider soft tissue grafting either before tooth extraction or at any time point prior to finalisation of the prosthetic procedures.

17.6 Tips

- In cases with intact sockets with good interproximal height of bone and intact buccal plates within 3–4 mm of the facial gingival margin of the tooth to be extracted with no gingival recession, immediate implant placement should be considered.
- Compromised sites require precise management and an overall evaluation of the aesthetic sensitivity of the case should be performed.

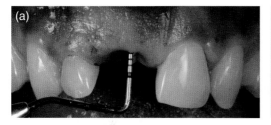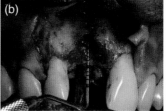

Figure 17.9. (a) Pre-operative bone sounding of the buccal plate reveals probing depths in excess of 10 mm. (b) Intra-surgical view showing complete absence of the buccal plate.

- In cases with significant facial tissue recession and buccal plate dehiscenses a less experienced clinician should consider extracting the tooth and augmenting the site prior to implant placement.
- In cases where there is compromise of the interproximal height of bone, interdisciplinary treatment such as pink porcelain, restoration of the adjacent teeth, or orthodontic extrusion should be considered prior to tooth extraction.

17.7 Conclusion

Evaluation of the anatomy around teeth prior to extraction in the aesthetic zone is of critical importance. A clinician should be aware of the sensitivity of tooth extraction in the aesthetic zone and should attempt to avoid any complications prior to them occurring.

References

1 Buser, D., Chappuis, V., Belser, U.C., and Chen, S. (2017). Implant placement post extraction in esthetic single tooth sites: when immediate, when early, when late? *Periodontology 2000* 73 (1): 84–102.

2 Linkevicius, T., Apse, P., Grybauskas, S., and Puisys, A. (2009). The influence of soft tissue thickness on crestal bone changes around implants: a 1-year prospective controlled clinical trial. *International Journal of Oral and Maxillofacial Implants* 24 (4): 712–719.

3 Grunder, U., Gracis, S., and Capelli, M. (2005). Influence of the 3-D bone-to-implant relationship on esthetics. *Int J Periodontics Restorative Dent* 25 (2): 113–119.

4 Belser, U.C., Grütter, L., Vailati, F. et al. (2009). Outcome evaluation of early placed maxillary anterior single-tooth implants using objective esthetic criteria: a cross-sectional, retrospective study in 45 patients with a 2- to 4-year follow-up using pink and white esthetic scores. *J Periodontol* 80 (1): 140–151.

5 Tettamanti, S., Millen, C., Gavric, J. et al. (2016). Esthetic evaluation of implant crowns and Peri-implant soft tissue in the anterior maxilla: comparison and reproducibility of three different indices. *Clinical Implant Dentistry and Related Research* 18 (3): 517–526. https://doi.org/10.1111/cid.12306.

6 Spray, J.R., Black, C.G., Morris, H.F., and Ochi, S. (2000). The influence of bone thickness on facial marginal bone response: stage 1 placement through stage 2 uncovering. *Annals of Periodontology* 5 (1): 119–128. https://doi.org/10.1902/annals.2000.5.1.119.

7 Grunder, U. (2000). Stability of the mucosal topography around single-tooth implants and adjacent teeth: 1-year results. *International Journal of Periodontics and Restorative Dentistry* 20 (1): 11–17.

8 Grunder, U. (2011). Crestal ridge width changes when placing implants at the time of tooth extraction with and without soft tissue augmentation after a healing period of 6 months: report of 24 consecutive cases. *International Journal of Periodontics and Restorative Dentistry* 31 (1): 9.

9 Braut, V., Bornstein, M.M., Belser, U., and Buser, D. (2011). Thickness of the anterior maxillary facial bone wall-a retrospective radiographic study using cone beam computed tomography. *International Journal of Periodontics and Restorative Dentistry* 31 (2): 125–131.

10 Araújo, M.G., Sukekava, F., Wennström, J.L., and Lindhe, J. (2006). Tissue modeling following implant placement in fresh extraction sockets. *Clinical Oral Implants Research* 17 (6): 615–624. https://doi.org/10.1111/j.1600-0501.2006.01317.x.

11 Araujo, M., Linder, E., Wennström, J., and Lindhe, J. (2008). The influence of Bio-Oss Collagen on healing of an extraction socket: an experimental study in the dog. *International Journal of Periodontics and Restorative Dentistry* 28 (2): 123–135.

12 Funato, A., Salama, M.A., Ishikawa, T. et al. (2007). Timing, positioning, and sequential staging in esthetic implant therapy: a four-dimensional perspective. *International Journal of Periodontics and Restorative Dentistry* 27 (4): 313–323.

13 Chu, S.J., Salama, M.A., Salama, H. et al. (2012). The dual-zone therapeutic concept of managing immediate implant placement and provisional restoration in anterior extraction sockets. *The Compendium of Continuing Education in Dentistry* 33 (7): 524–532, 534.

14 Gastaldo, J.F., Cury, P.R., and Sendyk, W.R. (2004). Effect of the vertical and horizontal distances between adjacent implants and between a tooth and an implant on the incidence of interproximal papilla. *Journal of Periodontology* 75 (9): 1242–1246. https://doi.org/10.1902/jop.2004.75.9.1242.

15 Kan, J.Y., Roe, P., Rungcharassaeng, K. et al. (2011). Classification of sagittal root position in relation to the anterior maxillary osseous housing for immediate implant placement: a cone beam computed tomography study. *The International Journal of Oral & Maxillofacial Implants* 26 (4): 873–876.

18

Surgical Protocols for Implant Placement

Christopher C.K. Ho

18.1   Principles

The surgical placement of implants can be performed by using a flapless approach or alternatively raising a full-thickness mucoperiosoteal flap to visualise and access the alveolar ridge for implant insertion. The flapless approach is used mainly as a guided approach with digital planning merging cone beam computed tomography (CBCT) imaging along with diagnostic models (digital intra-oral scan or conventional) selecting the diameter, length, and alignment of the implant to be virtually planned. The planning and guided approach allows the implant to be surgically inserted through the surgical guide using an access through the soft tissues achieved with a tissue punch. The tissue punch effectively removes a disc-shaped piece of gingival tissue corresponding to the implant selected. This approach is not only time efficient but also results in minimal morbidity as no flap is raised, along with the shortened duration of surgical procedure. The limitations with the use of guided surgery is that the punch can remove keratinised tissue, so in cases of minimal or insufficient keratinised tissue the elevation of the flap to maintain keratinised tissue is recommended. An additional limitation is when patients have limited opening; this technique may be contraindicated as the use of guided drills are normally 8–12 mm longer than a normal drill, and there may be insufficient space to allow the drills to be used safely.

Conventional surgical implant placement involves raising a full-thickness flap, ensuring adequate visibility and access to the alveolar ridge, as well as identification of anatomical landmarks and vital structures. Vital structures should be avoided by at least 2 mm to allow for the extended length of the tip of the drill as well as allowing for possible errors on drilling and imaging.

The objective when placing implants is to ensure safe and predictable placement. Using a surgical guide may assist in optimal placement. The surgeon should perform the osteotomy in an atraumatic technique, ensuring no overheating of the bone, which may cause necrosis of the bony ridge. This should be achieved by cooling the drills with fluid irrigation, as well as the use of an intermittent pumping motion whereby drills are inserted intermittently so bone is not constantly under pressure and heat generation.

Practical Procedures in Implant Dentistry, First Edition. Edited by Christopher C.K. Ho.
© 2022 John Wiley & Sons Ltd. Published 2022 by John Wiley & Sons Ltd.
Companion website: www.wiley.com/go/ho/implant-dentistry

Implant bed preparation also entails a determination of the type of bone present. Lekholm and Zarb [1] established a classification depending on the ratio of cortical and spongy bone from type 1 to type 4. Hard, dense bone with larger cortex is classified as bone type 1. Soft bone with lots of spongy low-density trabecular bone is classified as bone type 4. In type 1 dense bone it is suggested that the drilling is carried out with intermittent motion, and the use of dense bone drills or screw taps is required to minimise lateral pressure to the bone when inserting the implants. In the case of type 4 or soft bone, it is advisable to underprepare the osteotomy to ensure a higher primary stability. The density of the bone is not evident on the most commonly used radiographic examinations such as peri-apical radiographs and orthopantomograms, nor on CBCT imaging. The only radiographic imaging that will provide density information is medical computed tomography imaging through the Hounsfield unit scale, a qualitative scale for describing radiodensity.

The aim of implant placement is to achieve sufficient primary stability at insertion, which is normally a range of around 30–45 Ncm insertion torque. Sufficient primary stability may then allow for one-stage surgical placement with a healing abutment or even immediate loading contemplated. Exceeding the recommended insertion torque with dental implants may lead to bony necrosis, with bony remodelling, and it may be necessary to reverse the implant out and perform further preparation to ensure a more passive insertion.

18.1.1 Implant Positioning

The positioning of dental implants is often referred to as 'prosthodontically driven', requiring placement in the correct three-dimensional position allowing for optimal support and stability of the peri-implant bone and soft tissues. This will also ensure an aesthetic outcome for the patient.

Determining the size and length of the implant is based on the analysis of the bony anatomy as well as the functional forces a restoration will be subjected too. The position must be considered with the following guidelines:

- *Mesio-distal position*: The implant should not be closer than 1.5 mm to an adjacent tooth and not closer than 3.0 mm to an adjacent implant. Encroaching this space may lead to crestal bone loss with ensuing loss of soft tissue, leading to unaesthetic results (Figure 18.1).
- *Bucco-lingual/palatal position*:
    - Anterior region: The implant should be positioned palatal to a line taken from the point of emergence of the adjacent teeth. It has been shown that implants placed at or buccal to this line between the cervical margins of the adjacent teeth have 3x more recession [2]. The aim is to have sufficient bony envelope surrounding the implant with at least 1.5 mm bone on the labial side and 1 mm on the palatal (Figure 18.2).
    - Posterior region: The implant is positioned in the centre of the planned restoration. This allows forces to be centred directly and does not allow cantilever forces on the restoration.

(a)

(b)

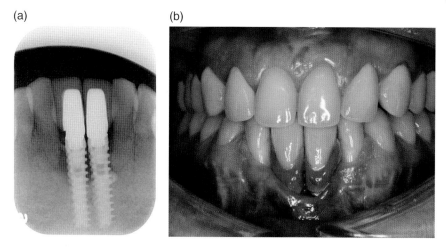

Figure 18.1 Incorrect placement of implants, with insufficient spacing between adjacent implants and insufficient space between teeth and implants, leads to severe bone loss and failure of the implant treatment.

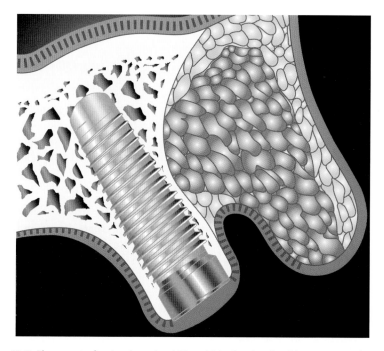

Figure 18.2 Placement of an implant should be within the alveolar ridge, ensuring there is at least 1 mm of bone palatally with 2 mm on the labial/buccal region to give long-term stability of the implant.

(a)   (b)

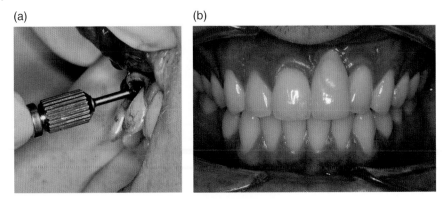

Figure 18.3 Placement of an implant too labially will lead to poor aesthetic outcomes with the appearance of a 'long tooth' with gingival recession.

- The placement of implants too labially in the anterior zone leads to gingival recession with a long tooth, thinner tissue, and the possibility of titanium shadowing (Figure 18.3).

- *Apico-coronal position*: The implant shoulder is positioned 3 mm apical to the emergence of the future restoration. Placing the implant too shallow may lead to metal show-through of componentry, and too deep may lead to a deep peri-implant pocket.

18.2 Procedures

After appropriate flap management to expose a surgical site, it is important to clear any soft tissue debris and granulation tissues from the alveolar ridge.

It is important to assess the site visually and compare this to the radiographic imaging to ensure that the planning the surgeon has performed is suitable for the site.

The following steps are performed during implant installation:

- *Osteotomy initiation*: According to the implant manufacturer system selected it is preferable to begin the osteotomy using a needle-shaped bur/Lindemann or round bur to initiate initial entry into the cortical bone. Using a needle-shaped or round bur ensures the bur does not on entry scatter uncontrollably on the harder cortical bone. These burs are also extremely useful in extraction sockets or sloping defects, where parallel-sided burs may slip as they drill. At this stage it is often a good idea to place guide pin or the same drill back into the osteotomy site to assess alignment, and if incorrect relocate the drill and start another osteotomy site. If the position or alignment is incorrect it is difficult to reorientate once the drilling has progressed to the larger drills.
- *Drill sequence*: Depending on the diameter and length of the implant chosen it is best to follow the manufacturer's instructions for the drilling protocols. The

drill speed ranges from 600 to 1500 rpm with markings on the drill laser-etched for depth markings. The drills often are colour coded depending on the diameters for easier identification. Drills can be either disposable or multi-use. Multi-use burs will have a maximum use of approximately 10 times. Caution: Drills are longer than their markings because they have sharp tips for drilling. They are normally 0.4–1.0 mm longer than labelled.

- *Direction and depth verification*: Once a drill has been removed from the handpiece the same drill or a directional indicator can be relocated into the osteotomy site to verify that the preparation is aligned correctly.
- *Use of thread former/screw tap*: In cases of dense bone it may be necessary to form threads within the bone to lessen the insertion torque. These thread formers are normally used at 25 rpm, and need to be reversed back once to depth.
- *Inserting implant*: The implant is inserted at a speed of 20–25 rpm and insertion torque registered is a gauge as to the initial primary stability of the implant. An alternative measurement of stability is resonance frequency analysis to assess the ISQ (implant stability quotient). This provides an objective measurement of the implant stability expressed as a number (<50 ISQ is questionable integration, 50–55 ISQ two-stage, possibly one-stage procedures, 55–60 ISQ one-stage procedures, 60–65 ISQ possible early loading, >65 ISQ immediate provisionalisation).

18.2.1 One-Stage versus Two-Stage Protocols

The Brånemark protocol involved strict surgical and prosthodontic criteria with a two-stage surgical procedure and an unloaded submerged healing period of about three to six months. A concern was that premature loading would lead to micro-motion and possible fibrous encapsulation of the implant with subsequent failure. One-stage healing was demonstrated in multiple studies to lead to similarly successful results [3, 4]. A healing abutment or provisional abutment/restoration could be used with a one-stage implant procedure. Even without occlusal loading, functional stresses on the implant with tongues, cheeks, lips, and indirect masticatory forces are a possibility. The use of provisional dentures similarly should be relieved to ensure no direct application of forces to the implant during the osseointegration period. The decision to use a two-stage approach is made when there is poorer bone quality or quantity with poorer primary stability. Furthermore, in patients with several health considerations or in those requiring regenerating bone with augmentation procedures a two-stage approach may be indicated.

18.2.2 Post-operative Management Protocols

The patient should be provided verbally and with a written instruction sheet on what to expect post-operatively, along with medications or restrictions that they should adhere to (Table 18.1). A follow up telephone call the next day is a welcome reassurance to the patient, with advice on any questions being a good practice builder.

Table 18.1 Post-operative instructions provided to the patient following implant surgery.

Oral hygiene	Begin your normal oral hygiene routine as soon as possible on day 2 or 3 after surgery. Soreness and swelling may not permit vigorous brushing of all areas, but please make every effort to clean your teeth *within the bounds of comfort*. Avoid, however, brushing near the gums/stitches
Diet	After your surgery, have food that can be eaten comfortably. The temperature of the food does not matter, but avoid extremely hot foods and liquids. We recommend that you only **consume soft foods during the first few days** to avoid food particles contaminating the wound
	After each meal **on day 2**, the mouth should be thoroughly rinsed with warm saline solution (*1/2 teaspoon of salt in a glass of warm water*) or chlorhexadine mouth rinse
Managing swelling	**On day 1** we recommend covered ice packs or a cold compress applied for a period of 15 minutes to the face over the surgery site to reduce any chance of swelling resulting from the surgery. We suggest that you apply 15 minutes on and 15 minutes off. If possible, elevate the head with an extra pillow during the **first nights** after surgery to reduce swelling
Managing bleeding	**On day 1** bite down softly on the gauze packs, making sure they remain in place. Continue to change the gauze packs every 30–40 minutes if there is continual bleeding. To replace gauze, fold a clean piece into a pad thick enough to bite on. Dampen the pad and place it directly on the surgical site. (A cool damp tea bag may also be used in its place if gauze is unavailable.) Bleeding should never be severe. If bleeding remains uncontrolled, please call us
Managing pain	The length of time you experience numbness varies, depending on the type of anaesthetic you've received. While your mouth is numb please be careful not to bite on your cheek, lip, or tongue. The numbness should subside within a few hours
	Tablets for pain relief should be taken as necessary and according to instructions. If pain persists for more than 72 hourrs, please call us
Managing infection	The mouth should be thoroughly rinsed with warm saline solution or mouthwash containing chlorhexidine after each meal to reduce the chance of infection for the first week. Place the solution in your mouth and gently rotate your head from side to side. Please do not swish aggressively
Antibiotics	It is essential that you complete the course of antibiotics prescribed. Post-operative infection may occur occasionally. You have been prescribed antibiotics depending on the type of surgery undertaken. These should be taken with food as directed and no alcohol should be consumed during this period
Prolonged numbness	Rarely, you may experience numbness in the lip, tongue, cheek, gum, or teeth for longer than 4 hours after surgery. This is normally temporary and rarely permanent. You should contact us if you are still numb after 24 hours
Healing	After an implant placement, a blood clot forms in the surgical area. This is an important part of the normal healing process. You should therefore avoid activities that might disturb the surgical area
	Do not rinse your mouth vigorously or probe the area with any objects or your fingers
	Do not smoke or drink through a straw for 72 hours following your surgery. These activities create suction in the mouth, which could dislodge the clot and delay healing
	If you do not care for the taste in your mouth, drink some fluids or use a wet washcloth and wipe your tongue, but please stay away from the surgical area
	Avoid strenuous activity for the first 24 hours after your procedure. This will reduce bleeding and help the blood clot to form

Table 18.1 (Continued)

Dentures	Where relevant, dentures will be refitted as soon as possible after the implant placement. However, inserting the dentures too early may jeopardise a successful healing process
Losing healing abutment	The purpose of the healing abutment is to shape the gum tissue and keep the gum open to receive your final implant crown. Occasionally the implant healing abutment can loosen from tongue movement and chewing during the osseointegration process. This does not mean the implant is compromised. If you notice that the healing abutment is loose or has come off please call us and we can re-tighten or replace the abutment
Contact us	If you are concerned over any matter regarding the surgery or recovery, please call us

18.3 Tips

- If required during surgery a peri-apical radiograph may be taken to ensure the correct alignment of implants. This is particularly important in narrow edentulous spaces where minimal dimensions are present between adjacent roots.
- When preparing the osteotomy it can be useful to insert a blunt round probe into the osteotomy site to ensure that no fenestration of the bone has been made, and to ensure that the osteotomy has not encroached on any anatomical landmarks.
- There may be situations where the cortical bone is very dense, yet the cancellous bone is type 4 soft bone. Although underpreparation can be made in the cancellous trabecular bone, because of the denser cortical plate it may still be necessary to undertake the final drill diameter of the implant you have selected and just drill through the cortical layer, i.e. the first 1–2 mm. Too much coronal pressure on the crest with an implant may lead to crestal bone remodelling with subsequent bone loss and exposed threads.
- Do not exceed the manufacturer's maximum insertion torque recommendations. This may lead to implant fracture or pressure necrosis with subsequent bone loss. If an implant is exceeding the maximum torque then it is advisable to back the implant out and replace it in its carrier before performing further preparation or screw tapping.

References

1 Lekholm, U. and Zarb, G.A. (1985). Patient selection and preparation. In: Proceedings of the Tissue Integrated Prostheses: Osseointegration in Clinical Dentistry (eds. P.I. Brånemark, G.A. Zarb and T.S. Albrektsson), 199–209. Chicago, IL: Quintessence Publishing.
2 Evans, C.D. and Chen, S.T. (2008 Jan). Esthetic outcomes of immediate implant placements. *Clin. Oral Implants Res.* 19 (1): 73–80.

3 Ericsson, I., Nilner, K., Klinge, B., and Glantz, P.O. (1996). Radiographic and histological characteristics of submerged and non-submerged titanium implants. An experimental study in the Labrador dog. *Clin. Oral Implants Res.* 7: 20–26.

4 Schroeder, A., Van Der Zypen, E., Stich, H. et al. (1981). The reaction of bone, connective tissue, and epithetlium to endosteal implants with titanium-sprayed surfaces. *J. Oral Maxillofac. Surg.* 9: 15–25.

19

Optimising the Peri-implant Emergence Profile

David Attia and Jess Liu

19.1 Principles

Successful implant-supported restorations closely resemble what once existed in nature both functionally and aesthetically. The primary goal in implant dentistry is to achieve complete functional and aesthetic harmony and integration of the restoration with the urrounding hard and soft tissues and natural dentition.

Having a thorough understanding of the individual elements that influence the peri-implant emergence profile is essential in predictably maintaining peri-implant health and achieving aesthetic outcomes. The purpose of this chapter is to outline the clinical factors and describe the surgical and prosthetic procedures that should be considered in order to develop an optimal peri-implant emergence profile.

19.1.1 The Peri-implant Emergence Profile

The peri-implant emergence profile is composed of a connective tissue cuff, a junctional epithelium, and a gingival sulcus. This zone of tissue that begins at the bone crest and extends to the free gingival margin differs in arrangement from the periodontium of the natural dentition [1]. More recently, the structures surrounding and supporting osseointegrated implants were defined as the 'peri-implant phenotype' and described both the soft tissue and osseous components (Figure 19.1) [2].

In order to predictably maintain peri-implant health and achieve aesthetic outcomes, clinicians must be able to develop the peri-implant architecture through a thorough understanding of these tissues [3].

In order to achieve an ideal peri-implant emergence profile, several factors ought to be considered prior to surgical placement of the dental implant in order to establish the foundation for a successful implant-supported restoration. These factors include the ideal hard tissue volume, soft tissue quantity and quality, and the subsequent three-dimensional implant position.

Practical Procedures in Implant Dentistry, First Edition. Edited by Christopher C.K. Ho.
© 2022 John Wiley & Sons Ltd. Published 2022 by John Wiley & Sons Ltd.
Companion website: www.wiley.com/go/ho/implant-dentistry

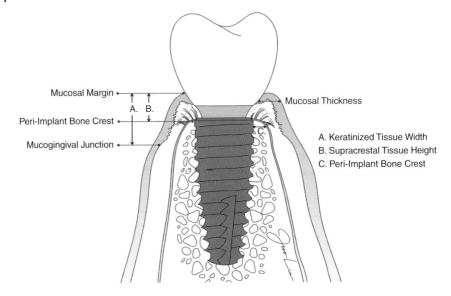

Mucosal Margin

Peri-Implant Bone Crest

Mucogingival Junction

A. B.

Mucosal Thickness

A. Keratinized Tissue Width
B. Supracrestal Tissue Height
C. Peri-Implant Bone Crest

Figure 19.1 The peri-implant phenotype.

Following osseointegration of dental implants and prior to implant restoration, the peri-implant tissues may require further modification or augmentation in order to achieve an ideal emergence profile, ensuring functional and aesthetic longevity of the implant-supported restoration.

19.2 Procedures

19.2.1 Single-Stage versus Two-Stage Implant Surgery

The decision to perform single-stage or two-stage implant surgery procedures is often influenced by the pre-existing clinical condition of the proposed implant site, or the primary stability achieved at the time of surgical implant placement. Sites that present with insufficient bone volume may require bone augmentation procedures prior to, or in conjunction with simultaneous implant placement. Similarly, sites that present with inadequate soft tissue quantity or quality may also require augmentation procedures prior to, or in conjunction with simultaneous implant placement. Furthermore, sites that present with poor bone quality result in lower implant primary stability and therefore a two-stage implant procedure may be considered.

Single-stage implant surgery allows the clinician to avoid the need for a second surgical procedure and therefore reducing patient morbidity. However, in certain clinical scenarios two-stage implant surgery may be considered as it can be advantageous; providing the clinician with an opportunity to manipulate or augment the soft tissues to improve the peri-implant emergence profile.

The timing of the second-stage surgery/implant exposure procedure varies from case to case and can be influenced by a number of factors, such as the primary stability achieved at the time of implant placement, the site-specific bone quality (e.g. maxilla or mandible), and patient medical history (e.g. diabetic patients).

Additionally, the implant exposure technique employed will vary depending on the presenting clinical situation. Correct clinical assessment of the site will help the clinician determine the appropriate technique required to improve and idealise the peri-implant emergence profile.

19.2.2 Buccal Roll Flap

Problem
- A mild to moderate horizontal buccal ridge deficiency (Figure 19.2).

Aim of Treatment
- Restore the horizontal buccal contour of the peri-implant soft tissues.

Indications
- Mild to moderate buccal horizontal morphological soft tissue defect exists.

Considerations
- A minimum of 3 mm of supracrestal soft tissue height
- A minimum of 2 mm of keratinised mucosa width remains both buccally and lingually following roll flap procedure.

Contraindications
- Insufficient keratinised mucosa width
- Supracrestal tissue height of less than 3 mm exists.

Steps

1) Using the tip of a No.15C blade, the dimensions of the flap are outlined on the edentulous crest. The flap consists of a full-thickness palatal/lingual paracrestal incision and a mesial and distal vertical incision (Figure 19.3d).
2) Using a No.15C blade or a high-speed diamond bur, remove the surface epithelium overlying the implant. Following complete removal of the surface

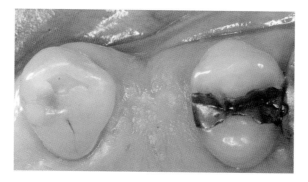

Figure 19.2 Missing first premolar site with mild to moderate horizontal buccal ridge deficiency.

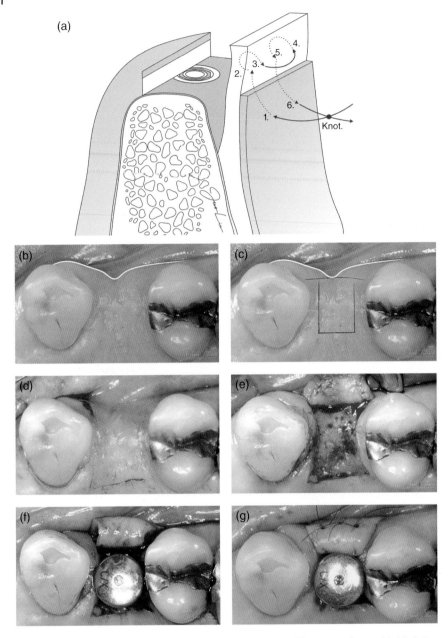

Figure 19.3 (a–i) Buccal roll flap suturing sequence. (b) Healed first premolar site highlighting deficient buccal contour. (c) Proposed incision outline. (d) Buccal roll flap outlined with tip of surgical blade. (e) Full-thickness mucoperiosteal flap reflected exposing underlying bone. Note bone has grown over implant cover screw. (f) Buccal pouch preparation, healing abutment installed and crestal aspect of flap has been de-epithelialised and rolled into position. (g) De-epithelialised aspect of the pedicled flap is secured into position using horizontal mattress and single interrupted sutures.

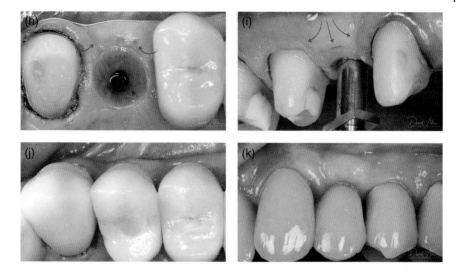

Figure 19.3 (Cont'd) (h) Healed peri-implant emergence profile (occlusal view); note improved buccal contour. Scarring present due to excessive tension from suture. (i) Healed peri-implant emergence profile (buccal view). Note scarring due to excessive tension from suture. (j) Final buccal contour following delivery of final restoration (occlusal view). (k) Final buccal contour following delivery of final restoration (buccal view). *Source:* Case by Dr. David Attia.

epithelium, the subepithelial tissue surface will be matte and non-reflective in appearance.

3) With the blade kept perpendicular to the tissue surface, following the mesial, distal, and palatal outline, the de-epithelialised area is cut palatal/lingually and extended mesially and distally, exposing the underlying bone and cover screw (Figure 19.3e). The palatal aspect of the flap should be placed level with the palatal aspect of the implant body, and should be the same mesio-distal length as the buccal fixed portion of the flap.

4) The mesial and distal incisions are placed a minimum of 1 mm from the sulcus of the adjacent teeth so as to not compromise the papilla. These two incisions should not extend beyond the buccal-occlusal line angle in order to avoid any visible scarring following healing (Figure 19.3e).

5) While maintaining a buccal pedicle, using the round end of a Buser mucoperiosteal elevator, reflect the full-thickness, de-epithelialised portion of the flap to expose the underlying bone and implant cover screw (Figure 19.3e).

6) Once the flap has been reflected, a buccal pouch is created using split-thickness dissection (Figure 19.3f). It is important to extend this pouch laterally towards the mesial and distal line angles of the adjacent teeth in order to ensure sufficient flap mobility, and provide enough space to accommodate the crestal de-epithelialised aspect of the pedicled buccal flap.

7) The de-epithelialised aspect of the pedicle flap is rolled and secured into the buccal pouch using a horizontal mattress suture (Figure 19.3g).
   a) The suture needle passes through mesial aspect of the buccal flap and is retrieved from within the pouch.

    b) Maintaining the same mesial position, the needle passes through the inner surface of the de-epithelialised flap and then moves distally, staying in the same horizontal plane.

    c) The needle is then passed back through the outer surface of the de-epithelialised flap, and enters the pouch.

    d) Maintaining the same distal position, the needle passes through the inner aspect of the buccal pouch, exiting through to the buccal aspect of the flap.

8) As both ends of the suture are pulled, the round end of a Buser mucoperiosteal elevator is used to aid in rolling the de-epithelialised aspect of the pedicled flap, into its final position within the buccal pouch.

9) The knot is tied.

10) The cover screw is removed from the implant and replaced with a healing abutment.

11) One mesial and one distal single interrupted suture may be added for extra security as required.

19.2.3 Pouch Roll Technique [4]

Problem
- A mild to moderate horizontal buccal ridge deficiency (Figure 19.4).

Aim of Treatment
- Restore the horizontal buccal contour of the peri-implant soft tissues.

Indications
- Mild to moderate buccal horizontal morphological soft tissue defect exists.

Considerations
- A minimum of 3 mm supracrestal soft tissue height.

Contraindications
- Insufficient keratinised mucosa width.
- Supracrestal tissue height of less than 3 mm exists.

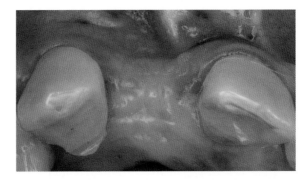

Figure 19.4 Healed lateral incisor site with mild to moderate horizontal buccal ridge deficiency.

Steps

1) Using a No.15C blade or a high-speed diamond bur, the soft tissue overlying the implant is de-epithelialised until it appears matte and non-reflective in appearance (Figure 19.5c).

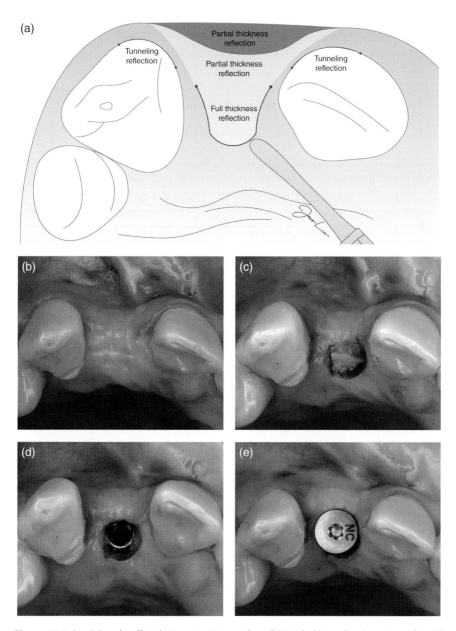

Figure 19.5 (a–e) Pouch roll technique incision outline. (b) Healed lateral incisor site with mild to moderate buccal deficiency. (c) Crestal tissue de-epithelialised. (d) Implant platform exposed and crestal tissue rolled into buccal pouch. (e) Healing abutment installed. *Source:* Case by Dr. Jess Liu.

2) With the blade kept perpendicular to the tissue surface, the No.15C blade is used to cut the de-epithelialised area palatally, mesially and distally, forming a 'U' shaped incision line. The buccal aspect is not cut to maintain a buccal pedicle (Figure 19.5c).
3) An intrasulcular incision is made around the teeth mesial and distal to the edentulous ridge with the buccal defect.
4) Microblades are used to dissect a partial-thickness flap on the buccal aspect of the edentulous area. The partial-thickness flap should be extended at least one tooth mesial and one tooth distal to the tap.
5) In order to achieve adequate flap mobility, the papillae of the teeth immediately adjacent to the edentulous ridge are dissected over the periosteum and incorporated into the overall flap.
6) While maintaining a buccal pedicle, using the round end of a Buser mucoperiosteal elevator, the full-thickness, de-epithelialised portion of the flap is reflected to expose the underlying bone and implant cover screw.
7) Once the flap has been reflected, the microblade is used to dissect the inner aspect of the flap from the underlying periosteum forming a buccal pouch. Following dissection, the buccal pouch and the buccal tunnel prepared through the sulcus of the adjacent teeth should now be connected.
8) The mobilised pedicled flap can now be rolled into the buccal pouch (Figure 19.5d).
9) The cover screw is removed and replaced with the appropriate healing abutment (Figure 19.5e).

19.2.4   Apically Repositioned Flap

Problem
- Shallow vestibular depth with associated mucosal pull on the peri-implant soft tissues (Figure 19.6)
- Insufficient buccal keratinised gingiva.

Aim of Treatment
- Restore the vestibular depth and eliminate mucosal pull on the peri-implant soft tissues.
- Augment the zone of the buccal keratinised gingiva.

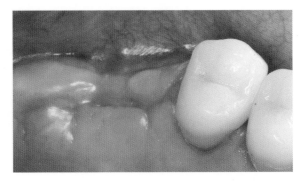

Figure 19.6 Healed first and second molar site with shallow vestibulum and lack of buccal keratinised gingiva.

Indication
- Increase the zone of keratinised and attached gingiva to a level that will resist gingival recession, enhance aesthetics and facilitate effective oral hygiene maintenance
- Increase vestibular depth.

Considerations
- Minimum of 2 mm of buccal keratinised and fixed gingiva required
- Vertical soft tissue thickness capable of undergoing split flap dissection.

Contraindications
- Aesthetically demanding cases.

Steps
1) Using the tip of a No.15C blade, an initial 1 mm deep crestal incision is made within the keratinised gingiva, perpendicular to the tissue surface. This initial incision should incorporate a minimum of 1 mm of keratinised tissue in the buccal partial-thickness flap.
2) Two partial-thickness vertical releasing incisions are made at each end of the crestal incision at the mesial and distal line angles of the adjacent teeth. The vertical releasing incisions should be:
   a) extended below the mucogingival junction in order to allow flap mobilisation
   b) placed a minimum of 1 mm from the sulcus of the adjacent teeth.
3) With the tip of the blade, continue to trace the original incision line from distal to mesial, successively increasing the angle of the blade in 30 degree increments until it is parallel with the overlying soft tissue surface.
4) In the same manner, the corners of the flap and the vertical releasing incisions are traced with the tip of the blade, being sure to stay within the same plane as the partial-thickness flap dissection performed in the crestal incision. The side of the blade is used to aid in elevating the corners of the flap.
5) The partial-thickness flap is completed by making an undermining incision that extends apical to the initial incision line, remaining parallel to the overlying flap. At all times, maintain visibility of the blade through the superficial overlying buccal flap, in order to minimise the risk of flap perforation. It is important to avoid handling or reflecting the flap to observe the blade from the internal aspect of the flap as this may increase the risk of flap perforation.
6) The partial-thickness flap is secured apically to the underlying periosteum (Figure 19.7c). The distance (x mm) from the healing abutments can be modified depending on the amount of desired keratinised gingiva gain (Figure 19.7a).
   a) First, the vertical releasing incisions are secured to the attached tissue apico-lateral to the flap using single interrupted sutures.
   b) The suture needle passes through the external surface of the partial thickness flap corner at 90 degrees while maintaining a distance of 3 mm from the flap margins.
   c) The needle then passes through the attached tissue apico-lateral to the flap from inside to outside, emerging 3 mm from the vertical incision line.

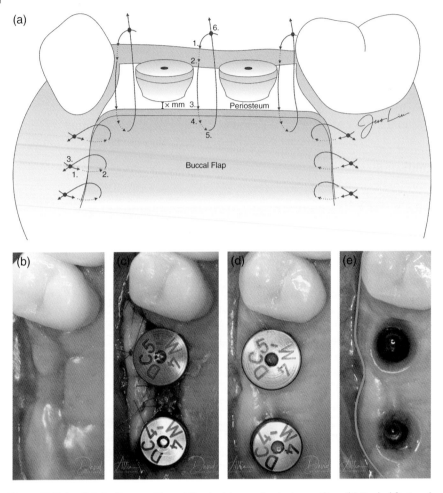

Figure 19.7 (a–d) Apically repositioned flap incision and suturing outline. (b) Healed first and second molar site with shallow vestibulum and lack of buccal keratinised gingiva. (c) Partial-thickness flap apically repositioned using single interrupted sutures. (d) Post-operative healing at two weeks. (e) Healed peri-implant emergence profile at four weeks. *Source:* Case by Dr. David Attia.

    d) The knot is secured on the attached tissue.
    e) Depending on the length of the vertical releasing incisions, additional single interrupted sutures are added, maintaining a minimum distance of 2 mm between each suture.
7) Following apical fixation of the vertical flap margins, the horizontal flap margin is secured to the underlying periosteum in an apical position using evenly spaced single interrupted sutures, maintaining a minimum distance of 2 mm between each suture.
8) The underlying periosteum is left exposed with the borders of the wound surrounded by keratinised tissue. Therefore, as the wound heals, the area of exposed periosteum heals with the formation of newly formed keratinised and attached tissue.

19.2.5 Buccally Repositioned Flap

Problem
- Buccal mucogingival defect (Figure 19.8)
- Insufficient buccal keratinised gingiva
- Site visible in the aesthetic zone.

Aim of Treatment
- Restore the vestibular depth and eliminate mucosal pull on the peri-implant soft tissues
- Augment the zone of the buccal keratinised gingiva
- Restore buccal ridge contour
- Improve aesthetics.

Indication
- Increase the zone of keratinised and attached gingiva to a level that will resist gingival recession, enhance aesthetics, and facilitate effective oral hygiene maintenance
- Increase vestibular depth
- Sites within the aesthetic zone where vertical releasing incisions are contraindicated.

Considerations
- Minimum of 2 mm of buccal keratinised and fixed gingiva required
- Vertical soft tissue thickness capable of undergoing split flap dissection.

Contraindications
- Insufficient vertical soft tissue thickness.

Steps

1) Using the tip of a No.15C blade, an initial 1 mm deep crestal incision is made within the keratinised gingiva, perpendicular to the tissue surface. This initial incision should incorporate a minimum of 1 mm of keratinised tissue in the buccal partial-thickness flap.
2) The split-thickness crestal incision is extended to the sulcus of the teeth mesial and distal to the edentulous ridge.

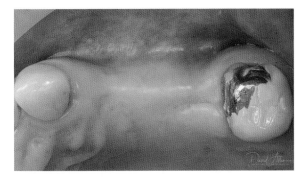

Figure 19.8 Healed first premolar, second premolar, and first molar site with shallow vestibulum and moderate buccal contour defect with deficient buccal keratinised gingiva.

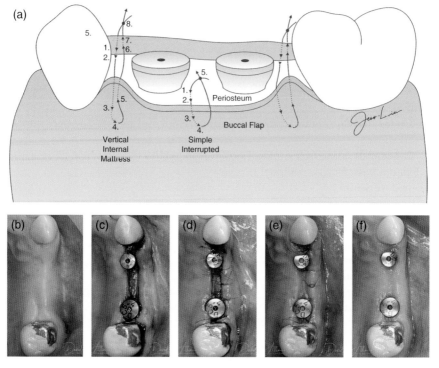

Figure 19.9 (a–f) Apically repositioned flap incision and suturing outline. (b) Healed first premolar, second premolar, and first molar site with shallow vestibulum and moderate buccal contour defect with deficient buccal keratinised gingiva. (c) Split-thickness flap preparation and installation of healing abutments. (d) Buccal fixation of the flap leaving exposed periosteum between implant healing abutments. (e) Post-operative healing at two weeks. (f) Post-operative healing at four weeks. *Source:* Case by Dr. David Attia.

3) With the tip of the blade, continue to trace the original incision line from distal to mesial, successively increasing the angle of the blade in 30 degree increments until it is parallel with the overlying soft tissue surface.

4) The partial-thickness flap is completed by making an undermining incision that extends apical to the initial incision line, remaining parallel to the overlying flap. At all times, maintain visibility of the blade through the superficial overlying buccal flap, in order to minimise the risk of flap perforation. It is important to avoid handling or reflecting the flap to observe the blade from the internal aspect of the flap as this may increase the risk of flap perforation (Figure 19.9c).

5) The partial thickness flap is secured buccally to the underlying periosteum (Figure 19.9d).

   a) First, the papillae are re-approximated using a vertical mattress suture.

   b) The suture needle passes through the external surface of the buccal partial-thickness flap at the mesial papilla at 90 degrees while maintaining a distance of 3 mm from the tip of the papilla.

c) The needle then passes through the internal surface of the palatal papilla, 3 mm from the tip of the papilla.
d) Next, the needle passes through the external surface of the palatal papilla, 1 mm from the tip of the papilla.
e) Finally, the needle passes through the internal surface of the buccal partial-thickness flap at the mesial papilla, 1 mm from the tip of the papilla.
f) The knot is secured.

6) Following re-approximation of the mesial and distal papillae, the horizontal flap margin is secured to the underlying periosteum in a buccal position using evenly spaced single interrupted sutures, maintaining a minimum distance of 2 mm between each suture.

7) The underlying periosteum is left exposed with the borders of the wound surrounded by keratinised tissue. Therefore, as the wound heals, the area of exposed periosteum heals with the formation of newly formed keratinised and attached tissue.

19.2.6 Free Gingival Graft

Problem
- Horizontal buccal soft tissue defect (Figure 19.10)
- Shallow vestibular depth with associated mucosal pull on the peri-implant soft tissues
- Insufficient buccal keratinised gingiva (1.5 mm) with a probing depth of 1 mm

  – Only 0.5 mm of buccal attached tissue.

Aim of Treatment
- Improve the horizontal buccal contour of the peri-implant soft tissues
- Restore the vestibular depth and eliminate mucosal pull on the peri-implant soft tissues
- Augment the zone of the buccal keratinised gingiva.

Indications
- Increase the zone of keratinised and attached gingiva to a level that will facilitate effective oral hygiene maintenance and resist gingival recession
- Increase vestibular depth.

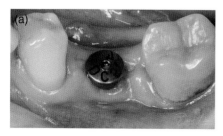
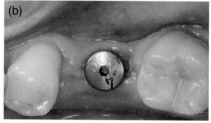

Figure 19.10 (a, b) Healed first molar site with shallow vestibulum, moderate buccal contour defect and deficient buccal keratinised gingiva.

Considerations
- Donor site
  - Hard palate
  - Maxillary tuberosity
  - Maxillary buccal keratinised gingiva
  - Edentulous ridges
- Local anatomical structures in the recipient (e.g. mental nerve) and donor site (e.g. greater palatine artery).

Contraindications
- The aesthetic zone where the appearance of the graft will not harmoniously integrate with the surrounding tissues.

Steps – Recipient Site Preparation
1) Using the tip of a No.15C blade, an initial 1 mm deep crestal incision is made at the mucogingival junction, perpendicular to the tissue surface.
2) Two partial-thickness vertical releasing incisions are made at the mesial and distal extent of the crestal incision. The releasing incisions should be:
   a) placed a minimum of 1 mm from the sulcus of the adjacent teeth to maintain a sufficient amount of keratinised gingiva on the adjacent teeth
   b) extended apically to allow a gain of 4–5 mm of immobile keratinised tissue with the free gingival graft, being mindful of local anatomical structures.
3) With the tip of the blade, continue to trace the original crestal and vertical incision lines from distal to mesial, successively increasing the angle of the blade in 30 degree increments until it is parallel with the overlying soft tissue surface. The side of the blade is used to aid in elevating the corners of the flap.
4) The partial-thickness mucosal flap is secured apically to the underlying periosteum using evenly spaced single interrupted sutures, maintaining a minimum distance of 2 mm between each suture.
5) The recipient bed is assessed by moving the cheek/lip and any mobile muscle tissue that is present over the recipient bed is carefully dissected using a fresh No.15C blade. This ensures that the final free gingival graft is secured to immobile periosteum.
6) A template of the recipient site is used to transfer the dimensions of the required graft to the donor site. This can be fabricated using a piece of sterile aluminium foil or the sterile suture packet.
   a) The template is often larger in dimensions than the desired graft size, taking into consideration graft shrinkage following harvesting.

Steps – Harvesting of the Free Gingival Graft

1) After sufficient local anaesthesia, place the graft template onto the proposed palatal donor site. Typically, the distal extent of the graft should not extend beyond the mesial border of the first molar and maintain a minimum distance of 2 mm from the palatal gingival margin of the teeth. Be mindful of local anatomical structures.
2) Using a new No.15C blade trace the coronal outline of pre-fabricated template. The tip of the blade should be kept perpendicular to the tissue surface.

3) With the template still in place and in the same manner, the mesial and distal vertical releasing incisions are made. In order to achieve a uniform thickness of the graft, the blade should be kept perpendicular to the tissue surface and the incision lines should overlap.

4) Continue to re-trace the coronal, mesial, and distal incision lines, gradually increasing the angle of the blade until it is parallel with the overlying tissues. The side of the blade is used to aid in elevating the corners of the flap and calibrate the desired thickness of the graft.

5) With the blade parallel to the overlying soft tissue surface, an undermining incision is made, maintaining the desired graft thickness. This incision should be extended past the apical extent of the vertical releasing incisions. The graft harvest is completed by making the final apical horizontal incision, separating the graft from the palatal tissues. To avoid prolonged bleeding from the donor site, this final apical horizontal incision is made at the end of the harvesting procedure.

6) The graft is placed in sterile saline solution while the donor site is closed.

7) A quick resorbing collagen sponge is used to stabilise the blood clot in the donor site, prior to suturing (Figure 19.11).

8) A crossed horizontal sling suture is used to close and compress the palatal donor site.
   a) First, the back of the needle is passed through the interdental space between the first and second premolar in a buccal to palatal direction without engaging any tissue.
   b) Next, the needle passes through the palatal tissue parallel to the most apical border of the donor site. The needle is inserted at the level of the interdental space between the first molar and second premolar and guided from distal to mesial so that it emerges in the space between the first and second premolars.
   c) The back of the needle is then passed back through the interdental space between the first molar and second premolar in a palatal to buccal direction.
   d) The suture knot is tied on the buccal side and positioned coronal to the gingival margin of the tooth to prevent inadvertent trauma to the marginal periodontal tissues of the anchor tooth.

9) Compression sutures are added in a similar fashion to achieve sufficient compression of the donor site from distal to mesial.

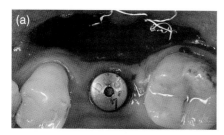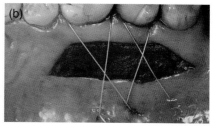

Figure 19.11 (a) Partial-thickness mucosal flap secured apically using single interrupted sutures. (b) Quick resorbing collagen sponge placed into donor site and stabilised with crossed sling compression sutures.

Steps – Preparation and Stabilisation of the Free Gingival Graft

1) Place the graft on a piece of wet sterile gauze with the subepithelial connective tissue surface face-up.
2) Using a new No.15C blade, remove all subepithelial adipose/glandular tissue from the graft. This ensures that the resulting graft is composed strictly of the surface epithelial layer and subepithelial connective tissue only.
3) Place the graft into position on the prepared recipient site ensuring that the borders of the graft are lined up with the borders of the recipient site (Figure 19.12c).
4) Approximate the coronal mesial and distal corners of the graft to the adjacent keratinised mucosa using simple interrupted sutures (Figure 19.12d).
5) Depending on the length of the vertical releasing incisions, approximate the mesial and distal boarders of the graft to the mesial and distal vertical releasing incisions using evenly spaced simple interrupted sutures, maintaining a minimum distance of 2 mm between each suture.
6) Next, a periosteal sling compression suture is used to compress the graft against the underlying periosteum. An intimate adaptation of the graft to the underlying periosteum is key to maintaining blood supply, and therefore integration of the free gingival graft. Visibility of the periosteum is gained by retracting the lip/cheek outwards, exposing the periosteal bed.
   a) The suture needle passes through lingual attached gingiva distal to the implant healing abutment from lingual to buccal.
   b) Next, the needle engages the periosteal bed from mesial to distal. The entry and exit point of the suture needle should be approximately 3–4 mm apart, ensuring an adequate bite of the underlying periosteum.
   c) The needle then passes through the lingual tissues mesial to the healing abutment, from buccal to lingual.
   d) The knot is secured on the lingual attached tissue.
   e) Depending on the size of the graft and the number of implants, additional periosteal sling compression sutures can be added to ensure sufficient compression of the graft against the recipient site.

19.3   Tips

- Thorough pre-surgical clinical assessment is paramount in achieving appropriate technique selection for each individual clinical scenario.
- Cone beam computed tomography (CBCT) assessment is vital for safe execution of surgical procedures, allowing the clinician to avoid trauma to vital anatomical structures.
- When taking CBCT scans, place a piece of gauze over the patient's tongue and a cotton roll in the vestibular area adjacent to the proposed surgical site. This will separate the patient's tongue from the palatal tissue, and the cheeks from the buccal soft tissues, allowing accurate measurement of the soft tissue thickness on the potential palatal donor site and the recipient site, respectively.

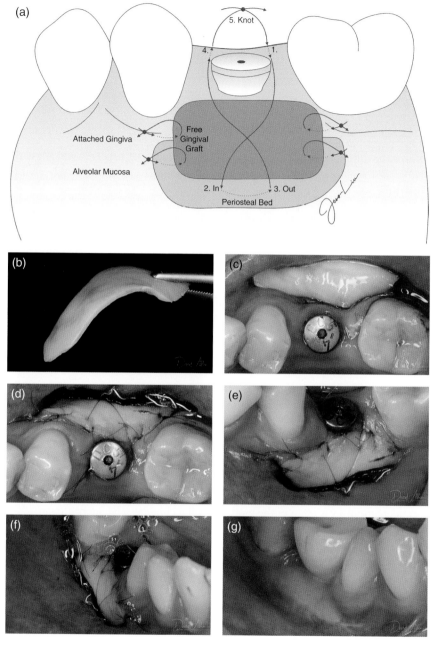

Figure 19.12 (a) Free gingival graft incision, graft, and suturing outline. (b) Harvested free gingival graft. (c) Free gingival graft positioned at recipient site. (d) Free gingival graft secured at recipient site to underlying periosteum using single interrupted and periosteal sling compression sutures (occlusal view). (e) Free gingival graft secured at recipient site to underlying periosteum using single interrupted and periosteal sling compression sutures (buccal view). (f) Free gingival graft secured at recipient site to underlying periosteum using single interrupted and periosteal sling compression sutures (lateral view). (g) Post-operative healing at three months. *Source:* Case by Dr. David Attia.

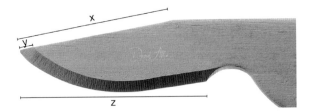

Figure 19.13 Surgical blade dimensions.

- Know the dimensions of your surgical blades (Figure 19.13). This will allow the clinician to make precise incisions, without the need to continuously change instruments.
- Measure twice and cut once! After harvesting autogenous grafts, a certain degree of graft shrinkage can be expected. Harvest slightly larger autogenous grafts to compensate for the expected shrinkage.
- During split-thickness flap dissection, maintain visibility of the blade through the superficial overlying buccal flap at all times, in order to minimise the risk of flap perforation.
- Handle soft tissues with the appropriate armamentarium to avoid tissue trauma (e.g. microsurgical instrumentation).

References

1 Chu, S.J., Kan, J.Y., Lee, E.A. et al. (2019). Restorative emergence profile for single-tooth implants in healthy periodontal patients: clinical guidelines and decision-making strategies. *The International Journal of Periodontics & Restorative Dentistry* 40 (1): 19–29.

2 Avila-Ortiz, G., Gonzalez-Martin, O., Couso-Queiruga, E., and Wang, H.L. (2020). The peri-implant phenotype. *Journal of Periodontology* 91 (3): 283–288.

3 Park, S.H. and Wang, H.L. (2012). Pouch roll technique for implant soft tissue augmentation: a variation of the modified roll technique. *The International Journal of Periodontics & Restorative Dentistry* 32 (3): e116–e121.

4 Schoenbaum, T. (2015). Abutment emergence profile and its effect on peri-implant tissues. *Compendium of Continuing Education in Dentistry* 36: 474–479.

20

Soft Tissue Augmentation

Michel Azer

20.1 Principles

Modern day implant aesthetics focus on soft tissue, often referred to as 'pink aesthetics' and teeth referred to as 'white aesthetics'. Finding a balance between these two can be challenging. After teeth extractions bone healing events take place. Numerous studies have shown that bone remodelling leads to unfavourable loss of ridge dimensions. These changes often lead to unpleasant aesthetic outcomes with high lip line, a non-hygenic prosthetic design, or loss of peri-implant protective function. Fortunately, soft tissue management techniques can be used to prevent excessive loss of ridge dimension and to treat complications as they occur. There are a variety of soft tissue augmentation techniques that can be used during the course of implant therapy. Case selection is of great importance when a clinician opts to utilize a specific soft tissue augmentation technique. In this chapter we are going to review some of these techniques and common indications.

20.1.1 Types of Oral Soft Tissue

In the oral cavity there are two types of soft tissue: (i) keratinised tissue and (ii) non-keratinised tissue. The clinician must understand the differences in oral soft tissue types, which helps in determining the purpose of soft tissue grafting and choosing the right harvesting site. In 1975, Karring and co-authors showed in an experimental model that the origin of connective tissue underneath the epithelium dictates the fate of more superficial layers along the course of healing. This means connective tissue grafts harvested from palate will evolve into keratinised tissue in the future at the recipient site, whereas connective tissue harvested from the soft palate will give rise to non-keratinised movable mucosa upon healing. Therefore it is important to use the keratinised tissue sites as donor tissue, because it is primarily dense connective tissue that is rich in collagen (Figure 20.1) [1]. Commonly used areas include the following:

- Keratinised attached gingiva around the teeth
- Hard palate

Practical Procedures in Implant Dentistry, First Edition. Edited by Christopher C.K. Ho.
© 2022 John Wiley & Sons Ltd. Published 2022 by John Wiley & Sons Ltd.
Companion website: www.wiley.com/go/ho/implant-dentistry

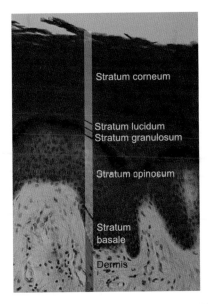

Figure 20.1 Histology: Oral keratinised tissue epithelium consists of four layers.

- Retromolar area
- Tuberosity
- Edentulous spaces.

Other areas in the mouth are non-keratinised and should be avoided if at all possible as they possess vital structures and lack the genetic code to turn into dense connective tissue around implants and teeth. This type of tissue is located in:

- Inner lips and inner cheeks
- Soft palate
- Floor of the mouth
- Ventral surface of the tongue.

20.1.2 Anatomical Considerations for Harvesting Autogenous Soft Tissue Grafts

20.1.2.1 Hard Palate
The hard palate is the most common donor site for day-to-day soft tissue augmentation procedures. While harvesting connective tissue the clinician should be able to identify the greater palatine foramen (GPF) and greater palatine artery (GPA). Three types of palatal vaults have been identified: shallow, moderate, and deep. The deeper the palatal vault the further apical the GPA was found. This allows a better chance of harvesting bigger connective tissue grafts without injury to the artery [2].

20.1.2.2 Tuberosity
The tuberosity is a popular donor site due to the thickness that can be harvested as well as high percentage of collagen present. This quality makes it attractive

for soft tissue augmentation in the pontic area because it hardly undergoes secondary shrinkage.

20.1.2.3 Buccal Attached Gingiva of Maxillary Molars

Buccal attached gingiva from the maxillary molar area has been used for the purpose of free gingival only graft. Some clinicians claim that it provides a better blending compared to palatal grafts.

20.1.3 Soft Tissue Substitutes

20.1.3.1 Allogenic Origin
- *Acellular dermal matrix*: Cadaver skin that is processed to remove the epithelium, immune cells, and other organic matter that can lead to tissue rejection, while preserving the dermal matrix (dermis).
- *Market brands*: Alloderm (Biohorizon), ADM allograft dermal matrix (Straumann).

20.1.3.2 Xenograft Origin
Mucograft: This is a porcine collagen matrix, used in open healing to substitute free gingival grafts or protected healing like a connective tissue graft.

20.1.4 Purpose of Soft Tissue Graft (Periodontal Plastic Surgery)

20.1.4.1 Aesthetic Purpose
- Root coverage
- Cover gingival discolouration from root or implant
- Soft tissue augmentation to improve pink-to-white aesthetic tissue balance.

20.1.4.2 Functional Purpose
- To protect tissue from brushing trauma
- To prevent further recession
- Better adaptation around implants abutments and crowns
- Caries prevention
- Sensitivity.

20.2 Procedures

20.2.1 Techniques

20.2.1.1 Harvesting the Palatal Tissue Graft as a Free Gingival Graft and Connective Tissue Graft
Clinicians should be aware of anatomical location of critical landmarks such as the GPF and GPA. Ninety percent of the time the GPF opens distal to the middle aspect of second molars and then gives a main branch GPA that runs in an ascending fashion with the farthest section at the molar and closest at the canine (Figures 20.2–20.4) [3].

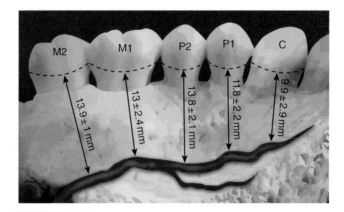

Figure 20.2 Schematic drawing showing the distance between the cemento-enamel junction of the maxillary teeth and greater palatine artery. *Source:* Source: Figure was adapted with permission from primary author Dr. L. Tavelli from Tavelli, L., et al., What is the safety zone for palatal soft tissue graft harvesting based on the locations of the greater palatine artery and foramen? A systematic review. J. Oral Maxillofac. Surg., 2018. DOI-https://doi.org/10.1016/j.joms.2018.10.002.

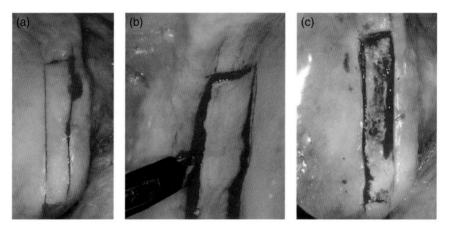

Figure 20.3 (a) The desired outline is cut with a blade. (b) Undermining the soft tissue altogether with the epithelium and connective tissue. (c) The donor site after harvesting. *Source:* Courtesy of Dr. Ehab Moussa.

20.2.1.2 Root Coverage

Root coverage procedures are a great option for patients who have recession, causing unaesthetic result or sensitivity (Figure 20.5).

20.2.1.3 Soft Tissue Augmentation Prior to Bone Grafting

This technique is particularly helpful if previous bone grafts have caused mucogingival scarring or epithelial encleftation (Figures 20.6–20.10). In this case the goal is to eliminate any epithelial encleftation that occurred due to unfavourable healing of previous bone graft. The second goal is to increase the thickness of soft tissue to achieve primary closure on second attempt at bone augmentation. The

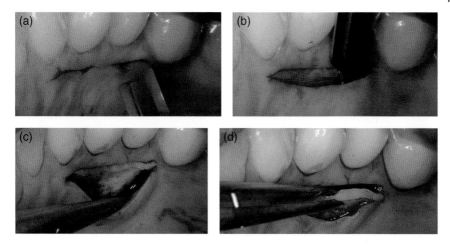

Figure 20.4 (a) A deeper, more coronal incision down to osseous is made. (b) Followed by a shallower and apical incision line. (c) The split-thickness incision is then extended to the desired graft size. (d) The graft is then elevated in full thickness or split thickness until released from the bone. Two vertical incisions are then made mesial and distal to the desired graft edges. *Source:* Case is courtesy of Dr. Sherif Said.

technique is used where the patient has had a previously failed attempt to perform guided bone regeneration with tenting screws.

- *Initial presentation*: Figure 20.3 shows soft tissue deformity due to presence of epithelial pockets in the edentulous site.

  The steps used are as follows:

1) Trace the encleftation of tissue with a probe (Figures 20.3–20.8).
2) Decide whether a flap is needed or not. In most cases a tunnel approach is preferred for better adaptation.
3) Refresh the epithelial lining with a bur or a blade. In this step we remove the epithelial lining and expose the microvessels underneath.
4) Measure the graft dimensions.
5) Harvest the connective tissue graft from the palate.
6) In this case the graft was split to make it longer and to provide adequate coverage for all the deficient area.
7) Stabilise the graft with minimum tension.

20.2.1.4   Soft Tissue Graft to Gain Keratinised Tissue

The goal of this procedure is to correct mucogingival line displacement after extensive bone augmentation (Figures 20.9–20.17).

  The steps used are as follows:

1) Initial examination and following bone augmentation protocol done. Steps are discussed in next chapter.
2) A common finding is mucogingival distortion due to flap advancement. In this case mucogingival surgery has to be done, as shown in Figures 20.9–20.14.

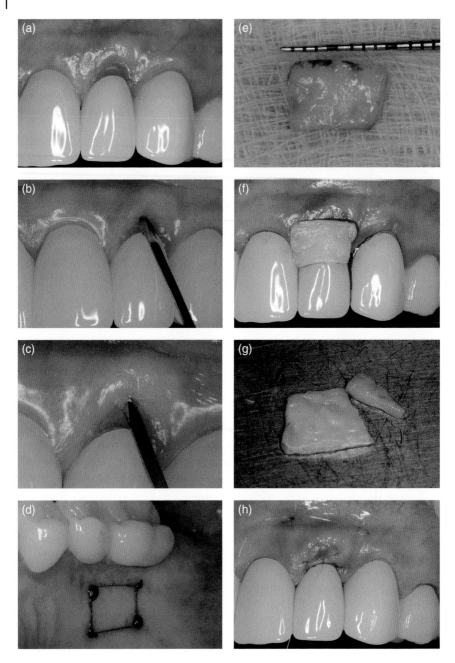

Figure 20.5 (a) Initial presentation showing recession on lateral incisor. (b, c) Tunneling approach via microsurgical blade started from the sulcus of the tooth reaching all the way to the mucogingival junction. (d, e) Free gingival graft harvesting. (f) Trial fitting of the harvested graft. (g) De-epithelialisation of the graft. (h) Suturing with 7-0 polypropylene. *Note:* Some of the graft margin can be left exposed for future epithelialisation. This can be done when adequate graft size is harvested to ensure good blood supply. The general rule is leave no more than 20% of the graft site exposed. *Source:* Courtsey of Dr. Jonathan Dutoit.

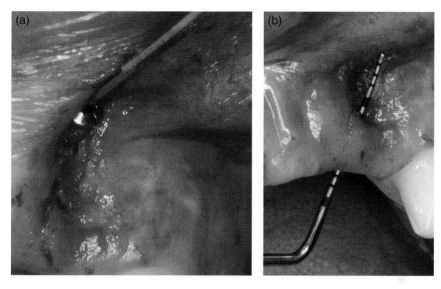

Figure 20.6 (a) The previous block fixation screw was exposed and removed to allow for uneventful soft tissue healing. (b) The epithelial cleating was traced with a probe.

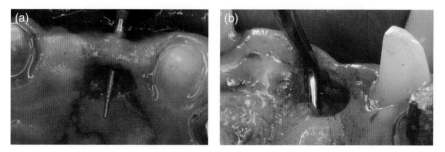

Figure 20.7 (a) The inside of the tissue was de-epithelialised using a finishing bur on a low speed setting. (b) The epithelial lining was curetted using grace curettes. *Tip:* Keep use of the cutting end of the grace curette toward the tissues on both sides.

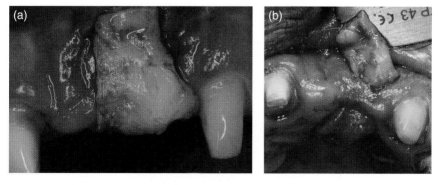

Figure 20.8 (a) Connective tissue graft was harvested from the palate and pre-fitted on the crest. (b) Insertion of the connective tissue in the prepared tunnel buccal and palatal and underneath the tissue bridge on the crest.

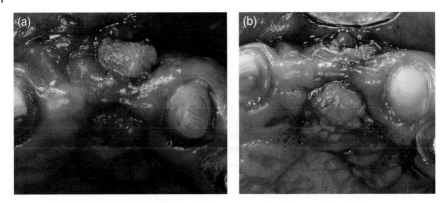

Figure 20.9 (a) Insertion of the connective tissue in the prepared tunnel buccal and palatal and underneath the tissue bridge on the crest. (b) Suturing of the graft, ensuring stable site and minimal tension.

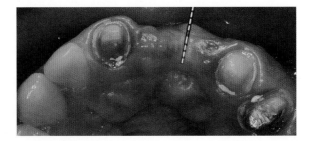

Figure 20.10 Three months post-operative showing gain in soft tissue thickness and elimination of epithelial tissue clefts.

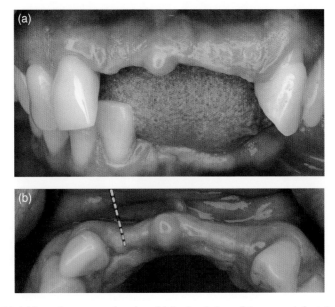

Figure 20.11 (a) Buccal pre-operative view. (b) Occlusal view of the same defect showing massive loss of the bucco-lingual dimension.

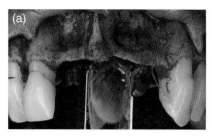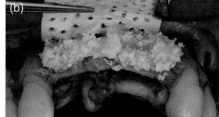

Figure 20.12 (a) Pre-augmentation bone view. (b) Augmentation with rhBMP-2-soaked collagen sponge and coated with xenograft particles. The graft material was covered with perforated dPTFE membrane. A titanium mesh can also be used in this combination of graft material.

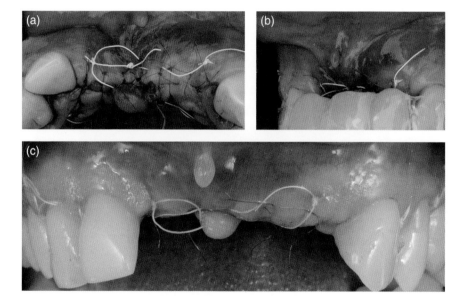

Figure 20.13 (a) Immediately post-operation 4-0 PTFE and 6-0 proline sutures. (b) Immediate post-operative side view shot. Note distortion of the muco-gingival junction over the crest. (c) Three-week follow-up after bone augmentation.

3) The recipient bed prepared via a split-thickness flap. Care should be taken to remove all muscle pull attached to the periosteum.
4) Two free gingival strip grafts harvested and fitted prior to trimming.
5) The graft stabilised prior to the flap in the apical position to allow access with the needle to the more apical layers of periosteum.
6) The apical flap repositioned using chromic gut suture. A resorbable material is recommended to prevent discomfort for the patient during suture removal and also to prevent entrapment of the suture material in the process of graft maturation.

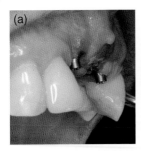
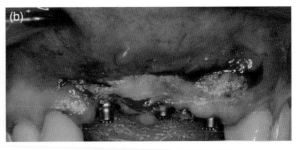

Figure 20.14 (a) After implant placement and uncovers. Note the frenum and mucosal pull reaching all the way to the crest. (b) Insertion of the connective tissue in the prepared tunnel buccal and palatal and underneath the tissue bridge on the crest.

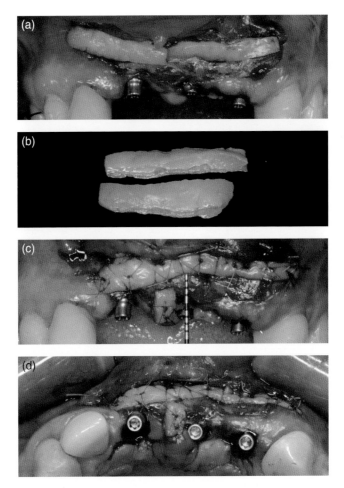

Figure 20.15 (a, b) Two strip free gingival grafts harvested from the palate and fitted on the recipient bed preparation site. (c, d) Graft sutured to the recipient site with horizontal sutures. A small piece of the graft was sutured to the nasopalatine after epithelialisation of the buccal side to give the illusion of the papilla.

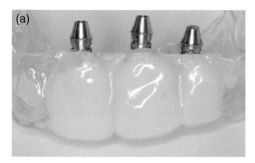
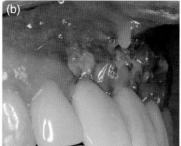

Figure 20.16 (a) An essex shell was prepared off the wax-up followed by implant temporisation via a direct pick-up technique. (b) One-week follow-up showing deepened vestibule and no muscle pull as well as keratinisation of the tissue.

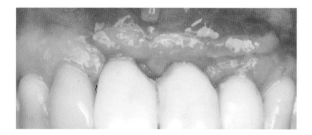

Figure 20.17 Two months after soft tissue procedure.

20.3 Tips

When preparing the recipient site the bed should be as close as possible to the periosteum to assure minimal bed movement. If the bed has any movement, the blood supply to the tissue overlying the graft may be compromised, leading to graft shrinkage.

Graft stability can be obtained by suturing the connective tissue graft to the inner side of the flap or over the periosteum.

Suturing should be done with 6-0/7-0 Prolene or Vicryl for any periodontal plastic surgery for optimal healing results. These are fine sutures that have been known to break before the tissue tears while tying the knots. They are good quality and very safe to use, avoiding crushing the tissues and the risk of ischaemia.

References

1 Karring, T., Lang, N.P., and Loe, H. (1975). The role of gingival connective tissue in determining epithelial differentiation. *J. Periodontal Res.* 10 (1): 1–11.
2 Reiser, G.M., Bruno, J.F., Mahan, P.E., and Larkin, L.H. (1996). The subepithelial connective tissue graft palatal donor site: anatomic considerations for surgeons. *Int J Periodontics Restorative Dent* 16 (2): 130–137.

3 Tavelli, L., Barootchi, S., Ravidà, A. et al. (2019). What is the safety zone for palatal soft tissue graft harvesting based on the locations of the greater palatine artery and foramen? A systematic review. *J. Oral Maxillofac. Surg.* 77 (2): 271.e1–271.e9.

Further Reading

Araujo, M.G., da Silva, J.C., de Mendonca, A.F., and Lindhe, J. (2015). Ridge alterations following grafting of fresh extraction sockets in man. A randomized clinical trial. *Clin Oral Implants Res* 26: 407–412.

Botticelli, D., Berglundh, T., and Lindhe, J. (2004). Hard-tissue alterations following immediate implant placement in extraction sites. *J Clin Periodontol* 31: 820–828.

Chappuis, V., Araújo, M.G., and Buser, D. (2017). Clinical relevance of dimensional bone and soft tissue alterations post-extraction in esthetic sites. *Periodontol* 73 (1): 73–83.

21

Bone Augmentation Procedures

Michel Azer

21.1   Principles

Interest in bone grafting began in the orthopaedic literature for the treatment of bone fractures and spinal injuries. In the 1970s it became a topic of interest in dentistry for regeneration around teeth. Multiple materials have been used, such as autogenous bone chips, coagulum, and bone substitutes. However, the results were not consistent until the discovery of the cell-occlusive properties of non-resorbable membranes in experimental jaw models.

21.1.1   Why is Bone Grafting Necessary?

The main objective of bone grafting is to reconstruct the biological requirements for implant success. The minimum requirements for implant success are to have 2 mm of surrounding bone. This is necessary to compensate for 1–1.5 mm of bone remodelling after the first year of loading, also called 'peri-implant biological width' [1]. Some authors suggest that in the aesthetic zone the peri-implant buccal bone should be 2–4 mm to maintain the labial gingival level [2].

21.1.2   Defect Topography Classification

Multiple classifications have been introduced in the literature to accurately describe an edentulous ridge and to give the clinician a better sense of the complexity of the situation. Traditionally, defects were classified as horizontal, vertical, or combined. However, a more comprehensive classification is the Cologne Classification of Alveolar Ridge Defects (CCARD), which categorises defects according to three aspects:

1) Defect orientation:
   H: Horizontal
   V: Vertical
   C: Combined
   S: Sinus

Practical Procedures in Implant Dentistry, First Edition. Edited by Christopher C.K. Ho.
© 2022 John Wiley & Sons Ltd. Published 2022 by John Wiley & Sons Ltd.
Companion website: www.wiley.com/go/ho/implant-dentistry

2) Reconstruction needs:
   1: Low <4 mm
   2: Medium 4–8 mm
   3: High >8 mm
3) Relation of augmentation to the surrounding bone:
   a: Internal: Inside the ridge contour
   b: External: Outside the ridge contour.

Two examples using this classification are:

H.2.b Medium horizontal defect outside the ridge contour.
H.1.a.S.1 Small horizontal defect inside the ridge contour with sinus defect requiring grafting <4 mm.

21.1.3 Requirements for Successful Tissue Grafting

A simple mnemonic to remember while undertaking bone grafting is 'PASS' [3]:

P – Primary wound healing
Non-interrupted healing for six to nine months is required. This can be fulfilled by good early healing resulting from appropriate flap management and prevention of bacterial and mechanical insult (e.g. pressure from denture or temporary pontics).

A – Angiogenesis
The healing process after bone augmentation begins with a blood clot that forms in the first 24 hours. This is then dissolved by macrophage and neutrophils to form granulation tissue, which is dense in blood vessels and helps in osteoid formation. The literature showed that increased blood vessels means better regeneration quality.

S – Space maintenance
The most important requirement for successful guided bone regeneration (GBR) is to allow space for the appropriate cells to repopulate. In GBR it is osteoprogenitor cells.

S – Stability
The membrane used in GBR has a triple function of space cell exclusion, space maintenance, and protection against the micro-movement of blood clots.

21.1.4 Materials Used for Augmentation

21.1.4.1 Autogenous Bone
Autogenous bone has been the gold standard in augmentation and an example of autogenous bone graft is shown in Figure 21.1.

21.1.4.2 Membranes
Resorbable membranes used in bone grafts include:

- long-lasting crosslinked collagen membranes (e.g. RCM6 by ACEsurgical®)
- fast-resorbing non-crosslinked collagen membranes (e.g. Bio-Gide by Geistlich®).

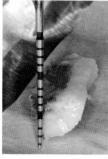
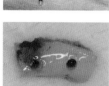
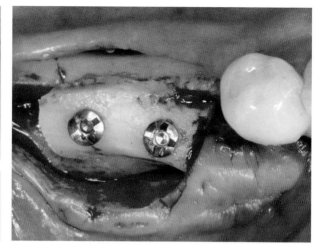

Figure 21.1 Onlay autogenous bone graft harvested and stabilised on the posterior mandible with the aim of vertical and horizontal bone augmentation. Two screws were used to fix it to minimise micromovement and rotation.

Non-resorbable membranes used include:

- unreinforced dense polytetrafluoroethylene (dPTFE), also known as cytoplast membrane (Osteogenics®)
- titanium-reinforced dPTFE
- titanium mesh.

21.1.4.3   Membrane Fixation Systems
- *Tacks*: Non-threaded pins, which work by tapping to fix the membrane. Recommended to be used with resorbable and non-resorbable membranes.
- *Screws*: Threaded fixation screws work by manual torquing. These are not recommended for resorbable collagen membranes as they may cause wrinkling of the membrane and sometimes tearing.
- Tenting screws.
- Block fixation screws.

21.2   Procedures

21.2.1   Bone Graft with Non-resorbable Membrane (Figures 21.2 and 21.3)

1) Perform full-thickness reflection and degranulation of any fibrous tissue or previously grafted particles. Care should be taken not to traumatise the flap or cause perforations.
2) Perform releasing incision and flap stretching.

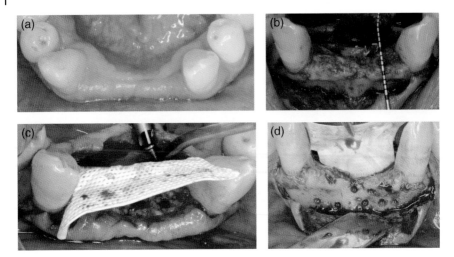

Figure 21.2 (a) Pre-operative view. (b) Initial situation prior to grafting. (c) d-PTFE with titanium mesh used for membrane fixation with a screw on the lingual side. (d) After membrane fixation with two screws on the lingual side.

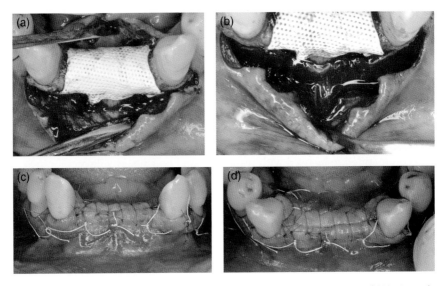

Figure 21.3 (a) Bone graft packed and stabilised on the buccal via two screws. (b) Horizontal releasing incision above the muscle layer. (c, d) Two layers of suturing is recommended: a horizontal mattresses with 4-0 cytoplast and 6-0 proline to approximate the edges.

3) Decorticate if needed as a source of blood supply and osteoprogenitor cells.
4) Measure the membrane dimensions.
5) Fix the palatal or buccal.
6) Pack the bone.
7) Use periosteal sutures to stabilise the membrane.
8) Use horizontal mattress suture to position the flap edges.
9) Use single interrupted suture to close the flap incision line.

21.2.2 Autogenous Bone Graft (Figures 21.4–21.10)

1) Perform full-thickness flap reflection with releasing incisions for better visibility and later on to achieve primary closure.
2) Measure the ridge defect mesiodistally and apico-coronally.
3) Harvest autogenous bone (Figure 21.5)
4) Split the block and scrape all irregularities with a bone scraper.
5) Fix the plate, starting with the buccal first.
6) Use a thin carbide/fissure drill to drill through the plate and into the native bone. The length is measured with a probe and the appropriate size fixation screw is used. Usually the appropriate screw length is 3–4 mm longer than this length.
7) Use a palatal drill in a similar fashion to stabilise the palatal plate.
8) Trim the excess grafting material to generate autogenous bone chips. Then pack in between the plate.
9) Use a platelet-rich fibrin (PRF) membrane prior to closure. If PRF is not available closure can be attained without a membrane.

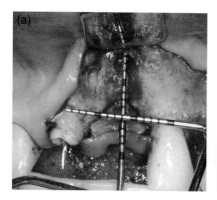
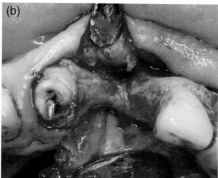

Figure 21.4 (a, b) Pre-operative view and initial situation prior to grafting.

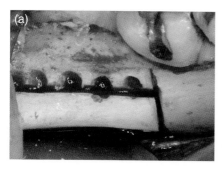
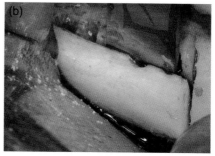

Figure 21.5 (a) Outlining the graft borders starting with medial and distal, followed by apical, and finally the coronal border. (b) A chisel is used with light pressure to greenstick fracture the bone and dislocate it from the mandible.

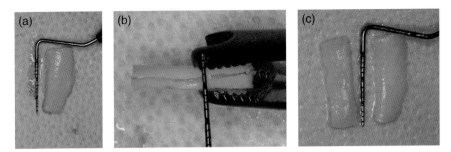

Figure 21.6 (a) Initial view of the graft. (b) The graft was split with piezo. A microsaw can also be used for this step. (c) After complete sectioning.

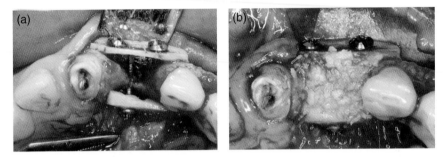

Figure 21.7 (a) Buccal plate is fixed first followed by palatal plate. Note: The palatal screw reaches all the way to the buccal plate for maximum stability. (b) Autogenous bone chips are packed into the prepared box.

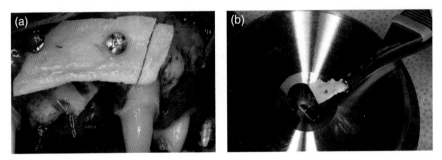

Figure 21.8 (a) We can benefit from excess bone by careful trimming and using it to generate more bone chips. (b) The excess bone prior to grinding via bone mill.

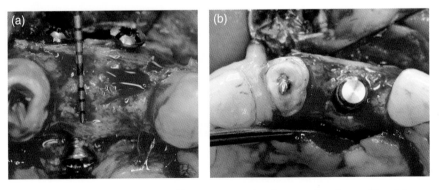

Figure 21.9 (a) Horizontal and vertical bone regeneration four months after grafting. (b) Implant placement in the ideal three-dimensional position.

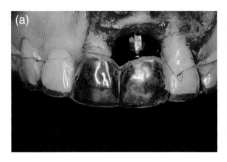
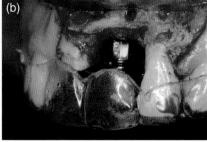

Figure 21.10 (a, b) Buccal view of the implant position showing implant placement at appropriate depth to allow for proper emergence profile.

21.3 Tips

Primary Closure
- Achieve tension-free primary closure using correct releasing incisions.
- Instruct the patient to avoid wearing removable dental prostheses for two to three weeks.
- If a fixed temporary prosthesis is used then this should to be relieved accordingly.
- Use proper pre-operative and post-operative protocols.
- At the beginning of the learning curve it is advisable to use resorbable collagen membranes as any complications may be less serious.

Angiogenesis
- A good clinician should assess the quality, not just the quantity of regeneration.
- Blood supply and final product is important for long-term stability of the graft.

Space Maintenance
- A titanium-reinforced membrane or titanium mesh will give superior results to collagen membrane when the defect is extensive.

References

1 Berglundh, T. and Lindhe, J. (1996). Dimension of the periimplant mucosa. Biological width revisited. *J. Clin. Periodontol.* 23 (10): 971–973.
2 Spray, J.R., Black, C.G., Morris, H.F., and Ochi, S. (2000). The influence of bone thickness on facial marginal bone response: stage 1 placement through stage 2 uncovering. *Ann. Periodontol.* 5 (1): 119–128.
3 Wang, H.L. and Boyapati, L. (2006). *"PASS" principles for predictable bone regeneration. Implant. Dent.* 15 (1): 8–17.

22

Impression Taking in Implant Dentistry

Christopher C.K. Ho

22.1   Principles

An impression is necessary to accurately transfer the position and design of an implant, or abutment to a master cast. This accuracy is required for passive fit of the final prosthesis, as misfit may increase the risk of biological and mechanical failures. Therefore, the fabrication of a definitive cast that exactly transfers the intra-oral position of an implant is essential for the long-term stability of the prosthesis. Additionally, the impression captures the soft tissue contours that frame the restoration, providing the pink aesthetic frame around the tooth.

An impression is usually made at the implant level or abutment level with an elastomeric impression material such as polyether or polyvinyl siloxane. In recent times, chairside intra-oral scanning or digital impressions have been introduced. These digital impression techniques involve the use of scan markers with the patient scanned for a digital impression with the registration of the implant carried out concurrently. Digital impression techniques may offer several advantages, including patient comfort, removal of possible errors associated with elastic materials, and increased cost effectiveness.

A poor impression may lead to an inaccurately fitting prosthesis or compromised result, which may lead to future complications or failure. This can add to costs incurred as well as leading to extended treatment times and inconvenience for the patient. The accuracy of definitive casts may be influenced by the impression technique used, the parallel or non-parallel placement of implants, depth of implant position, type of impression material used, dimensional stability of the gypsum used to fabricate the cast, die system, and the length of the impression copings.

The implant impression will provide:

- Implant position
- Depth of implant
- Axis/angulation of implant
- Rotational position of the implant
- Soft tissue contour (emergence profile).

Practical Procedures in Implant Dentistry, First Edition. Edited by Christopher C.K. Ho.
© 2022 John Wiley & Sons Ltd. Published 2022 by John Wiley & Sons Ltd.
Companion website: www.wiley.com/go/ho/implant-dentistry

The requirements of the elastomeric impression materials include:

- Accuracy
- Rigidity yet resilient properties
- Ability to be removed from undercuts
- Dimensional stability.

The use of polyether or addition polyvinyl siloxanes have been recommended to fulfil the impression material requirements. Silicone impression materials have better biomechanical stability than polyether, which are susceptible to moisture and sunlight. They tend to have a favourable modulus of elasticity that allows simpler removal from the mouth, especially for soft tissue undercuts.

The fit of implant prostheses requires extreme accuracy because of the precise machine fit along with the rigid connection to bone. Implants do not possess a periodontal ligament, which makes allowance for minor inaccuracies such as in teeth. Impressions for multiple implants restorations are even more critical. Passive fit is the objective, as misfit may lead to stress placed on the implants leading to bone loss and even loss of integration.

22.1.1 Impression Techniques Used in Implant Dentistry

- Abutment level impressions:
  - Direct
  - Indirect
- Implant level impressions:
  - Pick up (open tray)
  - Transfer (closed tray).

22.1.1.1 Abutment Level Impressions

Direct abutment level impressions require the placement of the abutment and then preparation and impression similar to that of a conventional crown preparation.

Indirect abutment level impressions require the use of snap-on abutments, such as Snappy Abutments (Nobel Biocare) or Solid Abutments (Straumann), which involve placing a standard abutment with impression cap that gets picked up within the impression. An analogue to fit this abutment is then inserted and a model made.

22.1.1.2 Implant Level Impressions

- *Indirect transfer (closed tray)*: The impression coping remains in the mouth following removal of the set impression. An analogue is then placed onto the impression coping and the coping is replaced back into the impression. These copings are normally tapered to allow removal.
- *Direct pick up (open tray)*: Direct techniques are also described as open tray impression techniques because the tray has an open window for unscrewing the guide pins of the impression copings (Table 22.1). These techniques can be subdivided into splinted and non-splinted techniques. The coping is incorporated within the impression and the guide pin unscrewed then

Table 22.1 Comparison between open and closed tray implant impression taking.

Factors	Transfer (closed tray) coping	Pick up (open tray) coping
Ease of use	Simpler, may be better for gagging patients	More steps involved
Tray preparation	None	Tray must be perforated where the impression coping is situated
Inter-occlusal space	Less space required. Simpler in posterior region	More space is required to access screw to insert and remove coping
Multiple unit splinting	Not possible	Possible
Precision of impression	Possible inaccuracy due to having to reinsert the coping back into the impression	Less inaccuracy due to coping remaining in the impression
Divergent implants	Difficult to remove impression	Simpler to remove impression
Depth of implants	Deeper placement may preclude use of a closed tray coping as it may not engage the impression material sufficiently	Impression coping is square and can engage impression material and can be modified if required

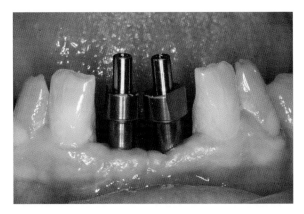

Figure 22.1 Open tray impression copings. Notice the square form of the coping which is picked up in the impression.

subsequently removed upon setting of the impression. The tray needs to be open to allow access to the retaining screw so that it can be released to remove the impression. The copings are normally square, allowing locking of the coping within the impression (Figure 22.1).

In a systematic review, Kim et al. [1] critically appraised the literature to assess the impression accuracy achieved with direct and indirect techniques. They reported that the direct (open tray) impression and splinted techniques are more accurate. Other authors have reported that the pick-up type impression coping is the more accurate type of impression as errors occur on removal and replacement of the transfer type impression copings, especially in the occluso-gingival direction [2, 3]. There may be certain indications for closed tray techniques when access is difficult, as in the posterior regions of the mouth or when mouth opening is limited or in cases of patients with an exaggerated gag reflex when impression may need to be removed as quickly as possible [4].

22.1.2 Customised Impression Copings

Manufacturers' impression copings are standardised and do not take into account the varying soft tissue profiles that may be formed by provisional restorations or contoured healing abutments [5]. Impression copings may be customised to accurately record soft tissue using two methods. The first is by placing an impression coping and flowing composite resin into the subgingival regions and light curing. This cures the composite resin that has flowed into the tissues, not allowing collapse of the soft tissues. The second method is to insert an analogue into a provisional restoration and form an impression of the provisional crown and analogue assembly by placing this into impression material covering up to the submucosal portion of the provisional restoration. Once it is set, the provisional restoration is removed leaving the analogue within the impression material and the contours of the provisional crown left as a negative for an impression coping to be then placed onto the analogue. The negative space can be filled with acrylic or flowable composite resin, giving a customised impression coping that can be then used intra-orally to capture the provisional crown contours (Figure 22.2).

22.1.3 Multiple Unit Impressions

Because of the machine fit of implant componentry impressions are needed to achieve passive fit of a prosthesis or, put simply, to 'create as accurate a fit as is clinically possible to avoid bone strain resulting from uncontrolled loading of the

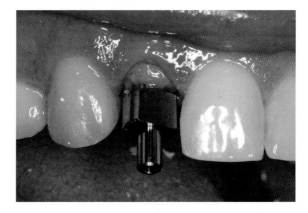

Figure 22.2 Customised impression coping in place, supporting and reproducing the gingival architecture developed by the provisional restoration. This has been customised by inserting flowable composite resin in the submergence region and polymerising the material so that it sets in the profile of the developed submergence profile.

implants through the superstructure'. This becomes more critical when there are two or more implants in implant-supported bridgework because the misfit stress may be amplified, leading to clinical complications.

Sorrentino et al. [6] evaluated the effect of implant alignments (parallel versus non-parallel) and coping engagement lengths (1 mm versus 2 mm) in internal connection implants. They reported more accurate casts were produced when implants were parallel rather than non-parallel alignments and that short engagement length produced more accurate results when the implants were not parallel. Mpikos et al. [7] report in external connection implants that neither impression technique nor implant parallelism influenced impression accuracy; conversely, in internal connection implants accuracy was significantly influenced by the implant parallelism. This is likely due to internal connection implants having longer or broader implant/abutment connections than external connection implants. The longer or broader connection area can cause displacement of the impression copings during the removal of the impression, increasing the amount of distortion in non-parallel implant cases. Impression copings have been developed for single restorations that possess an internal engaging part similar to the abutment supporting the restorations. This is normally a long engaging hex registering and transferring the position. However, in a fixed dental prosthesis a long hex may preclude passive retrieval of the impression coping from the implant, especially if the implant is tilted, as it may bind and forces generated upon removal may introduce distortion into the impression. To avoid or reduce distortion in the impression the use of non-hexed (non-engaging) open tray impression copings are recommended (Figure 22.3).

To increase the accuracy of multiple unit impressions it has been suggested that there is improved precision of fit when impression copings are splinted prior to taking the impression. The majority of studies in the systematic review by Lee

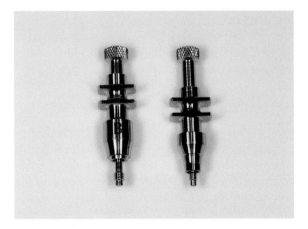

Figure 22.3 Engaging and non-engaging impression copings. Single restorations possess an internal long engaging hex similar to the abutment supporting the restorations. In multiple units such as a fixed dental prosthesis the long hexes may preclude passive retrieval of the impression coping from implants, distorting the impression. The use of non-hexed (non-engaging) impression copings are thus advised.

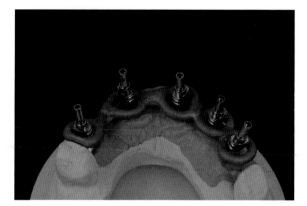

Figure 22.4 Impression jig constructed in the laboratory for intra-oral pick-up by splinting of copings to the jig. This has been fabricated with metal, although many clinicians would construct this from pattern resin.

et al. [8] found increased accuracy for splinting and no study reported that non-splinted techniques were more accurate than splinted.

In a recent systematic review by Papaspyridakos et al. [9], it was found that the splinted impression technique was more accurate for both partially and completely edentulous patients. The open tray technique is more accurate than the closed tray for completely edentulous patients (Figure 22.4), but for partially edentulous patients there seems to be no difference. If you have multiple implants but plan on restoring them as single units, you may choose to use closed tray impression copings for ease of use, but note that you cannot splint closed tray impression copings as there is no way of removing them when removing the final impression.

22.2 Procedures

The procedures are demonstrated in the videos included within the book and readers are encouraged to view these videos for more detail.

22.2.1 Implant Level Impression

1) After removal of the healing abutment or provisional restoration the impression coping should be inserted without delay as soft tissue may collapse inwards, making it more difficult to insert the coping.
2) Insert either an open or closed tray impression coping. If taking a multiple unit impression, consider splinting the impressions with wire, resin, or another framework with an open tray technique.
3) Take a peri-apical radiograph. A paralleling technique is utilised so as to visualise the complete seating of the copings. The use of a film holder is encouraged (Figure 22.5).
4) Try in the tray and prepare the tray by perforating the tray in the region of the impression coping if utilising an open tray technique.

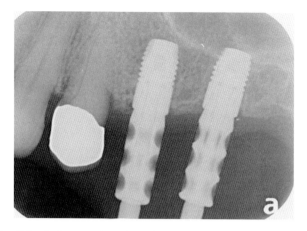

Figure 22.5 Parallel technique used to take radiograph of implant and impression coping. Note that there has been complete seating of the impression coping.

5) Be aware of undercuts, or existing crown and bridgework that may need to be blocked out to ensure ease of displacement of the impression from the mouth.
6) Proceed to take the impression. Inspect to see that the impression is accurate and extends to all teeth required. Additional attention should be made to assess that the coping fits into the impression if a closed tray technique is used, and if an open tray technique is used ensure that the coping is sitting firmly within the material with no chance of dislodgement.
7) Reinsert the healing abutment or provisional restoration.

22.2.2 Digital Impressions

The development of chairside intra-oral scanning has allowed digital impression-taking, which enables the clinician to accurately impress implants with the same level of accuracy as conventional impressions in single-tooth and partially edentulous implant cases up to four units. However, in fully edentulous cases where there is cross-arch implant placement differing views in relation to accuracy are reported in the literature. At this time, it may be prudent to consider conventional impressions for full arch implant reconstructions, or if digital impressions are to be used then physical verification should be performed to ensure accuracy of fit. Evolving developments in photogrammetry and continuing innovations in intra-oral scanning with different length-calibrated scan bodies may soon enable accurate digital intra-oral scanning for full arch implant cases.

22.3 Tips

- Take a periapical radiograph to check fit and seating of copings which may be below the mucosa and not visible. The radiograph should be taken perpendicular to the implant to ensure that threads are sharp and not blurred, providing a diagnostic radiograph that allows comparative assessment over time.

- If implants are in close proximity to each other, it may be impossible to place the impression copings together. If this happens you may wish to modify the impression copings with a bur to allow complete seating. Another solution may be to use an adjusted engaging temporary cylinder or other abutment that can be used like a pick-up coping.
- In splinting of multiple unit impressions when implants are spaced some distance apart, there may be inaccuracy because of the polymerisation contraction that resins undergo. The use of stiff wire and resin may be substituted to minimise this effect.

References

1 Kim, J.H., Kim, K.R., and Kim, S. (2015). Critical appraisal of implant impression accuracies: a systematic review. *J. Prosthet. Dent.* 114: 185–192.
2 Liou, A.D., Nicholls, J.I., Yuodelis, R.A., and Brudvik, J.S. (1993). Accuracy of replacing three tapered transfer impression copings in two elastomeric impression materials. *Int J Prosthodont* 6: 377–383.
3 Assif, D., Fenton, A., Zarb, G., and Schmitt, A. (1992). Comparative accuracy of implant impression procedures. *Int J Perio Rest Dent* 12: 112–121.
4 Chee, W. and Jivraj, S. (2006 Oct 7). Impression techniques for implant dentistry. *Br. Dent. J.* 201 (7): 429–432.
5 Buskin, R. and Salinas, T. (1998). Transferring emergence profile created from provisional to definitive restoration. *Pract. Periodontics Aesthet. Dent.* 10: 1171–1179.
6 Sorrentino, R., Gherlone, E.F., Calesini, G., and Zarone, F. (2010). Effect of implant angulation, connection length, and impression material on the dimensional accuracy of implant impressions: an in vitro; comparative study. *Clin. Implant. Dent. Relat. Res.* 12 (suppl 1): e63–e76.
7 Mpikos, P., Tortopidis, D., Galanis, C. et al. (2012). The effect of impression technique and implant angulation on the impression accuracy of external- and internal-connection implants. *Int. J. Oral Maxillofac. Implants* 27: 1422–1428.
8 Lee, H., So, J.S., Hochstedler, J.L., and Ercoli, C. (2008). The accuracy of implant impressions: a systematic review. *J Prosthet Dent.* 100 (4): 285–291.
9 Papaspyridakos, P., Chen, C.J., Gallucci, G.O. et al. (2014). Chronopoulos accuracy of implant impressions for partially and completely edentulous patients: a systematic review. *Int. J. Oral Maxillofac. Implants* 29 (4): 836–845.

23

Implant Treatment in the Aesthetic Zone

Christopher C.K. Ho

23.1 Principles

Historically, success in implant therapy has been defined as a functioning implant with healthy peri-implant tissues and stable crestal bone levels. More recently, aesthetics has become as important a criterion for successful implant rehabilitation. Patients require both 'white' and 'pink' aesthetics in areas visible in a smile to provide harmony and balance. Providing an aesthetic outcome requires understanding of the criteria related to hard and soft tissue aesthetics. The clinician must be aware of parameters related to gingival morphology, form, and dimension, characterisation, surface texture, and colour. Ceramists may fabricate restorations that match adjacent teeth in terms of colour, but if the surrounding soft tissues are not harmonious, an aesthetic outcome is not likely. Furthermore, it is important to understand the aesthetic risk to treatment outcomes by establishing the patients' treatment expectations.

Comprehensive planning of implant rehabilitations involves a prosthodontically driven approach so that precise surgical and prosthodontic treatment results in an optimal aesthetic and functional result. Correct three-dimensional implant placement is vital to an aesthetic outcome. Respecting spatial requirements to ensure that the implant shoulder is located in an ideal position allows an optimal aesthetic outcome with stable, long-term peri-implant tissues. As part of the consultation, discussions should be had with patients to determine whether they have any dento-facial aesthetic concerns. An overall smile evaluation may be conducted to enhance the aesthetic display of teeth in conjunction with implant rehabilitation. This may involve adjacent restorative procedures such as composite resin addition or porcelain veneers/crowns, orthodontic tooth movement, periodontal procedures, and implant site development to meet the patient's requirements.

23.1.1 General Considerations

Analysing a smile involves integration of dento-facial and dento-labial form which may influence the overall attractiveness of the face. Digital smile evaluation is a design and communication tool that allows a technician to create a

Practical Procedures in Implant Dentistry, First Edition. Edited by Christopher C.K. Ho.
© 2022 John Wiley & Sons Ltd. Published 2022 by John Wiley & Sons Ltd.
Companion website: www.wiley.com/go/ho/implant-dentistry

three-dimensional (3D) diagnostic wax-up or mock-up on articulated casts based on the two-dimensional (2D) elements prescribed by the digital design. It also permits a virtual wax-up by placement of tooth-coloured forms on a photograph to simulate an intra-oral mock-up. The final smile design elements may be constrained by functional relationships such as eating and talking. In this chapter we will not attempt to explain smile design in detail, but to emphasise particular factors that need careful assessment related to implant treatment in the aesthetic zone.

23.1.1.1 Lip Contour and Length

The anterior teeth and supporting structures support the lip contour, and removal of these teeth and the associated resorption may lead to loss of lip contour with a sunken lower face. The average lip length is estimated to be 20–24 mm from the edge of the upper lip to the base of the nose [1], with lip mobility of about 7–8 mm [2].

23.1.1.2 Tooth Display at Repose and in Broad Smile

The average 30-year-old female at repose displays 3.4 mm of tooth structure, while males display 1.9 mm [3]. The starting point for any aesthetic rehabilitation is the face and assessment of the maxillary incisal edges in relation to the patient's face provides the roadmap to set teeth for an aesthetic display. Depending on lip mobility the length of teeth may be modified to provide an attractive smile.

23.1.1.3 Smile Line

The smile line is carefully assessed by asking the patient to smile broadly to see how the maxillary lip moves. This can be classified as low, average, or high. In a low smile line, <75% of the maxillary incisors in the full smile are displayed; for the average smile 75–100% of the upper incisors and interdental papillae are displayed; and a high smile is where the complete length of the incisors is visible with some amount of gingival display (Figure 23.1).

Two different smiles have been described. The *social/posed smile* is reproducible voluntarily. The lips part due to moderate muscular contraction of the lip elevator muscles, and the teeth and sometimes the gingival scaffold are displayed. In contrast, the *enjoyment/unposed smile/Duchenne smile* is an

(a)   (b)   (c)

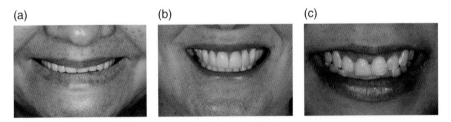

Figure 23.1 (a) With a low smile line <75% of the maxillary incisors in the full smile are displayed. (b) In the average smile 75–100% of upper incisors and interdental papillae are displayed. (c) A high smile is where the complete length of the incisors is visible with some amount of gingival display.

involuntary smile and is elicited by laughter or great pleasure and results from maximal contraction of the elevator and depressor muscles, causing full expansion of the lips, gingival show, and maximum anterior tooth display. Patients do not often give their most natural smile in the dental office; asking them to give you their 'biggest' smile will reveal if they expose the gingival margins in their smile. If it is difficult to attain a smile, an alternative is to ask the patient to say 'eeee'.

A low smile line may be less critical because the implant restoration interface will be hidden under the upper lip, with problems such as deficiencies in hard and soft tissue or poor gingival contour and colour hidden covered by the lip. However, it cannot be assumed that this is not a concern for the patient and their input should be sought to find out whether this is problematic. A high smile line will make these problems visible and may require intervention to provide an aesthetic result. During a broad smile the majority of the maxillary anterior teeth are displayed with 2 mm considered by dental clinicians and laypersons as aesthetically pleasing [4].

23.1.1.4   Teeth Length, Shape, Alignment, Contour, and Colour

Tooth shapes can be classified as square, ovoid, or triangular. Triangular tooth shapes with high gingiva scalloping are often more difficult procedures to manage due to the possible loss of papilla height, and the resultant 'black hole' from the missing papilla.

23.1.1.5   Gingival Display, Gingival Zeniths, and Papillae of Maxillary Anterior Teeth

'Pink aesthetics' involves several important features including papilla height, position of the mucosal margin, as well as the texture, colour, and contour of the peri-implant mucosa [5–7]. To achieve a natural appearance the peri-implant soft tissues should closely mimic those of the adjacent dentition. The re-creation of papilla-like tissue is one of the most challenging goals of implant therapy in the aesthetic zone. The principal factor determining the presence of a papilla is the distance between the bone crest and the proximal contact point. A seminal study by Tarnow et al. [8] in natural teeth found that when the distance from the contact point to the crestal bone was 5 mm or less, the papilla between teeth was present nearly 100% of the time. However, when this distance was increased to 6 and 7 mm, the papilla was only present 56 and 27% of the time, respectively. Similarly, the regeneration of papillae adjacent to single implants is not predictable when the distance from the bone crest to contact point is above 5 mm [9]. Moreover, the papilla level associated with single-implant restorations is related to the bone crest at the adjacent teeth and is independent of the bone level at the implant [9, 10]. A minimum safe lateral distance of 1.5 mm has been suggested to preserve the papilla, as positioning the implant too close to the adjacent tooth can result in loss of the proximal bone [11]. Recent studies suggest that a greater potential for complete papilla fill may be achieved if the distance from the adjacent teeth is increased to 3 mm or more [12–14]. However, this minimum distance may be less important when using implants with a platform-switched design [15]. Even though spontaneous improvement in papilla fill has been observed adjacent to single-implant restorations [7, 14], this is rarely achieved between multiple adjacent implants.

23.1.1.6 Width of Edentulous Space

There is higher aesthetic risk in cases where two or more teeth are missing in an edentulous space when creating an aesthetic soft tissue profile with normal gingival scalloping. Findings by Tarnow et al. [16] suggest a mean soft tissue height of 3.4 mm can be expected above the crestal bone between two implants. Loss of interdental papillae is an adverse event due to the aesthetic deformity or 'black hole disease'. This can lead to food impaction and phonetic deficiencies. Due to this deficiency in papilla height, it may be necessary to modify the shape of the teeth to provide a longer contact areas and smaller embrasure space. With severe deficiencies, the papilla can be recreated prosthetically with pink porcelain, acrylic or composite resin.

23.1.1.7 Gingival Biotype

The gingival biotype can have a significant influence on the outcome of implant treatment. Gingival thickness can be broadly categorised into either a thin or thick biotype. The thin gingival biotype has been associated with long narrow teeth and a highly scalloped gingival margin, whereas the thick biotype is associated with short wide square tooth forms and a flat, low-scalloped gingival margin with apically positioned interdental contacts [17]. Thin gingival biotypes have been reported to be present in one-third of the population with higher prevalence in females [18]. Appreciation of the gingival biotype is important since it can influence the aesthetic risk and complexity of treatment. The thick gingival biotype are normally characterised by a wide band of attached keratinised tissue and represents robust tissues with a lower risk of mucosal recession. In contrast, a thin gingival biotype is often characterised by minimal keratinised attached gingiva, fenestrations, and dehiscence of the labial bone over roots and thin mucoperiosteium. This thin tissue is more susceptible to surgical trauma due to reduced vascularisation, which can lead to a greater risk of recession and aesthetic failure [19, 20].

23.1.2 Major Deficiencies in Hard and Soft Tissues

Patients may be reluctant to undergo multiple extensive surgical procedures to rebuild lost hard and soft tissues, as these may entail extended periods of treatment and healing, surgical morbidity, as well as cost. Even with surgical augmentation, reconstruction of lost tissues may not be able to achieve perfect natural aesthetics. It may be difficult to attain perfect soft tissue architecture with missing interproximal papilla, resulting in long contact points. Furthermore, lost vertical height of alveolar ridges may be difficult to reconstruct, leading to long crown heights and unaesthetic appearance, especially in high smile line patients. In these patients, use of artificial materials such as pink porcelain, composite resin, or acrylic resin may be considered (Figure 23.2). Reconstruction of lost tissues in these artificial materials may be aesthetic as long as the transition zone is hidden. For example, a removable dental prosthesis could be used for a

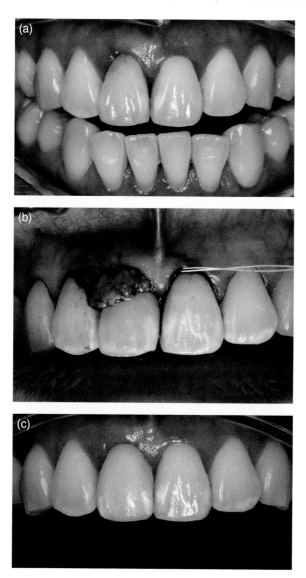

Figure 23.2 (a) Tooth 11 suffering from external resorption. The patient has several aesthetic risk factors including triangular-shaped teeth with thin biotype and deficient papilla.
(b) A connective tissue graft was used to increase the volume of soft tissue and rebuild lost papilla. (c) Completed final implant-supported crown.

major defect in the maxillary anterior region (class IV Kennedy), with the prosthesis and flange replacing missing lip support and soft tissue. Retainers can be minimised by using a dual path of insertion.

Dental implants and removable prostheses can also work in combination providing cost-effective solutions where implants provide additional retention, while the acrylic flange can provide appropriate contour and support for lips as well as hiding any aesthetic deformities. These overdenture solutions also ensure that access for hygiene is simplified and the number of implants needed is often less because of the mucosal support provided by the denture base.

23.2 Procedures

Kois [21] published five diagnostic keys for predictable single-tooth peri-implant aesthetics. He wrote that the predictability of peri-implant aesthetic outcomes may be ultimately determined by the patient's own presenting anatomy rather than the clinician's ability to manage state-of-the-art procedures. These five keys are the relative tooth position/free gingival margin, the form of the periodontium, gingival biotype, tooth shape, and position of the osseous crest. Understanding these five keys may enable the clinician to develop treatment options and clinical procedures specific to the patient (Table 23.1).

23.2.1 Assessment of Gingival Biotype

Several methods to assess the gingival biotype have been described, including a visual evaluation, although this is not reliable because there is no means of visually assessing the gingival thickness or labial bone plate. Other methods include sounding to bone with an injection needle with a silicone stop to mark the depth. A thick biotype will show a thickness of >2 mm. However, this method is dependent on the angle of the needle. Another non-invasive method is to place a periodontal probe within the gingival sulcus, and if the probe tip is visible through the gingiva it is considered thin. A cone beam computed tomography (CBCT) scan can be used to measure the cross-section. The scan must have the lips separated from the ridge by cotton rolls; measurements can be made of both the labial bone and the soft tissues.

23.2.2 Clinical Management

Assessment of the gingival biotype allows the clinician to better manage the hard and soft tissues using appropriate techniques to compensate for any possible soft tissue shrinkage and bone resorption that may occur in patients with thin, highly scalloped gingival tissues.

Table 23.1 Five diagnostic keys for predictable single-tooth peri-implant aesthetics.

	Favourable	Unfavourable
Tooth position/free gingival margin	Coronal	Ideal
Gingival form	Flat scallop	High scallop
Biotype	Thick	Thin
Tooth shape	Square	Triangular
Position of osseous crest <3 mm from adjacent teeth and facially	High crest	Low crest

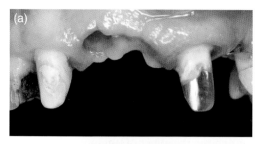
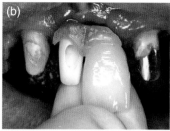
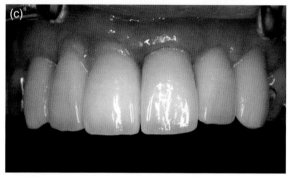

Figure 23.3 (a) The use of pink soft tissue replacement and a large soft tissue deformity. (b) Artificial pink with the use of porcelain or composite to simulate lost soft tissue. (c) Final implant-supported restoration.

Evans and Chen [19] found there was increased risk of mucosal recession in patients with thin biotypes after implant placement and provisionalisation. Hence in these patients it may be prudent to not place implants in a supracrestal level to account for any possible recession; furthermore, it may be possible to enhance the biotype by performing a subepithelial connective tissue graft (Figure 23.3).

23.2.3 Timing of Implant Placement

It has been proposed that immediate implant placement minimises bone resorption, particularly in the buccal bone plate. However, following removal of a tooth, the evidence demonstrates there is resorption of both the buccal and lingual bone plates irrespective of whether an immediate implant is placed, delayed placement is used, or a socket augmentation is performed. This bony resorption is thought to be due to the reduction in vascularisation upon removal of a tooth. The periodontal ligament supplies vascularity to the bundle bone in the ridge, and when a tooth is removed this compromises the vascularity significantly.

Immediate implants may assist in retaining the level of interdental papilla especially when supported with a provisional restoration or customised healing abutment. However, immediate implantation is suitable only when there is sufficient bony alveolus for placement. Patients presenting with periodontal disease or endodontic infections are often not suitable for immediate placement due to the compromised blood supply and possible infection. A staged placement protocol will be a better option in these cases.

23.2.4 Thickness of Soft Tissues

The colour of the peri-implant tissues can influence the final aesthetic outcome. Jung et al. [22] performed an *in vitro* study on the colour changes of soft tissues caused by different materials. They analysed the effect of titanium and zirconia with and without veneering ceramic on the colour of mucosa of three different thicknesses. To simulate different mucosa thicknesses, connective tissue grafts, 0.5 and 1.0 mm thick, were harvested from three jaws. Defined mucosa thicknesses were created by placing the grafts under a palatal mucosa flap. The colour of the tissue was evaluated with a spectrophotometer for three different soft tissue thicknesses (1.5, 2.0, and 3.0 mm). All restorative materials induced overall colour changes which diminished with increases in soft tissue thickness. Titanium induced the most prominent colour change. Zirconia did not induce visible colour changes in mucosa 2.0 and 3.0 mm thick, regardless of whether it was veneered. However, with a mucosa thickness of 3.0 mm, no change in colour could be distinguished by the human eye on any specimen. Mucosa thickness is a crucial factor in terms of discoloration caused by different restorative materials. In patients with thinner mucosa, zirconia will show the least colour change.

23.3 Tips

- Consider the use of zirconia abutments in the anterior zone as this will provide the best aesthetics; however, this may be contraindicated when the thickness of the abutment is less than 0.8 mm or where the abutment height is too short <3 mm. The dimensions of mandibular incisors and maxillary lateral incisors are often narrow, and in these situations use of metal abutments may be better.
- The use of vertical incisions in the aesthetic zone may lead to scarring and it may be advisable to move these vertical incisions to more posterior areas to hide any incision line.
- Use of microsurgical techniques (e.g. magnification, small elevators, microsurgical needle holders) can improve soft tissue healing by reducing tissue trauma and allowing precise flap adaptation and wound closure without tension.
- Clinical experience has shown that 5-0 and 6-0 monofilament suture materials are suitable for implant therapy in the aesthetic zone. Thinner suture (6-0 and smaller) risks thread breakage rather than tissue tearing under excessive tension, with the potential to reduce wound dehiscence. Finer suture diameters can achieve passive wound closure more predictably, although the selection of thicker suture (such as 5-0) is still necessary for repositioned flaps and when interproximal suturing dictates a larger needle size.

References

1 Rifkin, R. (2000 Nov-Dec). Facial analysis: a comprehensive approach to treatment planning in aesthetic dentistry. *Pract. Periodontics Aesthet. Dent.* 12 (9): 865–871.

2 McLaren, E.A. and Rifkin, R. (2002 Nov). Macroesthetics: facial and dentofacial analysis. *J. Calif. Dent. Assoc.* 30 (11): 839–846.

3 Vig, R.G. and Brundo, G.C. (1978). The kinetics of anterior tooth display. *J. Prosthet. Dent.* 39 (5): 502–504.

4 Kokich, V.O. Jr., Kiyak, H.A., and Shapiro, P.A. (1999). Comparing the perception of dentists and lay people to altered dental esthetics. *J. Esthet. Dent.* 11 (6): 311–324.

5 Belser, U.C., Grütter, L., Vailati, F. et al. (2008). Outcome evaluation of early placed maxillary anterior single-tooth implants using objective esthetic criteria: a cross-sectional, retrospective study in 45 patients with a 2- to 4-year follow-up using pink and white esthetic scores. *J. Periodontol.* 80: 140–151.

6 Fürhauser, R., Florescu, D., Benesch, T. et al. (2005). Evaluation of soft tissue around single-tooth implant crowns: the pink esthetic score. *Clin. Oral Implants Res.* 16: 639–644.

7 Jemt, T. (1997). Regeneration of gingival papillae after single-implant treatment. *Int J Periodontics Restorative Dent* 17: 326–333.

8 Tarnow, D.P., Magner, A.W., and Fletcher, P. (1992). The effect of the distance from the contact point to the crest of bone on the presence or absence of the interproximal dental papilla. *J. Periodontol.* 63: 995–996.

9 Choquet, V., Hermans, M., Adriaenssens, P. et al. (2001). Clinical and radiographic evaluation of the papilla level adjacent to single-tooth dental implants. A retrospective study in the maxillary anterior region. *J. Periodontol.* 72: 1364–1371.

10 Kan, J.Y.K., Rungcharassaeng, K., Umezu, K., and Kois, J.C. (2003). Dimensions of peri-implant mucosa: an evaluation of maxillary anterior single implants in humans. *J. Periodontol.* 74: 557–562.

11 Esposito, M., Ekestubbe, A., and Gröndahl, K. (1993). Radiological evaluation of marginal bone loss at tooth surfaces facing single Brånemark implants. *Clin. Oral Implants Res.* 4: 151–157.

12 Cosyn, J., Sabzevar, M.M., and De Bruyn, H. (2012). Predictors of inter-proximal and midfacial recession following single implant treatment in the anterior maxilla: a multivariate analysis. *J. Clin. Periodontol.* 39: 895–903.

13 Gastaldo, J.F., Cury, P.R., and Sendyk, W.R. (2004). Effect of the vertical and horizontal distances between adjacent implants and between a tooth and an implant on the incidence of interproximal papilla. *J. Periodontol.* 75: 1242–1246.

14 Schropp, L. and Isidor, F. (2015). Papilla dimension and soft tissue level after early vs. delayed placement of single-tooth implants: 10-year results from a randomized controlled clinical trial. *Clin. Oral Implants Res.* 26: 278–286.

15 Vela, X., Mendez, V., Rodriguez, X. et al. (2012). Crestal bone changes on platform-switched implants and adjacent teeth when the tooth-implant distance is less than 1.5 mm. *Int. J. Oral Maxillofac. Implants* 32: 149–155.

16 Tarnow, D., Elian, N., Fletcher, P. et al. (2003). Vertical distance from the crest of bone to the height of the interproximal papilla between adjacent implants. *J. Periodontol.* 74: 1785–1788.

17 Olsson, M. and Lindhe, J. (1991 Jan). Periodontal characteristics in individuals with varying form of the upper central incisors. *Journal of clinical periodontology.* 18 (1): 78–82.

18 De Rouck, T., Eghbali, R., Collys, K. et al. (2009 May). The gingival biotype revisited: transparency of the periodontal probe through the gingival margin as a method to discriminate thin from thick gingiva. *J. Clin. Periodontol.* 36 (5): 428–433.

19 Evans, C.D.J. and Chen, S.T. (2008). Esthetic outcomes of immediate implant placements. *Clin. Oral Implants Res.* 19: 73–80.

20 Kan, J.Y.K., Rungcharassaeng, K., and Lozada, J. (2003). Immediate placement and provisionalization of maxillary anterior single implants: 1-year prospective study. *Int. J. Oral Maxillofac. Implants* 18: 31–39.

21 Kois, J.C. (2004 Nov). Predictable single-tooth peri-implant esthetics: five diagnostic keys. *Compendium* 25 (11): 895.

22 Jung, R.E., Sailer, I., Hämmerle, C.H. et al. (2007). in vitro color changes of soft tissues caused by restorative materials. *Int. J. Periodontics Restorative Dent.* 27 (3): 251.

24

The Use of Provisionalisation in Implantology

Christopher C.K. Ho

24.1   Principles

A provisional restoration is defined as a fixed or removable dental prosthesis designed to enhance aesthetics, stabilisation, and/or function for a limited period of time, after which it is to be replaced by a definitive dental prosthesis.

Provisionals may serve the following functions in implant dentistry:

- They provide temporary aesthetic and masticatory function during grafting procedures or during the osseointegration phase.
- They help prosthetic guidance of soft tissue maturation for optimal gingival architecture.
- *Occlusion and positional stability*: Inter-arch and intra-arch relationships are maintained through both proximal and occlusal contacts, preventing tipping, drifting, and supra-eruption during integration procedures.
- *Diagnostic tool*: Through the duplication of the wax-up (analogue or digital) a preview of intended aesthetic, occlusal, phonetic, and occlusal vertical dimension changes is provided. This allows adequate opportunity for the patient to receive a trial prototype to gain acceptance and approval. This is an important step when preparing multiple anterior implant or full arch restorations, as the patient may need time to get used to the changes planned. It is the author's opinion the patient should be given time to assess before any modifications that may be required are undertaken.

The objective of this chapter is to outline the use of provisionals to prosthetically guide soft tissue healing and to improve the soft tissue aesthetics around implant restorations.

24.1.1   Prosthetically Guided Tissue Healing

In non-submerged healing, traditional healing abutments with a circular diameter result in a soft tissue profile that is not natural compared to teeth, which have either triangular or oval cross-sectional profiles. The use of

Practical Procedures in Implant Dentistry, First Edition. Edited by Christopher C.K. Ho.
© 2022 John Wiley & Sons Ltd. Published 2022 by John Wiley & Sons Ltd.
Companion website: www.wiley.com/go/ho/implant-dentistry

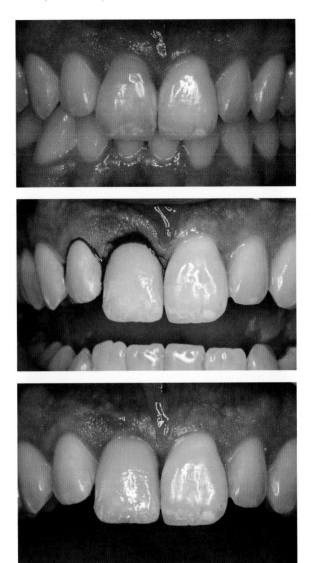

Figure 24.1 Immediate implant placement and provisionalisation. The maxillary central incisor was atraumatically extracted followed by immediate provisionalisation. This was slightly under-contoured on the labial to allow coronal creep of the mid-labial margin. The soft tissue architecture was maintained for an aesthetic final restoration with natural appearing peri-implant tissues.

provisional restorations may enhance the peri-implant architecture by establishing the proper contours, and provide an emergence allowing proper support of the interdental tissues and the labial tissue contour. It is possible to modify provisional restoration contours by adding or subtracting material to the provisional, and moulding the soft tissue into the form required. The peri-implant soft tissues can be likened to a balloon filled with fluid; placing pressure on one region of the balloon will displace fluid into another region, helping to shape the contours into the desired form. In cases where there is an abundance of gingival tissue, adding to the labial contour of the restoration may cause the tissue to recede; conversely, if the mid-labial gingival margin is more apical, the clinician may reduce the contour by slightly under-contouring the restoration, allowing tissues to creep coronally. Once the correct contours have been established, the final impression can be specially customised to replicate the contours in the final restoration (Figure 24.1).

Su et al. [1] describes the importance of correctly contoured restorations transitioning from the implant prosthetic connection to the anatomically correct dimensions of the tooth. Implant restorations can be described as over-contoured, flat, or under-contoured. They describe two distinct zones within the implant abutment and crown defined as critical contour and subcritical contour. The *critical contour* is the most superficial area influencing the gingival level and zenith location, whereas the *subcritical contour* corresponds to the deeper area and influences the peri-implant soft tissue support and, consequently, the gingival colour (Table 24.1). Over-contouring the critical contour will generally cause apical positioning of the gingival margin, while under-contouring will may allow the opposite effect of allowing coronal movement of the margin. In contrast, alteration of the subcritical contour within a physiological range may not affect the gingival margin level. However, there may be the opportunity with minor to moderate ridge concavities of 1.5–2 mm to compensate for the concavity by increasing facial convexity of this subcritical contour by adding materials to this region. It is important to ensure thorough polishing of this subcritical contour to minimise contamination and plaque accumulation which may enhance epithelial cell adhesion. The adding of restorative material can be performed sequentially as required, allowing an interval of greater than two weeks to allow healing and revascularisation. If required, further modifications can be made until a time that the restorative clinician is happy.

The interdental papilla is an anatomic feature that is difficult to recreate surgically, especially once lost or with adjacent implants. Numerous surgical techniques have been developed, but it remains an elusive task to recreate papillae with any predictability. Adjusting the subcritical contour by adding a convex contour interproximally can be used to enhance the papillary height by 0.5–1.0 mm (Table 24.2). If it is not possible to achieve complete fill of the

Table 24.1 Clinical guidelines for contour management of facial tissues around provisional restorations.

Facial tissues	Coronal gingival margin level	Ideal gingival margin level	Apical gingival margin level
Critical contour	Over-contour in facial/apical direction	Maintain same as natural tooth	Under-contour in a facial direction
Subcritical contour	Flat or slightly concave	Flat or slightly concave	Increase convexity

Source: Adapted from González-Martín, O., Lee, E., Weisgold, A. et al. (2020). Contour management of implant restorations for optimal emergence profiles: Guidelines for immediate and delayed provisional restorations. Int. J. Periodontics Restorative Dent. 40(1): 61–70.

Table 24.2 Clinical guidelines for height management of interdental papilla tissues around provisional restorations.

Interproximal papilla	Preserved	Slightly deficient
Critical contour	Equal to natural tooth	Equal to natural tooth
Subcritical contour	Equal to natural tooth	Increase convexity

Source: Adapted from Gonzalez-Martin et al. (2020).

interdental papilla it may be possible to add restorative material on adjacent teeth, as well as making the implant restoration with a longer contact point and squarer emergence profile, effectively closing the interdental space.

24.2 Procedures

Provisional restorations can be fabricated directly chairside or indirectly in a laboratory.

There is a diverse spectrum of materials used for the fabrication of provisional restorations including:

- Preformed crowns (resin, plastic or metal)
- Self-cured or light-cured resin
- Self-cured or heat-cured acrylic
- Metal, e.g. Iso-Form® crowns – tin/silver alloy; stainless steel crowns – nickel chrome.

24.2.1 Direct Techniques

The majority of provisional restorations are fabricated chairside directly in the patient's mouth. The techniques commonly used include the following:

- Shell crowns can be made from custom or stock shells relined with resin and trimmed and polished.
- Matrices are the most common provisionals as they duplicate the external contours of teeth that are being prepared or from a diagnostic wax-up. They are usually formed by alginate, or silicone, or vacuum-formed thermoplastic materials (Figure 24.2).
- Use of denture teeth or existing restorations.
- Direct freehand buildup may be possible by adding material and sculpting and trimming/polishing.

24.2.2 Indirect Techniques

It is possible to make an impression of the implant and have the model poured up to make a provisional. This adds to the cost but has several advantages, including using a material that may be stronger and more durable. It may be also used in multiple restorations and where an increase in vertical dimension or changes in occlusal scheme is planned.

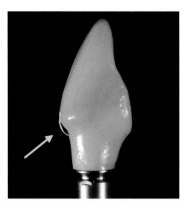

Figure 24.2 Adding resin (yellow) in this critical contour region to over-contour may displace the gingival margin apically.

24.3 Tips

- The use of provisional restorations when treating all anterior teeth in the arch is an opportunity to provide the patient with a 'trial smile'. Hence, it is clinically significant to have a range of shades for your provisional material of choice, in order to demonstrate the shade selected for approval.
- It is advisable to inform the patient of the correct 'flossing technique' around a provisional restorations to ensure optimal peri-implant soft tissue health prior to final impressions.
- In cases lacking volume of interdental papillae, it may be possible to modify the contact points of the restoration by elongating them and bringing the contact point more apically. Additionally, the dental ceramist may be able to use porcelain wings on the restoration, shading them darker to give the illusion that the tooth still has the same line angles and dimensions as a natural tooth (Figure 24.3).

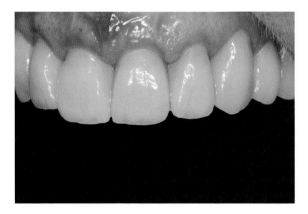

Figure 24.3 Patient with missing interdental papillae. Note the interproximal staining undertaken to close any embrasure space and minimising 'black holes', with staining accentuating the line angles visually, ensuring teeth appear the correct shape.

Reference

1 Su, H., Gonzalez-Martin, O., Weisgold, A., and Lee, E. (2010). Considerations of implant abutment and crown contour: critical contour and subcritical contour. *Int J Periodontics Restorative Dent.* 30 (4): 335–343.

25

Abutment Selection

Christopher C.K. Ho

25.1 Principles

An abutment is an intermediary component inserted onto the implant, with the restoration then seated over the abutment. It is retained in place with an abutment screw. An abutment provides the retention, support, and final position of a restoration (Figure 25.1).

The abutment can be constructed as a two-piece combination consisting of the abutment and restoration, with the latter being cemented into place, or as a one-piece type consisting of an abutment/restoration screwed into place as one unit. Abutments are generally available either as prefabricated (stock) abutments from the implant manufacturers or customised for the patient using computer-aided-design/computer-aided-manufacturing (CAD/CAM) or alternatively cast in a dental laboratory (Figure 25.2). Prefabricated abutments are less expensive and relatively easy to use, but have limitations because they are not customised. A customised abutment is made to specifically fit to the implant position, taking into consideration the adjacent teeth, soft tissues, and general contours.

Situations that may require a custom abutment include the following:

- Angle correction is greater than 15 degrees, then the abutment can be used to correct the implant angulation.
- There is minimal inter-occlusal space. The abutment height should not exceed the space required for the restorative material.
- Splinted multiple units are being used to allow parallelism.
- There is a requirement to replicate the anatomical cross-sectional profile of teeth.
- Collar height greater than 1 mm above the largest collar height of a stock abutment is needed. This allows easier clearance of cement. Abutment margins should be supragingival in non-aesthetic zones and slightly subgingival in the aesthetic zone.
- Interproximal distance is required. The abutment width must be sufficient to support the crown but must also possess adequate interproximal access for hygiene maintenance.

Practical Procedures in Implant Dentistry, First Edition. Edited by Christopher C.K. Ho.
© 2022 John Wiley & Sons Ltd. Published 2022 by John Wiley & Sons Ltd.
Companion website: www.wiley.com/go/ho/implant-dentistry

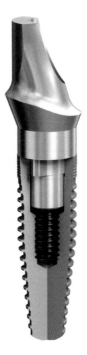

Figure 25.1 Implant and prefabricated titanium abutment (Esthetic Abutment, Nobel Biocare). Note that the margins are available with different collar heights to fit to the various marginal positioning. *Source:* Esthetic abutment, Nobel Biocare Services AG.

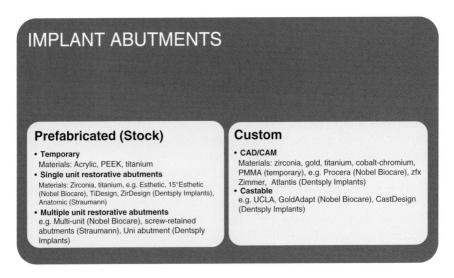

IMPLANT ABUTMENTS

Prefabricated (Stock)

- **Temporary**
  Materials: Acrylic, PEEK, titanium
- **Single unit restorative abutments**
  Materials: Zirconia, titanium, e.g. Esthetic, 15°Esthetic (Nobel Biocare), TiDesign, ZirDesign (Dentsply Implants), Anatomic (Straumann)
- **Multiple unit restorative abutments**
  e.g. Multi-unit (Nobel Biocare), screw-retained abutments (Straumann), Uni abutment (Dentsply Implants)

Custom

- **CAD/CAM**
  Materials: zirconia, gold, titanium, cobalt-chromium, PMMA (temporary), e.g. Procera (Nobel Biocare), zfx Zimmer, Atlantis (Dentsply Implants)
- **Castable**
  e.g. UCLA, GoldAdapt (Nobel Biocare), CastDesign (Dentsply Implants)

Figure 25.2 Descriptions of the various implant abutments available.

The final choice between a custom abutment and prefabricated abutment depends on the clinical situation, the practitioner's experience, and preference [1].

25.1.1   Custom Abutments

Custom abutments are used in situations where stock abutments cannot be used to correct angulations, and to provide an ideal anatomical profile and customised marginal position of a restoration.

These are fabricated using either wax-ups and casting or computer-generated designs:

- Castable abutments are waxed up to the required contours and customised for the restorative space. These techniques require waxing, investing, and casting with alloys at high temperature. This is labour intensive and subsequently costly. Custom abutments made of gold alloy, known as UCLA abutments, were very popular and widely used. Technicians used the lost wax technique to wax up the abutment to the correct contours and then cast it in gold, with the final finishing performed manually.
- Computer-generated abutments (Figure 25.3), e.g. NobelProcera® (Nobel Biocare), Atlantis® (Dentsply), CARES® (Straumann). The use of CAD/CAM technology was developed in the 1980s. Further developments have allowed digital impression taking, scanning, milling abutments, and restorations with great accuracy and precision. Conventional techniques rely on the accuracy of many steps, with impression taking, investment materials, wax, and casting, all of which can lead to errors. CAD/CAM abutments have the potential to provide the most accurate fit due to minimal manipulation after milling. This is particularly useful in implant dentistry where precision is crucial for fit, longevity, distribution of stress, ease of insertion, and long-term success.

25.1.2   Prefabricated (Stock) Abutments

Prefabricated (stock) abutments are available from implant manufacturers and are either used intact or further modified by the dentist or dental technician. They are available with various anatomical cross-sections and alignment for common clinical scenarios. It is advised to place the marginal design of an

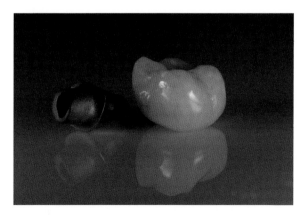

Figure 25.3 Customised titanium abutment with monolithic all ceramic (zirconia) crown.

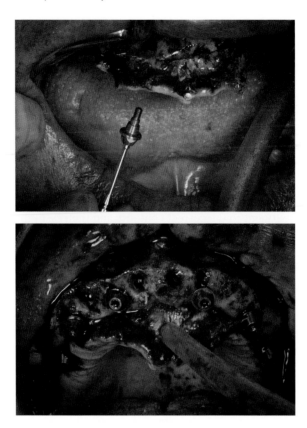

Figure 25.4 Multi-unit abutments (Screw-Retained Abutments; Straumann) are often used for partially and fully edentulous solutions). This allows the prosthetic platform to be located supracrestally as well as allowing for any divergence in implant positioning due to the 20 degree taper that allows implants to be divergent even up to 40 degrees.

abutment equigingival, or in a position that can be accessed if cementing a restoration due to the possibility of cement being left and undetected when a margin is placed deep subgingivally. Linkevicius et al. [2] reported that the amount of residual cement left is increased as margins are located more subgingivally, and at 2–3 mm subgingival the residual cement is 10x that of margins that are either equigingival or 1 mm subgingival.

Available prefabricated abutments include:

- Temporary abutments made of plastic, polyether ether ketone (PEEK), or titanium materials. These are often used to prosthetically guide soft tissue healing for improved soft tissue contours, progressive and immediate loading, or for assessing occlusion and phonetics in a more complex rehabilitation.
- Multiple unit abutments, e.g. Multi-Unit Abutments (Nobel Biocare), Uni Abutments (Dentsply Implants), are used in partially or fully edentulous patients (Figure 25.4). These components may allow movement of the restorative platform to a location that is not so deep subgingivally, allowing simpler insertion and removal of a prosthesis. In addition, these multiple

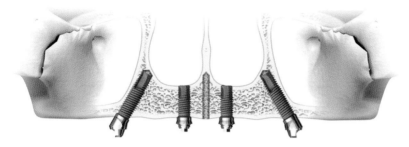

Figure 25.5 All on Four® Treatment concept (Nobel Biocare). Anterior implants have straight multi-unit abutments while posterior implants have angulated abutments correcting the access for the prosthetic screws. *Source:* Nobel Biocare Services AG.

unit abutments have a taper that allows for divergent implant alignments such as seen in the fully edentulous maxilla, where implants may be splayed buccall. For example, if the multi-unit abutments have a taper of 20 degrees, then using two multi-unit abutments may allow up to 40 degrees divergence between the implants. Inserting and removing an implant without use of these more tapered abutments may be difficult due to the nature of the internal connections.

- Angulated abutments are used to correct angulations in cases where implants are inserted intentionally at an angle, as in All on Four® Treatment Concept (Nobel Biocare) (Figure 25.5), or to allow for screw access in multiple unit cases. They are available in a number of different angulations allowing for correction of the prosthetic screw access.

25.1.3   Material Selection

Materials commonly used for abutments are zirconia, titanium, and gold. Other materials used are PEEK and other metals, such as cobalt-chrome. Historically, gold abutments were the 'gold standard' and considered to be aesthetically acceptable with good mechanical properties. However, it is now known that gold alloys are difficult to cast precisely and have poorer biocompatibility along with high costs. Welander et al. [3] found that epithelium did not attach to a gold alloy abutment, resulting in bone loss and recession. Gold abutments are fabricated using casting procedures whereas zirconia and titanium abutments are milled to the correct shape and contours. The success of these materials is dependent on the correct handling and case selection. Sailer et al. [4], in a systematic review of 29 studies on single and fixed partial dentures, found the estimated five-year survival for ceramic and metal abutments was 99.1% and 97.4%, respectively. In a randomised controlled trial comparing zirconia and titanium abutments in canine and posterior areas, Zembic et al. [5] found survival rates for both materials at 100% after five years in function.

A study by Abrahamson et al. [6] found abutments made of commercially pure titanium or ceramic allowed the formation of a mucosal attachment which included epithelial and connective tissue portions that were about 2 mm and 1–1.5 mm high, respectively. At sites where abutments were made of gold alloy or dental porcelain, no proper attachment formed at the abutment level, but the soft tissue margin receded and bone resorption occurred. The abutment fixture junction was thus occasionally exposed with the mucosal barrier established to the implant and not the abutment. This was confirmed by Welander et al. [3], who demonstrated that the soft tissue dimensions at Ti and ZrO_2 abutments remained stable between two and five months of healing. At Au/Pt alloy abutment sites, however, an apical shift of the barrier epithelium and the marginal bone occurred between two and five months of healing. Studies have shown that there is no significant difference between the two abutment materials in relation to collagen fibre orientation and mucosal attachment. Surface roughness of materials should be around $0.2\,\mu m$ [7], which is a similar roughness to that found on machined surfaces.

Zirconia is an inert, structurally stable material and recommended in the anterior zone for optimal aesthetics, improving both the optical characteristics of the white and pink aesthetics especially when the gingival thickness is <2 mm (Figure 25.6). Furthermore, zirconia abutments provide excellent biocompatibility and mechanical properties [8]. A minimal wall thickness of 0.8 mm is recommended to avoid fractures. If the access hole of the restoration is in closer proximity to the adjacent teeth, the weaker the walls and the greater the possibility of a fracture. In addition, zirconia materials are less prone to bacterial adhesion [9, 10], which may benefit from less peri-implant problems. Review of the selected articles [4, 5] suggests that zirconia abutments are reliable in the

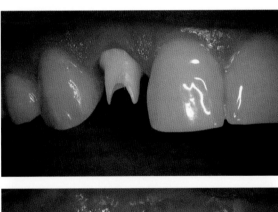

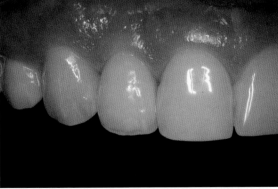

Figure 25.6 Zirconia abutment inserted and final all-ceramic crown.

anterior region both biologically and mechanically. Furthermore, zirconia abutments may represent a material surface less attractive for early plaque retention compared to titanium [11]. This has been thought to be due to zirconia having a very low surface free energy compared with other materials, which is why bacteria do not adhere to the surface [12].

There has been recent controversy regarding how smooth the zirconia abutment should be within the soft tissues, with both fibroblast and epithelial cells behaving differently on smooth and rough substrates. Nothdurft et al. [13] found that polished zirconia surfaces provide better adhesion for epithelial cells compared to titanium surfaces. Epithelial cells adhere to zirconia with hemi-desmosomal attachments but do not adhere to glazed porcelain surfaces, and it is recommended that no glazing is used on the subgingival portion of the prosthetic restoration. It is best to leave the subgingival portions of a zirconia abutment as polished zirconia without any veneering material.

25.1.4 Abutment Design

The fabrication of an abutment retaining the restoration is crucial to provide support for pink aesthetics framing the restoration and an integral factor in providing ideal white aesthetics. The submucosal portion of the prosthesis shapes the soft tissue contour and emergence profile. Historically, abutment design was oversized around the implant–abutment interface. This can place excessive pressure on the surrounding tissues and may lead to crestal bone loss. Contemporary concepts of abutment design are to create an abutment that is as narrow as possible without weakening the properties of the abutment. This narrower emergence from the implants would be more concave and divergent transmucosally, widening out coronally to the emergence that replicates the diameter of the tooth being replaced (Figure 25.7). The 'o-ring' or 'donut' of soft tissue allows thicker tissue around an abutment, providing better stability. It is often termed an 'S-shaped' contour, running from the implant platform to the

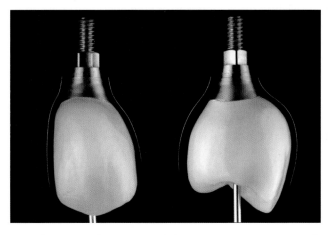

Figure 25.7 Correctly contoured emergence of abutments are more concave, allowing increased tissue thickness for stability, aesthetics, and tissue health. *Source:* Photograph courtesy of Dr. David Attia.

emergence profile. Furthermore, platform switching of implants along with the concave shape at the implant–abutment interface ensures greater peri-implant tissue thickness and tissue stability.

25.2 Procedures

1) After the impression has been taken a model is constructed within the laboratory or, if a digital impression is taken, the file is exported as an STL for a model to be fabricated.
2) The dentist and dental technician must decide whether to use a custom or a prefabricated abutment.
3) The use of a prefabricated abutment requires information on the size of the implant platform, and also a decision on the profile of the abutment. Many different shaped profiles are offered by manufacturers to allow for different emergence profiles. These abutments may also have different angulations to allow for different alignments of implant positions. Additionally, many of these abutments have different collar heights, placing the margin in a more appropriate position for cementation.
4) Preparation of prefabricated abutments can be performed for the most part extra-orally, although some clinicians prefer to place the prefabricated abutment onto an implant and prepare the abutment intra-orally, placing a retraction cord and then taking an impression as in a conventional crown preparation (i.e. abutment level impression).
5) Insertion of the abutment or a screw-retained one-piece abutment/crown requires removal of the healing abutment and irrigation of the implant connection. The author advises the use of a chlorhexidine gel to disinfect the connection before placing the abutment onto the implant. It is prudent to warn the patient that there may be some pressure on the soft tissues as the restoration is inserted, especially if there has been no guiding or moulding of the tissues with a provisional restoration. This is the result of tissue compression from the transition from a circular healing abutment to a correctly profiled restoration. This discomfort will gradually resolve over a few minutes, but if there is excessive tissue impingement then the subgingival profile of the abutment may require adjustment if it is over-contoured. If left, this could lead to tissue necrosis and gingival recession with possible bone loss.
6) After the abutment has been hand tightened it is customary to take a radiograph to ensure complete seating of the abutment.
7) Once it has been confirmed that the abutment is completely seated the abutment is torqued to the correct level as recommended by the implant manufacturer with the appropriate instrumentation.

25.3 Tips

- In the aesthetic zone where the tissue is a thin or the implant is superficially placed it may be advisable to use a zirconia abutment to allow improved aesthetics, especially if there is any tissue recession [14].

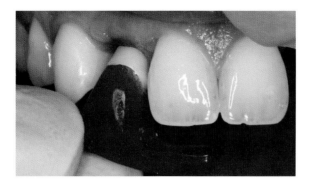

Figure 25.8 Location jig to allow correct placement of the implant abutment. This may be useful when dealing with multiple abutments with different positions when using cemented restoration.

- The insertion of abutments for a cemented restoration may be simpler with the use of an insertion jig, which orientates the correct position of the abutment in relation to the adjacent teeth (Figure 25.8).
- Zirconia abutments have certain dimensional requirements for sufficient mechanical properties. If an abutment is <0.8 mm or where the abutment height is too short <3 mm zirconia materials may be contraindicated. The dimensions of mandibular incisors and maxillary lateral incisors are often narrow, and in these situations metal abutments may be indicated. Furthermore, a clinician must plan treatment to use these ceramic abutments appropriately; if there is excessive parafunction or crown:implant ratio a metal abutment may be selected.
- Full zirconia abutments engaging into internal connection implants have been reported to be more susceptible to fracture; hence titanium bases have been developed to minimise fracture, reducing the potential for zirconia to be placed into tension within the conus of internal connection implants.
- Additional care should be exercised when using titanium bases. The restoration should be checked for proper contacts and occlusion prior to final torquing. Tight proximal contacts may hold the crown in a position that does not allow it to fully seat onto the implant. When the torque driver is used, it pulls the titanium base down with the screw, essentially pulling the abutment from the crown and breaking the cement bond. This may lead to failure of the restoration either immediately or, more often, at a later date. The dentist may not be aware and the restoration may loosen over time.
- Over-contouring of an abutment has the effect of placing pressure on soft tissues; this may subsequently result in recession. Special caution should be undertaken in design of the labial region of anterior abutments to ensure that there are no deleterious consequences. The contour is more concave to allow more soft tissue thickness and stability around the abutments.

References

1 Giglio, G. (1999). Abutment selection in implant supported fixed prosthodontics. *Int J Periodontics Restorative Dent* 19: 233–241.

2 Linkevicius, T., Vindasiute, E., Puisys, A., and Peciuliene, V. (2011). The influence of margin location on the amount of undetected cement excess after delivery of cement-retained implant restorations. *Clin. Oral Implants Res.* 22 (12): 1379–1384.

3 Welander, M., Abrahamsson, I., and Berglundh, T. (2008). The mucosal barrier at implant abutments of different materials. *Clin. Oral Implants Res.* 19 (7): 635–641.

4 Sailer, I., Philipp, A., Zembic, A. et al. (2009 Sep). A systematic review of the performance of ceramic and metal implant abutments supporting fixed implant reconstructions. *Clin. Oral Implants Res.* 20 (Suppl 4): 4–31.

5 Zembic, A., Philipp, A.O., Hämmerle, C.H. et al. (2015 Oct). Eleven-year follow-up of a prospective study of zirconia implant abutments supporting single all-ceramic crowns in anterior and premolar regions. *Clin. Implant. Dent. Relat. Res.* 17 (Suppl 2): e417–e426.

6 Abrahamsson, I., Berglundh, T., Glantz, P.O., and Lindhe, J. (1998). The mucosal attachment at different abutments. An experimental study in dogs. *J. Clin. Periodontol.* 25 (9): 721–727.

7 Happe, A. and Körner, G. (2011). Biologic interfaces in esthetic dentistry. Part II: the peri-implant/restorative interface. *Eur. J. Esthet. Dent.* 6 (2): 226–251.

8 Nakamura, K., Kanno, T., Milleding, P., and Ortengren, U. (2010). Zirconia as a dental implant abutment material: a systematic review. *Int. J. Prosthodont.* 23 (4): 299–309.

9 Scarano, A., Piattelli, M., Caputi, S. et al. (2004). Bacterial adhesion on commercially pure titanium and zirconium oxide disks: an in vivo human study. *J. Periodontol.* 75 (2): 292–296.

10 Rimondini, L., Cerroni, L., Carrassi, A., and Torriceni, P. (2002 Nov 1). Bacterial colonization of zirconia ceramic surfaces: an in vitro and in vivo study. *Int. J. Oral Maxillofac. Implants* 17 (6).

11 van Brakel, R., Cune, M.S., van Winkelhoff, A.J. et al. (2011 Jun). Early bacterial colonization and soft tissue health around zirconia and titanium abutments: an in vivo study in man. *Clin. Oral Implants Res.* 22 (6): 571–577.

12 Poortinga, A.T., Bos, R., and Busscher, H.J. (2001). Charge transfer during staphylococcal adhesion to TiNOX® coatings with different specific resistivity. *Biophys. Chem.* 91 (3): 273–279.

13 Nothdurft, F.P., Fontana, D., Ruppenthal, S. et al. (2015). Differential behavior of fibroblasts and epithelial cells on structured implant abutment materials: a comparison of materials and surface topographies. *Clin. Implants Dent. Res.* 17 (6): 1237–1249.

14 Jung, R.E., Sailer, I., Hämmerle, C.H. et al. (2007). in vitro color changes of soft tissues caused by restorative materials. *Int J Periodontics Restorative Dent* 27 (3): 251–257.

26

Screw versus Cemented Implant-Supported Restorations

Christopher C.K. Ho

26.1 Principles

An implant-supported restoration can be inserted onto an implant either by attaching it with screws or by cementing it onto abutments that have been secured by screws. There are advantages and disadvantages of both types of retention, and the decision whether to screw-retain or cement a restoration is often dependent on the implant position and clinician preference [1].

The factors that determine the decision on whether to screw-retain or cement a restoration are outlined in this chapter.

26.1.1 Retrievability

Screw retention allows the restoration to be removed for repair, prosthetic modifications, or soft tissue inspection, and creates access for hygiene if required. Many clinicians prefer to treat implant restorations in the same way as conventional crown and bridgework, cementing the final restoration and then, if there is any maintenance required, such as screw loosening, the restoration can be removed and replaced accordingly. The incidence of screw loosening has diminished with improved screw joint mechanics and connections; however, it may still occur. When abutment screws loosen, cement-retained restorations are not always predictably removed from abutments to allow screws to be re-tightened, and hence the restoration may need removal. This would destroy the restoration and render it unusable. Thus, it would be prudent and simpler to manage if the restorations were planned for screw retention so that if a problem did occur the restoration could be accessed through the screw hole, removed, and tightened. Additionally, as the complexity of the restoration increases along with the number of units, the expense of remaking an extensive restoration becomes untenable for the patient. This makes retrievability paramount.

Practical Procedures in Implant Dentistry, First Edition. Edited by Christopher C.K. Ho.
© 2022 John Wiley & Sons Ltd. Published 2022 by John Wiley & Sons Ltd.
Companion website: www.wiley.com/go/ho/implant-dentistry

26.1.2 Aesthetics

Screw retention requires a screw access hole to be made through the restoration. This is normally filled with composite resin once the restoration is in place (Figure 26.1). In the anterior region, screw retention may not be possible due to implant position, because having a screw access in a visible area, such as the labial surface of a maxillary incisor, is unacceptable. When screw access sites are in aesthetic areas, they can be realigned with use of angulated abutments or angulated screws. Alternatively the restoration should be retained with custom abutments and cemented. Screw-retained restorations can only be used when the trajectory of the implant allows the screw access to be in non-aesthetic areas. Some clinicians prefer to avoid having a hole in the restoration that is restored with composite resin, as this may wear and discolour over time. Furthermore, to achieve screw retention in the anterior region often involves aligning the implant slightly more palatally in the anterior maxilla to allow screw access in the cingulum area, which often leaves a ridge lap or unaesthetic crown.

26.1.3 Passivity

A passive fit is desirable for implant restorations as stress on an implant may overload the prosthesis, causing a technical complication. This may also lead to strain between the bone interface and the implant, resulting in peri-implant bony changes. It is said that one of the advantages of cement-retained restorations is that frameworks are more passive because the abutments are individually retained to the implants by screws and the restoration is cemented over the abutments. This cement space is said to allow for passivity because the cement

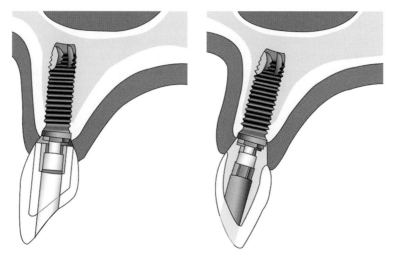

Figure 26.1 Screw-retained crowns need an access hole on the cingulum area to enable access to the screw. The image on the right shows alignment of the implant with the screw access leaving a hole on the labial surface of the crown. This would not be acceptable and would necessitate a cement-on crown.

acts as a shock absorber and reduces stress on the bone and implant interface. There is very little evidence to support this theory. Impression taking and handling of the casts are crucial to minimise errors and the advent of computer-aided-design/computer-aided-manufacturing (CAD/CAM) milling has eliminated many of the errors from casting and metalwork. Due to the passive fit with cemented restorations, there is a belief that there is less fatigue and fracture of componentry. It is believed that if there are overloading forces on the restoration then the cement layer fails first, thereby saving the implant and restoration from failure.

26.1.4   Hygiene (Emergence Profile)

To achieve screw access in maxillary anterior implant restorations it may be necessary to align an implant in a more palatal trajectory. This may leave the implant more palatally placed, especially in a resorbed alveolar ridge, and may give the final restoration a ridge lap which makes it more difficult to clean effectively or may lead to an unaesthetic appearance (Figure 26.2).

26.1.5   Reduced Occlusal Material Fracture

A screw-retained restoration will have a screw access hole, which disrupts the structural continuity of the porcelain, leaving some unsupported porcelain at the screw access hole. Cemented restorations are one-piece without any weakening of the structure of the crown. However, if veneering porcelain chips or fractures off an implant restoration in a screw-retained restoration, it would be a relatively simple procedure to remove and carry out an indirect repair on the implant restoration.

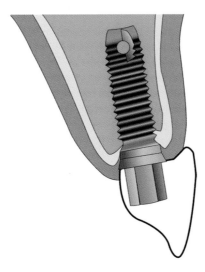

Figure 26.2 To achieve screw retention in the anterior region may involve aligning the implant slightly more palatally in the anterior maxilla to allow screw access in the cingulum area, which may leave a ridge lap or unaesthetic crown.

26.1.6 Inter-arch Space

A cemented restoration requires sufficient axial wall height to allow for retention form, and in those situations where there is limited inter-arch space it may not be possible to achieve adequate retention for a cemented restoration. However, screw-retained restorations can be secured to implants with as little as 4 mm of space from the platform of the implant to the opposing teeth.

26.1.7 Occlusion

In a cement-retained restoration there are no screw access holes that may interfere with occlusal stops or excursive movements. Often composite resin is used to cover access channels and these materials are susceptible to wear under functional forces. Occlusal contacts are preserved with cement-retained restorations.

26.1.8 Health of Peri-Implant Tissue

Incomplete removal of cement may result in peri-implant inflammation, soft tissue swelling, bleeding, and/or suppuration and eventual resorption of peri-implant bone [2]. It has been shown that even experienced practitioners can leave a surprising amount of cement remnants and scratching of abutments are observed when removing cement from subgingival margins around implants [3]. The use of screw retention or a customised abutment with the margins placed supra-gingivally or equi-gingivally is recommended to minimise trapping of cement. Linkevicius et al. [4] noted that the deeper the position of the margin, the greater the amount of undetected cement in a cemented restoration. They also reported that dental radiographs should not be considered a reliable method for detecting cement.

26.1.9 Provisionalisation

Provisional restorations may be used for immediate loading, as well as to achieve better aesthetics by developing a proper emergence profile by guiding soft tissue contours during healing. It is preferred to use a screw-retained rather than a cement-retained restoration as the screw can be used to seat the provisional restoration and expand the peri-implant mucosa. It can also be very difficult to remove excess cement and manage bleeding while seating a cemented provisional crown during implant surgery.

26.1.10 Clinical Performance

Sailer et al. [5] conducted a systematic review on the five-year survival and complication rates of cemented and screw-retained implant reconstructions and found that cement-retained reconstructions exhibited more serious biological complications. They found that 2.8% of patients had a marginal bone loss of >2 mm in cement-retained crowns as compared with 0% for screw-retained crowns. However, the screw-retained reconstructions exhibited more technical problems, with an estimated five-year incidence of technical complications of 24.4% compared with 11.9% for cement-retained crowns. They concluded that cemented reconstructions exhibited more serious biological complications (implant loss, bone loss >2 mm), while screw-retained reconstructions exhibited more technical problems. Screw-retained reconstructions are easier to retrieve than cemented reconstructions and, therefore, technical and eventually biological complications can be treated more easily.

Wittneben et al. [6] in a longer systematic review over 12 years found no statistical difference between cement and screw-retained reconstructions for survival or failure rates, although screw-retained reconstructions exhibited fewer technical and biologic complications overall.

26.2 Procedures

There has been a shift towards screw-retained restorations and away from cement-retained restorations (Table 26.1), mainly because of *in vitro* and clinical studies showing that it was impossible to remove all the cement around subgingival margins, with the deeper the margin the more cement left. This may be an additional predisposing factor for peri-implantitis. Retrievability is a key advantage of screw-retained restorations. They allow prosthodontic components to be adjusted, screws to be re-tightened, and fractured ceramics to be repaired, while removing cement-retained prostheses normally leads to destruction of the prosthesis. Cemented restorations are considered to fit more passively because the cement layer compensates for discrepancies and absorbs the strain of the deformation generated by any mismatch between the abutment and the implant.

26.2.1 Screw-Retained Restoration

There are two types of screw-retained restorations used in recent times: a hybrid cement/screw-retained restoration (titanium base) and a pure screw-retained restoration (single-piece assembly with no abutment). The hybrid cement/

Table 26.1 A comparison between cement- and screw-retained resorations.

Comparison	Cement	Screw
Retrievability	?	++
Aesthetics	+	
Passive casting	+	
Hygiene (emergence profile in anterior)	+	
Reduced occlusal material fracture	+	
Decreased fatigue/fracture of components	+	
Limited inter-arch space: low profile retention		+
No cement in sulcus		+

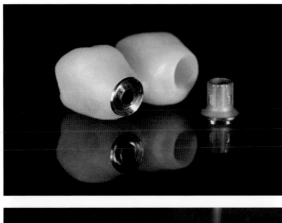

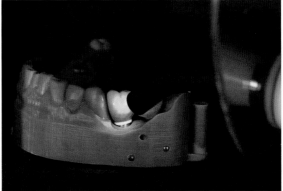

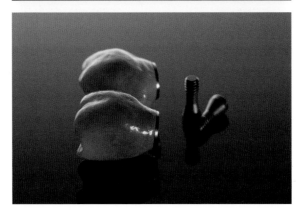

Figure 26.3 The hybrid cement/screw restorations involve a restoration being cemented onto a titanium base.

screw-retained crown combines features of both cement and screw-retained restorations; the restoration is finished by cementing it to a titanium base on the laboratory cast and is then screw-retained intra-orally (Figure 26.3). This ensures a passive fit because there is a layer of cement and yet still allows retrievability due to the access screw. This method is becoming increasingly popular with

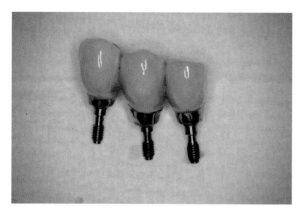

Figure 26.4 One-piece screw-retained restorations with the veneering porcelain built up on a customised gold abutments.

reduced economic costs and time-saving reductions of CAD/CAM production. Nevertheless, it must be remembered that the hybrid model is similar to a cement-retained prosthesis in that the cement holds the restoration to the titanium base. There are conflicting reports on surface treatment. Some authors recommend that the titanium bases should be micromechanically roughened with particle abrasion using aluminium oxide particles [7]; others suggest that the airborne particle abrasion decreases the retentive strength of the zirconia copings [8]. The use of 10-methacryloyloxydecyl dihydrogen phosphate (MDP) monomer may increase retention of zirconia to the titanium bases [7], enhancing the strength of the chemical bond. There have been reports of the titanium base debonding from the restoration and there may be contraindications to their use in some cases, such as a long crown restoration where there may be a biomechanical disadvantage because it acts as a long lever arm. In comparison, a screw-retained restoration is a single piece with the veneering porcelain applied directly onto the abutment with the screw responsible for retention (Figure 26.4).

1) Remove one-piece abutment and crown from the model and disinfect restoration prior to insertion.
2) Remove healing abutment or provisional restoration from the mouth and clean implant platform with disinfectant/water spray. Insert the crown without delay to prevent the soft tissue collapsing and making it more difficult to insert.
3) Try-in restoration by hand-tightening restoration until the screw fully seats. The restoration may not seat fully because of:
   a) Tight inter-proximal contacts
   b) Lack of seating into internal/external connection
   c) Soft tissue impingement. Ensure no soft tissue tags are caught within the connection. If there is too much tissue blanching where the emergence profile of the subgingival contours are over-contoured then this may be adjusted. Usually within five minutes the tissue blanching should disappear, however if there is still blanching then this will require adjustment. This principle also applies to pontic spaces for implant-supported bridgework.

4) Check the functional occlusion and confirm with the patient that they are happy with the aesthetics of the restoration.
5) Once the screw is hand tightened, take a paralleling peri-apical radiograph to check that the restoration is fully seated onto the implant platform.
6) Tighten the restoration to the manufacturer's instructions to the appropriate torque using a torque wrench or other device.
7) Insert a cotton wool pellet, gutta percha, or Teflon tape into the screw access hole on top of the head of the screw to ensure that access can be made through the crown in the future without damage to the head of the screw.
8) Seal off the access hole with a restorative material. In most cases this would be composite resin.
9) Check the final occlusion and function.

26.2.2 Cement-Retained Restoration

1) Remove the separate abutment and crown from the model and disinfect restoration prior to insertion.
2) Remove healing abutment or provisional restoration from the mouth and clean implant platform with disinfectant/water spray.
3) Seat the abutment by ensuring that orientation is correct. If the restoration does not seat fully this may be due to not engaging the connection (often a hex) correctly. Loosen the abutment, carry out a slight rotation to seat, and hand tighten the screw. If there is too much tissue blanching that does not dissipate over five minutes adjust the contours of the abutment accordingly.
4) Once the restoration is fully seated take a radiograph to ensure that there is complete seating.
5) Tighten the abutment to the manufacturer's instructions to the appropriate torque using a torque wrench or other device.
6) Ensure that the restoration is seated completely around the margins. If a restoration does not seat completely it is often tight inter-proximal contacts or soft tissue impingement.
7) Check the functional occlusion and confirm with the patient that they are happy with the aesthetics of the restoration.
8) Cover the access hole in the abutment with a cotton wool pellet, gutta percha, or Teflon tape so that when cementing the restoration no cement gets inadvertently trapped in the screw.
9) Cement the restoration. It is extremely important to stop cement being trapped in the peri-implant sulcus. Ensure that there are no remnants. This is crucial as it may predispose the implant to biological problems.
10) It is recommended the margins of the abutments are placed 1–2 mm subgingivally so that the cement is accessible for removal. The margin should be deep enough to hide the margin, and shallow enough to provide access to keep the cement clean. In an *in vitro* study with abutments designed with various restorative margins, Linkevicius et al. [9] found that it difficult to remove all excess cement after cementation if the margins are located subgingivally, with the deeper the margin the greater the amount of undetected cement. The greatest amount of cement was left when the crown

margin was 2 or 3 mm below the gingival level. Techniques to minimise excess cement trapping subgingivally include the use of retraction cords and use of minimal cement and vent holes in the lingual of the restoration. It may also be difficult to seat a restoration if margins are subgingival as the restoration may not seat fully due to the hydraulic pressure that builds with cement not being able to escape.

11) In a natural tooth the perpendicular periodontal fibres may provide sufficient barrier to cement when cementing a crown, but in implant tissues with the circular fibre attachment this may not possess the protective mechanisms of natural teeth due to the parallel fibre arrangement. The peri-implant tissues may thus be less resistant to pressure and excess cement may be pushed further subgingivally upon cementation. Furthermore, it is difficult to use radiographic examination to detect cement remnants as only cement on the mesial or distal of the implant would be visible on radiographs; buccal and palatal/lingual surfaces are not visible radiographically.

26.2.3 Lateral Set-Screw (Cross-Pinning)

Lateral set-screws have been developed in an attempt to overcome the problems of unpredictable retention and retrievability of implant restorations (Figure 26.5). The screw engages threads in the restoration normally perpendicular to the long axis of the abutment by the set-screw located in a non-aesthetic region (usually lingual surface). This technique allows relatively easy retrieval of the restoration with the screw hole access in a non-aesthetic and/or functional area.

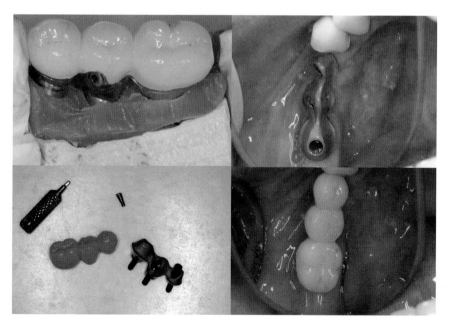

Figure 26.5 Use of lateral set-screw/cross-pin to allow a bridge to be temporarily cemented, enabling retrievability if required.

In some patients there can be difficulty in using this technique because of the angulation of the long axis of the tooth, such as lingual inclination, which may present a challenging access to the set-screw. Additionally, lingual walls of restorations are often thin, resulting in an insufficient number of screw threads to house the screw. This insufficient bulk in the restoration can also lead to distortion of the restoration or stripping of the screw threads when the set-screw is tightened. The use of cross-pins has diminished with the advent of bi-axial and angulated screws.

26.2.4   Angle Screw Correction/Bi-axial Screws

More recently, implant prosthodontics has benefited from the introduction of specially developed prosthetic screws that allow angle correction of up to 25–30 degrees (Figure 26.6). This makes screw access in the majority of anterior cases easier, avoiding the need for cement retention (Figure 26.7). These new screws

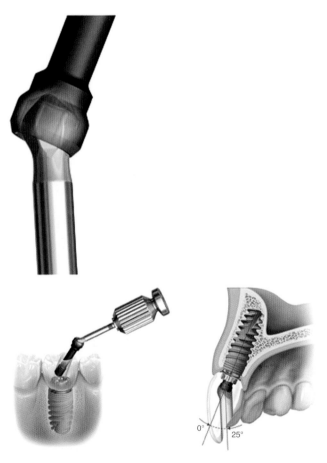

Figure 26.6 The use of specialised drivers with a unique head allows for angle correction of up to 25 degrees. *Source:* Courtesy of Nobel Biocare.

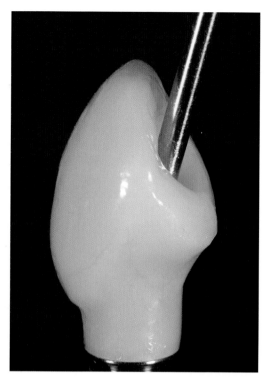

Figure 26.7 The ability to correct the angulation is useful to allow screw retention in the anterior zone.

necessitate the use of special drivers shaped like rhomboid/diamond heads, which allow access from infinite angles. Another advantage of angle screw correction is that it may help in posterior implant restoration of a patient with limited opening. The ability to access from the anterior part of the mouth at an angle can be useful when there is limited spacing.

26.3 Tips

- Chairside copy/replica abutment is a technique that minimises entrapped cement remnants in a cemented restoration. It involves duplicating an abutment by copying it with an impression material. Seating the restoration can be then carried out extra-orally on the duplicate abutment, removing all excess except a thin film that coats the internal surface of the restoration and then seating intra-orally. The technique ensures that there is an exact amount of cement on the restoration leaving minimal excess to clean up. Another technique is to use a small square of rubber dam with a hole punched in it the same size as the mesiodistal width of the edentulous area. The abutment is placed through the rubber dam with the dam below the gingival margin. This stops cement from being squeezed into the tissues.

- It has been shown that resin cements are the hardest to remove and if a restoration has sufficient retention it may be best to use cement that is easier to remove [3].
- Seating a restoration that is more anatomically correct than a healing abutment often flares the emergence profile, making insertion of the restoration uncomfortable for the patient. It is prudent to warn the patient on seating a restoration that there may be pressure pain on insertion and to reassure them that this disappears over a few moments. It would be good practice to seat this gently and slowly over a few moments to lessen the discomfort to patients.

References

1 Chee, W. and Jivraj, S. (2006 Oct 21). Screw versus cemented implant supported restorations. *Br. Dent. J.* 201 (8): 501–507.

2 Linkevicius, T., Puisys, A., Vindasiute, E. et al. (2013 Nov). Does residual cement around implant-supported restorations cause peri-implant disease? A retrospective case analysis. *Clin. Oral Implants Res.* 24 (11): 1179–1184.

3 Agar, J.R., Cameron, S.M., Hughbanks, J.C., and Parker, M.H. (1997 Jul). Cement removal from restorations luted to titanium abutments with simulated subgingival margins. *J. Prosthet. Dent.* 78 (1): 43–47.

4 Linkevicius, T., Vindasiute, E., Puisys, A. et al. (2013 Jan). The influence of the cementation margin position on the amount of undetected cement. A prospective clinical study. *Clin. Oral Implants Res.* 24 (1): 71–76.

5 Sailer, I., Muhlemann, S., Zwahlen, M. et al. (2012). Cemented and screw-retained implant reconstructions: a systematic review of the survival and complication rates. *Clin. Oral Implants Res.* 23 (Suppl 6): 163–201.

6 Wittneben, J.G., Millen, C., and Brägger, U. (2014). Clinical performance of screw- versus cement-retained fixed implant-supported reconstructions-a systematic review. *Int. J. Oral Maxillofac. Implants* 29 (Suppl): 84–98.

7 Linkevicius, T., Caplikas, A., Dumbryte, I. et al. (2019 Jun 1). Retention of zirconia copings over smooth and airborne-particle-abraded titanium bases with different resin cements. *J. Prosthet. Dent.* 121 (6): 949–954.

8 Papadopoulos, T., Tsetsekou, A., and Eliades, G. (1999 Mar). Effect of aluminium oxide sandblasting on cast commercially pure titanium surfaces. *Eur. J. Prosthodont. Restor. Dent.* 7 (1): 15.

9 Linkevicius, T., Vindasiute, E., Puisys, A., and Peciuliene, V. (2011). The influence of margin location on the amount of undetected cement excess after delivery of cement-retained implant restorations. *Clin. Oral Implants Res.* 22 (12): 1379–1384.

27

A Laboratory Perspective on Implant Dentistry

Lachlan Thompson

27.1 The Shift from Analogue to Digital

Over the past decade, and particularly in the last five years, the shift from analogue to digital laboratory protocols for implant restorations have been both instrumental and transformative in manufacturing and communication. This has ultimately provided improved prosthetic outcomes for patients.

Whereas porcelain fused to cast abutments were the standard 10 years ago, the shift to digital manufacturing is offering a wide range of design and material options for laboratory-manufactured implant restorations.

27.2 Standards in Manufacturing Today

Pre-manufactured titanium bases (Figure 27.1) or machined pre-milled titanium abutments (Figure 27.2) using a preface abutment holder (Figure 27.3) provide an interfacing structure for the laboratory to mill a secondary suprastructure in aesthetic zirconia or lithium disilicate, which is then in turn bonded to the chosen titanium abutment. These options provide the laboratory with the ability to produce these implant restorations locally, based on the requirements of the case while keeping the necessary genuine components.

Other materials used in digital manufacturing for implant restoration include:

- Cobalt chrome
- Lithium silicate (Ivoclar e.max, Hass Amber Mill, Vita Suprinity)
- Hybrid nano composites (Vita Enamic, Lava Ultimate, GC Ceramsart, Celtra Duo)
- PMMA (polymethylmethacrylate).

Practical Procedures in Implant Dentistry, First Edition. Edited by Christopher C.K. Ho.
© 2022 John Wiley & Sons Ltd. Published 2022 by John Wiley & Sons Ltd.
Companion website: www.wiley.com/go/ho/implant-dentistry

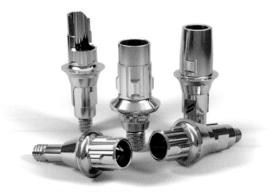

Figure 27.1 'Variobase' abutment.

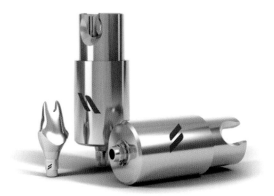

Figure 27.2 'Pre-milled' abutment.

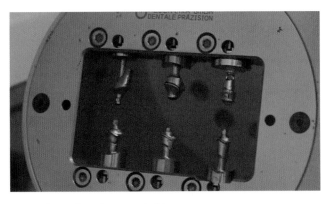

Figure 27.3 Medentika preface abutment holder.

27.3   The Importance of Implant Planning for the Laboratory

As discussed in previous chapters, implant planning (Figure 27.4) has become more accessible at a lower price point for both simple and complex cases. The point at which the laboratory is involved in implant cases has also changed. In the past, the laboratory would only see cases once impressions were submitted for fabrication. At times this would require a high level of problem solving in order to achieve an acceptable outcome. Today, the laboratory can share knowledge of abutment selection before surgery has taken place; coupled with the increased manufacturing options available this provides the ability to plan the ideal outcome.

This is increasingly advantageous in the aesthetic zone where biological reasons may affect the position of implant placement.

The prevalence of angled screw channel solutions (Figure 27.5) gives us the ability to compensate for implants placed into extractions sites that may require

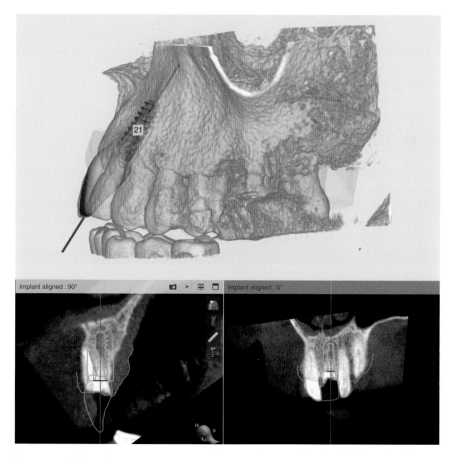

Figure 27.4 Planned case requiring angled screw channel.

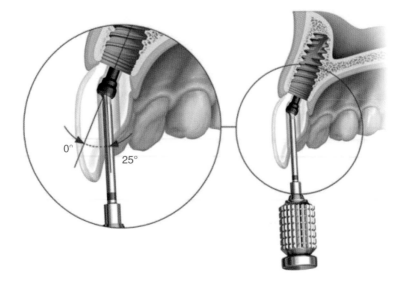

Figure 27.5 Nobel Biocare 'ASC' (angled screw channel).

a more tilted position to engage bone for primary stability. The abutment selection to restore these types of cases can be selected and communicated with the restoring clinician prior to surgery.

27.4   Digital Planning to Manage Aesthetic Cases

The advancement of digital technology also provides the ability to manufacture custom healing abutments to aid in the healing of implant sites. After the implant plan is confirmed, the laboratory can design a custom healing abutment (Figure 27.6) to support the tissue healing in an anatomical form (Figure 27.7). This design can later be scanned with an intra-oral scanner (Figure 27.8) to manufacture the final crown, effectively replacing the need to disrupt the tissue with impression copings or scan bodies.

27.5   Scanning for Implant Restorations

The workflow for restoring implants using intra-oral scanners makes use of markers known as scan abutments or scan bodies. These effectively replace impression copings and represent a known geometry in the restorative CAD software (Figure 27.9). The only difference is that with a scan body It is not possible for the laboratory to see the implant connection as with a traditional impression coping.

Every implant manufacturer and most third-party manufacturers supply scan abutments for certain implants. Often these parts have digital signatures (or

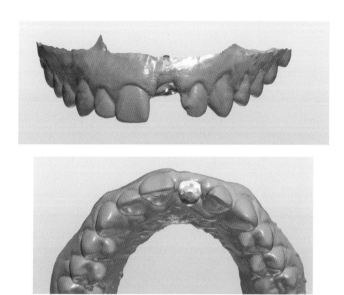

Figure 27.6 Digital design of healing abutment using implant planning data.

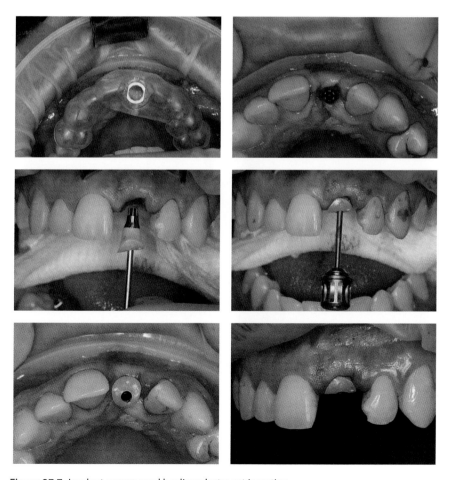

Figure 27.7 Implant surgery and healing abutment insertion.

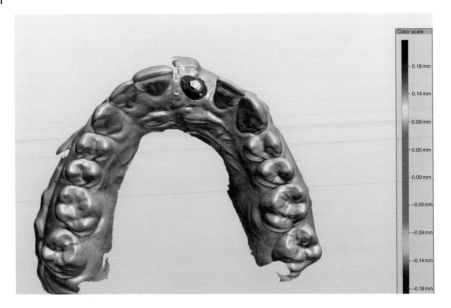

Figure 27.8 Alignment of healing abutment as scan body ready to design final restoration.

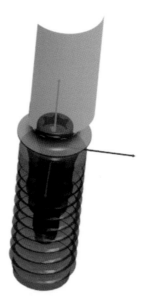

Figure 27.9 CAD implant library

locks) on the libraries; this often leaves a reduced number of options for manufacturing. In some cases to achieve the desired result the laboratory will have to work with other components that are not included in the library that the scan abutment belongs to. This can cause issues of rotation or height variation between the restoration and the fixture *in situ*.

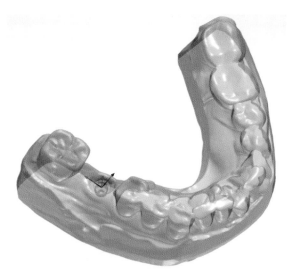

Figure 27.10 Implant coordinates after scan abutment alignment.

The multiple parts that make up the library include:

- Scan abutment
- Screw
- Abutment interface
- Digital analogue interface
- Visual representation of the implant.

The green, red, and blue lines represent the x, y, z positions of the implant library (Figure 27.10). Once the alignment is made in the CAD software using the scan abutment the position is not locked in place in these x, y, and z coordinates.

If any part of another implant library is used with this scan or the library is adjusted there is a chance errors will occur.

27.6 Digital Data Acquisition for Full Arch Cases

Prior to the shift into digital workflows, full arch restorations were for the most part limited to hybrid style acrylic titanium using CAD/CAM milled frameworks, porcelain fused to cast metal frameworks, and fully layered CAD/CAM zirconia frameworks. Outsourcing CAD/CAM framework milling was standard practice whereas today outsourcing in most labs is much reduced as the price of machinery and technology has fallen.

Some laboratories are now set up like small milling centres, offering fast turnaround on full arch cases. For example, an immediate acrylic/titanium hybrid can be delivered three days after surgery. Using intra-oral scanning technology as well as photogrammetry, such as Icam4D and PIC (Figure 27.11), makes this more predictable than ever.

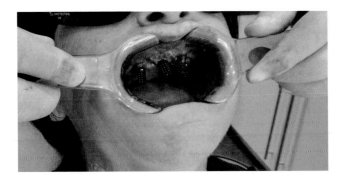

Figure 27.11 Icam4D scan locators.

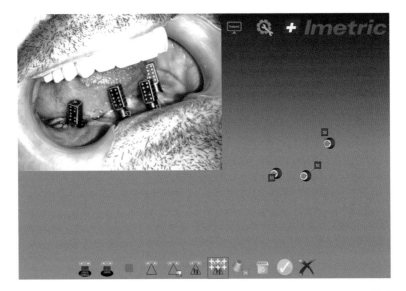

Figure 27.12 Acquisition of implant positions (Icam4D). *Source:* Imetric 4D Imaging Sàrl.

After surgery has taken place, records are taken of the implant positions using photogrammetry (Figure 27.12) and aligned with records of soft tissue and occlusion.

This design (Figure 27.13) can be 3D printed for try-in the day after surgery to confirm occlusion and aesthetics (Figure 27.14).

Utilising digital manufacturing, the laboratory compiles this data and manufactures with monolithic zirconia or polymers (Figure 27.15), providing stronger restorations while ensuring consistent accuracy across an arch that is not possible to achieve using traditional impression and stone model techniques.

27.7 Inserting Full Arch Cases at Surgery

Multiple systems have promised the possibility of inserting final restorations during surgery using guided surgery with various componentry to compensate for errors in systems. Taking these available workflows one step further it is

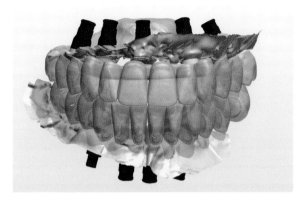

Figure 27.13 Design of restoration (3shape Dental System®). *Source:* 3Shape A/S.

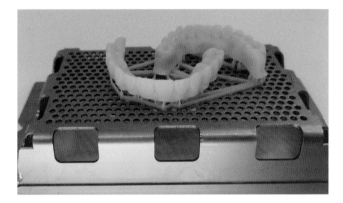

Figure 27.14 Printed try-in.

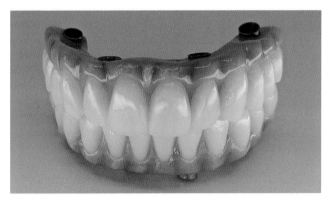

Figure 27.15 Final restoration ready for insertion three days post-surgery.

possible to plan and produce a final restoration that can be inserted directly during surgery using the Audentes protocol.

The surgical plan, intra-oral scans, and facial photos or face scans are aligned (Figure 27.16), and the prosthetic is designed based on the desire of the patient.

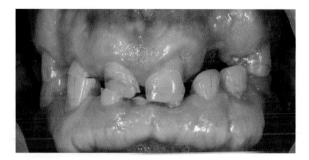

Figure 27.16 Pre-surgery situation.

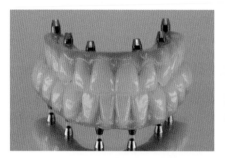
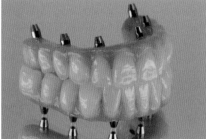

Figure 27.17 Audentes bridges manufactured for surgery.

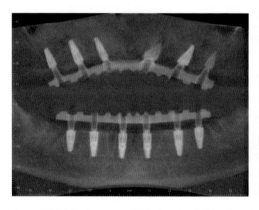
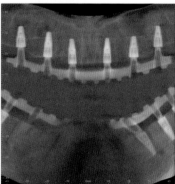

Figure 27.18 Post-surgery OPG showing bridge insert accuracy.

It is possible to share the outcome with the patient using CAD software to visualise the prosthetics in relation to their face.

Once the patient is satisfied with the planned result, the restoration is milled using titanium and graphene-strengthened polymer (Figure 27.17).

Using the Audentes technique, it is possible for the surgeon to perform implant placement and bridge insert in less than two hours (Figures 27.18–27.20), greatly increasing the comfort for the patient and increasing efficiency in the laboratory manufacturing while reducing clinical chair time.

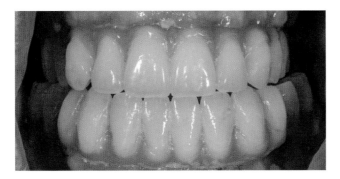

Figure 27.19 Intra-oral result one week post-surgery.

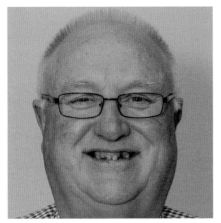 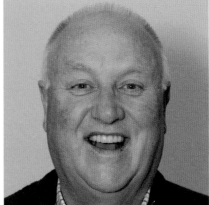

Figure 27.20 Before and after. One week post-surgery.

27.8 Tips

- Discuss restorative options with your laboratory during the implant planning stage. The ever-changing landscape is offering new solutions to simple and difficult cases alike. There is a good chance your laboratory will be on top of these options.
- Talk to your technician about which scan abutments they find easiest to integrate with their manufacturing. One type of scan body does not work for every situation.
- If the laboratory is unsure of the position of the scan abutment, send a photo showing the abutment connection and a landmark (usually a flat edge) on the scan abutment. This will verify the positioning of the crown is correct in the digital space.

28

Implant Biomechanics

Tom Giblin

28.1 Principles

A major frustration in the practice of dentistry is failure of our restorations. While there are many reasons for failure, biological or biomechanical reasons are the main aetiological problems in implant dentistry. In recent times there has been a large focus on peri-implant diseases, but very little on the biomechanical components of failure. When trying to understand the biomechanics of a system, we need to not only consider the restorations we place, but the whole masticatory system.

The jaws, teeth, and muscles are designed to break down food by shearing, crushing, and pulverising; by its very design it is an environment of destruction! We are expecting our restorations to replace lost tooth structure, to be aesthetic and biologically compatible, and to survive in a hostile environment. Teeth will break when the magnitude and nature of the forces needed to perform the function of chewing exceed those of the materials we use (Figure 28.1). It is therefore very important to understand and consider the forces involved in the masticatory process and engineer restorations to survive these extraordinary loads.

28.1.1 Forces and their Nature

Restorations do not simply fail on their own. While a tooth or restoration may be compromised with decay, or bone lost due to inflammation from periodontal disease, the forces that are applied to a tooth during function are what cause them to fail. It is therefore important to revise some basic physical principles.

Force is described as a push or pull on an object that can influence motion. If forces are balanced, the object will not move. If they are unbalanced, the object will move. In dentistry, there are several main principles we need to keep in mind. It is always valuable to assess forces as a combination of component vectors, as this allows us to better quantify and understand what is occurring (Figure 28.2).

Practical Procedures in Implant Dentistry, First Edition. Edited by Christopher C.K. Ho.
© 2022 John Wiley & Sons Ltd. Published 2022 by John Wiley & Sons Ltd.
Companion website: www.wiley.com/go/ho/implant-dentistry

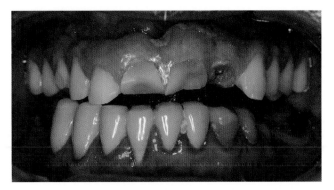

Figure 28.1 Poor biomechanical and occlusal planning can lead to rapid failure.

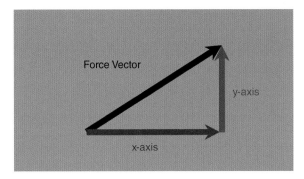

Figure 28.2 When examining forces on an object, it is important to be able to break it down to its component vectors to provide a better understanding of the situation.

28.1.1.1 Pressure = Force/Area

For any given force, the area that the force is distributed over will spread the load of the force and determine how much pressure is exerted on an object. For example, by having teeth in maximum intercuspal position (MIP), the force generated by muscles is distributed throughout all the teeth. Conversely, if one bites on a nut, for example, all the force is concentrated only on the teeth in contact with the nut, with the nut easily sheared as the force has been concentrated to exert maximum pressure with minimal force. Sharp cusps help with chewing efficiency in this way.

28.1.1.2 Impulse = Force/Time

Just as pressure is the area over which a force is applied, impulse is the time over which a given force is applied. In general, the shorter the period the force is delivered over, the more destructive it is. Reducing impulse force is the theory behind a crumple zone in a car; the force is dissipated over a longer time, absorbing the force and reducing its effect on the occupants. Another example would be the difference between two identical eggs dropped from the same height, one onto concrete and the other onto a soft pillow. The one hitting the concrete would break and the one on the pillow would be fine. They had the same kinetic energy, but in the case of the pillow, the time taken to dissipate the energy was longer, making the force transfer less destructive. The same occurs with teeth and implants: the periodontal ligaments in teeth act as shock absorbers and dissipate forces over a longer period, reducing damage. For this reason, the rigid connection of bone to implant in osseointegration can be disadvantageous as it can effectively amplify the destructive forces on restorations.

28.1.1.3 Compressive, Tensile, and Shear Forces
The way a force acts on an object has an influence on how the object will behave (Figure 28.3). Compressive forces occur when a force acts to compress or shorten an object. Tensile forces occur when forces act to stretch or lengthen an object. Both of these forces are reasonably well tolerated in dental materials and bone. Shear forces occur when unaligned forces push one part of a body in one direction and another part of a body in the opposite direction, causing deformation. This type of force is the most destructive and breaks things more readily.

28.1.1.4 Application to Materials and Occlusion
Materials such as ceramics and composites are good in compression and tension, but poor in shear forces, whereas metals, being malleable, perform well in all three types of force, making them more durable and a better choice in some high-load areas.

   Understanding the way these forces work should be applied when designing restorations as it may alter the material selection and occlusal schemes. For example, in ceramic restorations it is important to ensure occlusal contacts are in compression, and not in a shearing situation, like on an outer cusp or unsupported marginal ridge (Figure 28.4). This will also mean you need to potentially decrease the angles of cusps and reduce contacts on inclines. It may also entail a need to vary or modify the anatomy of a restoration depending on the material it is made from. Sometimes perfect anatomical form is not possible as the physical differences between dentine/enamel and ceramics mean they cannot be used in the same way.

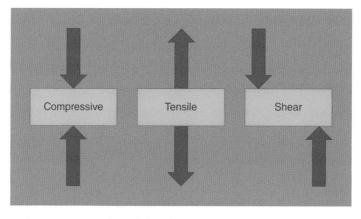

Figure 28.3 Compressive, tensile, and shear forces.

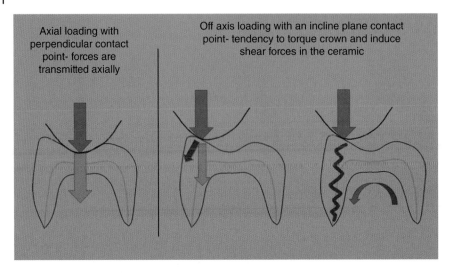

Figure 28.4 Correctly planned occlusions are important. Where you place your contact points may make the difference between loading your restoration in a compression, which is well tolerated, and inducing a shear force which may cause fractures or breakdown of bonding or cements. Contact points on incline planes will also cause a torque on a crown, potentially leading to breakages, tooth movement, or periodontal/pulpal symptoms.

Conversely, this shearing is how cusps cut food efficiently; without cusps to shear with, the teeth will only apply compressive forces and breaking down food will take a lot more force. These excess forces must then be borne by the restorations and the supporting structures (teeth, implants, bone, etc.), and may be detrimental.

28.1.1.5 Incline Plane Mechanics (Normal Force)

When a force is applied to an object, the equal and opposite force is applied perpendicular to the contact point. This means that even if a force is directed along the long axis of a tooth or implant, if the contact point is not perpendicular to that axis, it will generate lateral forces depending on the angle of the cusps (Figure 28.5). This lateral force is destructive and over many chewing cycles, may cause teeth or restorations to break, bonding to fail, the tooth to become sensitive, or the tooth to move orthodontically or lose bone and attachment.

28.1.2 Beams

Beams are a span bounded at both ends (Figure 28.6). They transfer load to their abutments by resisting bending – therefore the thickness and the material they are made of are important factors in resisting breakage. Beams are complex structures because they undergo compressive, tensile, and shear forces. A beam used regularly in dentistry is a bridge used to replace missing teeth by spanning an edentulous space. The longer the beam, the more flexure it undergoes and the less able it is to efficiently transfer loads. The flexure is generally related to the cube of the span: a two-unit bridge flexes eight times more than a one-unit bridge, and a three-unit

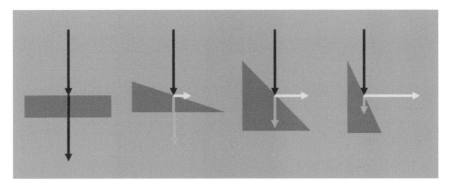

Figure 28.5 The resultant vectors when a force is applied to an incline plane can be unexpectedly destructive, inducing large lateral forces. For this reason, having tooth contacts on incline planes should be avoided as it will cause occlusal instability.

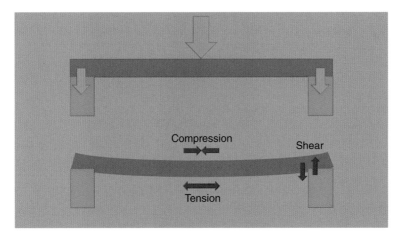

Figure 28.6 Beams transfer loads by resisting bending and are complex structures with the materials subjected to compressive, tensile, and shear forces. They must be thick enough to resist flexure and the effects of these forces.

bridge flexes 27 times a one-unit bridge. This flexure can lead to break down of abutments, or failure of the materials and fracture of the bridge.

28.1.3   Levers

A lever is a beam that pivots around a fulcrum and is used to apply a force. They are divided into three classes (Figure 28.7).

The mandible is a class 3 lever system as shown in Figure 28.8. It has a mobile joint with the TMJ, forces are exerted by the closure muscles, and the teeth do the work. An interesting feature of the jaws is that the further you get from the fulcrum and muscles, the greater the mechanical disadvantage is created, reducing the force that can be exerted on objects and teeth in the anterior. This is an important feature of anterior disclusion/canine guidance. It should also be noted that the occlusal plane is offset from the actual mechanical plane. This

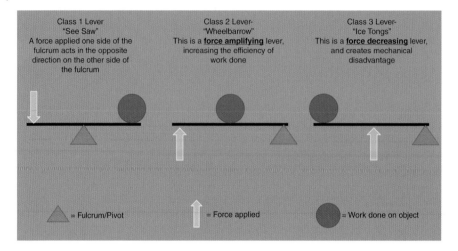

Figure 28.7 Class 1, 2, and 3 lever systems.

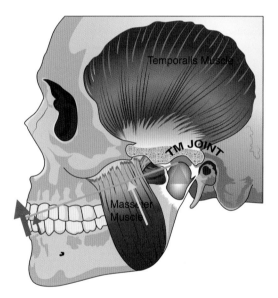

Figure 28.8 The mandible as a class 3 lever system. The occlusal forces are reduced the further forward you travel in the arch.

means that the lower teeth do not close straight up into the maxillary teeth, but rather travel upwards and forwards to meet the maxillary teeth, creating a shearing motion to increase the ability of the teeth to break down food.

28.1.4 Cantilevers

A cantilever is a beam that is only anchored at one end. Like a beam, they transfer load by resisting bending, but they will concentrate forces upon the anchor

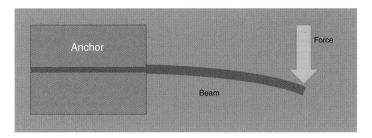

Figure 28.9 Cantilevers require rigid and strong anchorage to resist the forces created by the lever they support.

point, so it must be reinforced to tolerate the forces on it. A cantilever will always act as a lever and force amplifier and so should be approached with caution. In implants, the distal abutment of a cantilevered restoration will be the site that concentrates the greatest force, and as such is more prone to breakage (Figures 28.9 and 28.10).

Most dentists consider cantilevers in a mesio-distal direction, but often do not take vertical and buccolingual cantilevers into account. These can be just as detrimental. It should be remembered that ALL teeth are cantilevers, with the root as the anchor and crown as the cantilever (Figure 28.11). For this reason, crown-to-implant ratio is very important. Too long a crown and you will be increasing the cantilever and therefore concentrating more force onto the prosthetic connection and bone supporting the tooth. For the same reason it is important that implants are large enough to have enough surface area to dissipate these forces without overloading the bone. We see this also in natural teeth that have lost attachment due to periodontal disease. As bone is lost, the crown portion gets longer as the root/anchorage is reduced, leading to tooth mobility. Splinting is effective in reducing the cantilever effect and can be employed in implants to control forces more effectively.

28.1.5 Bone

If we address bone as a material, like many other materials it is good in compression, it is ok in tension, but it is poor at tolerating shear forces. Because of this, implants perform well when loaded axially, because this places the supporting bone into compression. Bone can be classified into types 1–4 according to Misch [1], with type 1 bone being the most dense and type 4 being quite soft and compressible. This will affect how forces are transmitted through the bone, but also how an implant will function. It must also be remembered that bone resorbs readily in the presence of inflammation. This can come about due to microbial infection (peri-implant mucositis or peri-implantitis), or from occlusal trauma. When you take into account that orthodontics induces bony resorption with only very light forces, you must anticipate that bone around implants will not tolerate unfavourable occlusal loads long term.

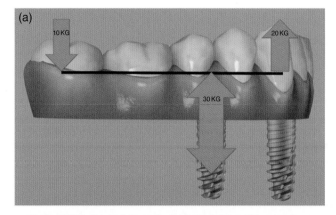

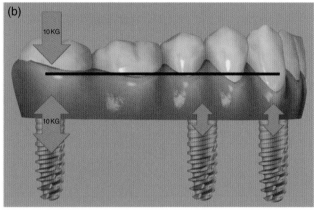

Figure 28.10 (a) Conceptual diagram showing a cantilever with a 2x A-P spread. We can see that merely by using a cantilever, we are amplifying the 10 kg load to 30 kg at the distal abutment. It must be remembered that this is not only 30 kg pressure on the implant and supporting bone, but the equal and opposite force in 30 kg upwards through the middle of the bridge. There is also a 20 kg force anteriorly that is trying to unseat the restoration. (b) All these excess forces are eliminated by placing an extra implant, eliminating the cantilever and its force-amplifying effects. *Source:* Adapted from Misch's Dental Implant Prosthetics.

When lateral forces are generated on implants due to prosthetic design or occlusal loads, this tends to concentrate forces on the crest of the ridge. Unlike natural teeth, which have a periodontal ligament that acts to dissipate the forces further down into the tooth and move the centre of rotation of the tooth apically, in implants the lateral forces cause the implant to load the crest of the bone. This bone is also generally cortical bone and has less give to it, and so the forces will concentrate, often causing bone loss. Traditionally, we have seen bone loss to the first thread, which is usually in cancellous bone and better able to dissipate these forces. Sub-crestal placement or implants that taper in at the top are designed to reduce the loading of the crest of the ridge and transmit the forces deeper into the bone, reducing crestal bone loss.

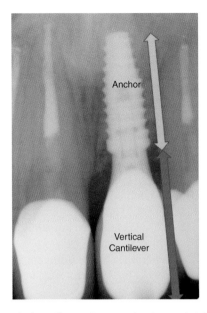

Figure 28.11 Teeth are vertical cantilevers. Crown to implant ratio is important to minimise the effects of a vertical cantilever. The larger the vertical cantilever, the larger the anchorage needs to be.

Reference

1 Misch, C.E. (2014). *Dental Implant Prosthetics*, 2e. St. Louis, MO: Elsevier.

Further Reading

Bahat, O. and Handelsman, M. (1996). Use of wide implants and double implants in the posterior jaw: a clinical report. *Int. J. Oral Maxillofac. Implants* 11: 379–386.

Bedi, S., Thomas, R., Shah, R., and Mehta, D.S. (2015). The effect of cuspal inclination on stress distribution and implant displacement in different bone qualities for a single tooth implant: a finite element study. *Int. J. Oral Health Sci.* 5: 80–86.

Benzing, U., Weber, H., Simonis, A., and Engel, E. (1994). Changes in chewing patterns after implantation in the edentulous mandible. *Int. J. Oral Maxillofac. Implants* 9 (2): 207–213.

Brunski, J.B., Puleo, D.A., and Nanci, A. (2000). Biomaterials and biomechanics of oral and maxillofacial implants: current status and future developments. *Int. J. Oral Maxillofac. Implants* 15 (1): 15–46.

Carlsson, G.E. (2008). Dental occlusion: modern concepts and their application in implant prosthodontics. *Odontology* 97: 8–17.

Falcón-Antenucci, R.M., Pellizzer, E.P., Perri de Carvalho, P.S. et al. (2010). Influence of cusp inclination on stress distribution in implant-supported prostheses. A three-dimensional finite element analysis. *J. Prosthodont.* 19 (5): 381–386.

Gibbs, C.H., Mahan, P., Lundeen, H. et al. (1981). Occlusal forces during chewing – influences of biting strength and food consistency. *J. Prosthet. Dent.* 46: 561–567.

Greenstein, G. and Cavallaro, J. (2010). Cantilevers extending from unilateral implant-supported fixed prostheses. *J. Am. Dent. Assoc.* 141: 1221–1230.

Katona, T.R., Goodacre, C.J., Brown, D.T., and Roberts, W.E. (1993). Force-moment systems on single maxillary anterior implants: effects of incisal guidance, fixture orientation, and loss of bone support. *Int. J. Oral Maxillofac. Implants* 8: 512–522.

McAlarney, M.E. and Stavropoulos, D.N. (1996). Determination of cantilever length—anterior/posterior spread ratio assuming failure criteria to be the compromise of the prosthesis retaining screw-prosthesis joint. *Int. J. Oral Maxillofac. Implants* 11: 331–339.

McGlumphy, E.A., Mendel, D.A., and Holloway, J.A. (1998). Implant screw mechanics. *Dent. Clin. N. Am.* 42 (1): 71–89.

McHorris, W.H. (1982). The importance of anterior teeth. *J. Gnathol.* 1 (1): 19–36.

Misch, C.E. and Bidez, M.W. (1994). Implant-protected occlusion: a biomechanical rationale. *Compendium* 15 (11): 1330–1334.

Misch, C.E., Goodacre, C.J., Finley, J.M. et al. (2005). Consensus conference panel report: crown-height space guidelines for implant dentistry-part 1. *Implant. Dent.* 14: 312–318.

Misch, C.E., Goodacre, C.J., Finley, J.M. et al. (2005). Consensus conference panel report: crown-height space guidelines for implant dentistry-part 2. *Implant. Dent.* 15: 113–121.

Rangert, B., Krogh, P.H., Langer, B., and Van Roekel, N. (1995). Bending overload and implant fracture: a retrospective clinical analysis. *Int. J. Oral Maxillofac. Implants* 10: 326–334.

Rangert, B.R., Sullivan, R.M., and Jemt, T.M. (1997). Load factor control for implants in the posterior partially edentulous segment. *Int. J. Oral Maxillofac. Implants* 12: 360–370.

Resnik, R.R. (2020). *Misch's Contemporary Implant Dentistry 4th Edition.* Elsevier.

Rodrigues, V.A., Tribst, J.P.M., Santis, L.R. et al. (2018). Biomechanical effect of inclined implants in fixed prosthesis: strain and stress analysis. *Rev. Odontol. UNESP* 47 (4): 237–243. Epub August 13, 2018.

Rodriguez, A., Aquilino, S., and Lund, P. (1994). Cantilever and implant biomechanics: a review of the literature, part I. *J. Prosthodont.* 3: 41–46.

Rodriguez, A., Aquilino, S., and Lund, P. (1994). Cantilever and implant biomechanics: a review of the literature, part II. *J. Prosthodont.* 3: 114–118.

Salama, H., Salama, M.A., Garber, D., and Adar, P. (1998). The interproximal height of bone: a guidepost to predictable aesthetic strategies and soft tissue contours in anterior tooth replacement. *Pract. Periodontics Aesthet. Dent.* 10 (9): 1131–1141.

Solnit, G.S. (1996). Occlusal considerations in the design of implant-assisted fixed prostheses. *Calif. Dent. Assoc. J.* 24 (1): 29–33.

Tan, B.F., Tan, K.B., and Nicholls, J.I. (2004). Critical bending moment of implant-abutment screw joint interfaces: effect of torque levels and implant diameter. *Int. J. Oral Maxillofac. Implants* 19 (5): 648–658.

Tarnow, D.P., Cho, S.C., and Wallace, S.S. (2000). The effect of inter-implant distance on the height of inter-implant bone crest. *J. Periodontol.* 71: 546–549.

Tarnow, D., Elian, N., Fletcher, P. et al. (2003). Vertical distance from the crest of bone to the height of the interproximal papilla between adjacent implants. *J. Periodontol.* 74 (12): 1785–1788.

Thornton, L.J. (1990). Anterior guidance: group function/canine guidance. A literature review. *J. Prosthet. Dent.* 64: 479–482.

Weinberg, L.A. and Kruger, B. (1996). An evaluation of torque (moment) on implant/prosthesis with staggered buccal and lingual offset. *Int. J. Periodontics Restorative Dent.* 16 (3): 252–265.

Zitzmann, N.U. and Marinello, C.P. (2000). Treatment outcomes of fixed or removable implant-supported prostheses in the edentulous maxilla. Part I: Patients' assessments. *J. Prosthet. Dent.* 83 (4): 424–433.

Zitzmann, N.U. and Marinello, C.P. (2000). Treatment outcomes of fixed or removable implant-supported prostheses in the edentulous maxilla. Part II: clinical findings. *J. Prosthet. Dent.* 83 (4): 434–442.

29

Delivering the Definitive Prosthesis

Aodhan Docherty and Christopher C.K. Ho

29.1 Principles

Screw-retained restorations have several advantages: they are retrievable, they may be used in clinical situations with limited inter-arch space, and they are easier to remove for hygiene or repairs. The disadvantages include greater cost, more difficulty in delivery if there is limited mouth opening, greater technique sensitivity, and more demanding laboratory procedures to attain passive fit. A screw-retained prosthesis requires a prosthetically driven treatment plan to ensure that the screw channel exits in an aesthetic manner.

Wittneben et al. [1] found that the five-year survival rate was similar for both cemented and screw-retained reconstructions, and that there was there no difference in their failure rates. Cement-retained prosthesis have a higher incidence of fistulae and suppuration, but all other biological complications, such as bone loss, recession, and peri-implant disease, occur at a similar rate. Cement-retained restorations had more technical complications than screw-retained prostheses except for ceramic fracture, which was higher for screw-retained prostheses.

When treatment planning, designing, and delivering, the definitive prosthesis should consider the following variables: soft tissue support, occlusal verification, aesthetic criteria, and prosthetic torque requirements.

29.1.1 Soft Tissue Support

The relationship between the implant prosthesis and the soft tissues is a key factor for success, particularly in the anterior zone [2]. Creating harmonious soft tissue architecture that mimics adjacent natural contours, providing both support and the illusion of natural emergence of the prosthesis is challenging. Planning involves selecting the type of implant, the proposed three-dimensional position (in relation to the adjacent teeth), and may include the use of prosthetically guided tissue healing with provisional restorations.

Many authors have recognised the role of the provisional restoration in creating the emergence profile and shaping the anatomy of the peri-implant soft tissues [3]. This is important because stock healing abutments do not mimic the

Practical Procedures in Implant Dentistry, First Edition. Edited by Christopher C.K. Ho.
© 2022 John Wiley & Sons Ltd. Published 2022 by John Wiley & Sons Ltd.
Companion website: www.wiley.com/go/ho/implant-dentistry

natural cross-section of teeth, particularly in the anterior zone where the natural root cross-section is oval or triangular in shape. Without developing the soft tissue profile the definitive prothesis may lack the appropriate emergence profile and soft tissue support (Table 29.1).

29.1.2 Occlusal Verification

There is insufficient evidence within the literature to provide any firm recommendations in terms of ideal occlusion for implant prosthesis [6–8]. However, basic prosthodontic principles should be applied when designing the occlusion for single-tooth implant prostheses, such as:

- Minimising lateral forces
- Reducing exaggerated cuspal inclines
- Ensuring minimal force on a single crown prosthesis upon intercuspal position.

A parallel periapical radiograph should be taken after manually torquing down the prosthesis to confirm it is seated correctly, and thereafter torquing to manufacturer's recommendation and closure of the access. Occlusion should be checked with articulating paper. Adjust the marked areas on the crown in intercuspal position and then excursions until there are no markings. Follow with shimstock to ensure total clearance and finally polish with finer grade diamond bur, followed by porcelain polishing burs.

For a full arch prosthesis we must consider that there is a reduction in proprioception and thus a reduced awareness of loading and function. It is important to ensure the laboratory does not design teeth with exaggerated cuspal inclines or excessively wide occlusal tables.

29.1.3 Aesthetic Evaluation

It is imperative to evaluate the aesthetics of the definitive restoration prior to cementation (if the prosthesis is cement-retained) or sealing the access (if the prosthesis is screw-retained). This evaluation should be done by both the clinician and the patient in order to provide consent for delivery.

At the tooth level, the following factors should be considered:

- Hue, value, and chroma
- Shape
- Surface texture
- Incisal edge position
- Emergence profile
- Aesthetics of the screw channel – for screw-retained prosthesis
- Emergence profile
- Level and contour of the gingival margin in comparison to corresponding tooth on the contralateral side of the arch
- Presence of black triangles.

Additional considerations for multi-unit prostheses such as implant bridges:

- Smile line and tooth display for the larger prosthesis
- Smile width and buccal corridors
- Midline

Table 29.1 Techniques for developing the soft tissue emergence profile [4].

Technique	Advantages	Disadvantages
Laboratory modification of soft tissue substitute on the master cast by the technician during construction of the definitive prosthesis	No chair time needed No additional cost	Unable to predict how the soft tissues will respond to the intended contour of the final restoration Does not take biotype or biology into consideration; it is a purely manual manipulation of the master cast Damage to soft tissues and bone may result from over-contouring the restoration Surgery may be required to seat the restoration
Direct surgical manipulation of soft tissues, prior to final impressions, e.g. at second-stage surgery: • Split-thickness flap with repositioning of soft tissues • Rotary handpiece and soft tissue trimming bur	There may be an opportunity to perform adjunctive surgical procedures at this time if required	Margin of unpredictability, as soft tissues still require time to heal In-chair time increased May be seen as invasive or causing trauma to peri-implant soft tissues
Custom healing abutment	Can be done chair-side by adding composite resin or light-cured acrylic to a abutment such as a temporary cylinder	Soft tissue collapse can occur during the time you are adding to the healing abutment Requires multiple reviews to evaluate the soft tissue response Not as predictable for emergence of the final restoration as using a provisional restoration
Provisional restoration – modification can be done in chair with addition of light-cured composite resin	Ability to incrementally influence the shape of the soft tissue, allowing progressive assessment of the changes to emergence and contour Under-contouring the restoration in the subgingival zone of the restoration may allow the tissues to coronally position, while over-contouring the restoration in the subgingival zone will make the tissues migrate/move apically [5] Peri-implant tissues have the opportunity to mature and both the patient and clinician can assess aesthetics and function prior to the definitive restoration being constructed; hence more predictable final result	Lengthy in-chair time may be required with multiple visits Soft tissues will collapse after the provisional restoration has been removed – hence a custom healing abutment should be placed while the restoration is being adjusted Risk of damage to peri-implant soft and hard tissues if over-contoured

Source: Modified from Alani, A. and Corson, M. (2011). Soft tissue manipulation for single implant restorations. Br. Dent. J. 211: 411–416.

- Lip position and fullness
- Transition line
- Occlusal plane.

Considerations for pink porcelain:

- Colour
- Texture
- Gingival margins and architecture
- Gingival zenith levels
- Stippling and characterisations.

29.1.4 Torque Requirement for Delivery

The clamping force holding the abutment to the implant is called the preload. The preload is developed when optimal torque is applied to the abutment screw, resulting in elongation of the screw with the resultant force pulling the components together in a clamping force. Several factors influence preload, including the torque applied to the abutment screw and also the material of the components, screw head design, screw thread design, and surface roughness.

Table 29.2 gives manufacturer-recommended torque guidelines for some common implant systems.

29.1.5 Cementation Technique and Material Selection – Cemented Crowns

According to Gultekin et al. [9], the ideal luting agent should:

- provide adequate retention for intra-oral use,
- allow for removal without damage to the restoration, abutment, or surrounding tissues, and
- be biocompatible.

The literature is inconclusive on the type of luting agent preferred for cementing restorations onto implant abutments. They are classed as either permanent or temporary (Table 29.3).

Some clinicians prefer to cement their implant-retained prostheses with temporary cement, such as zinc oxide eugenol (Temp Bond™) and zinc oxide (Temp Bond NE™). The advantages of temporary cements include: better retrievability, easier removal of excess cement, and, usually, sufficient retention. However, temporary cements are often more soluble than permanent cements, leading to gap formation, compromise of the margin of the restoration, issues with the health of peri-implant soft tissues, and debonding.

Nematollahi et al. [10] in a review found the retention of cement varied. Their results showed that the cements from least to most retentive were: zinc oxide (with or without eugenol), polycarboxylate, glass ionomer, resin-modified glass ionomer, zinc phosphate, and resin adhesive cements. Furthermore, the least to most difficult to clean up excess were: zinc phosphate, glass ionomer, and resin cements. Nematollahi et al. comment that there are no strict guidelines on how

Table 29.2 Prosthodontic torque guide for several implant manufacturers.

Manufacturer	Implant	Torque Ncm	Screwdriver
BioHorizons	Internal 3.5, 4.5, 5.7	30	0.050 (1.25 mm) hex screwdriver
	Tapered Internal 3.5, 4.5, 5.7	30	
	External implant 3.5, 4.0, 5.0	30	
Biomet 3i	Certain 3.25, 4.0, 4/3, 5.0, 5/4, 6.0	20	0.048 hex screwdriver
	Certain Prevail 3/4/3 (3.4), 4/5/4, 5/6/5, 4/3, 5/4, 6/5, Certain XP 4/5, 5/6	20	
	Miniplant 3.25	20	
	External	35	
Camlog	Screw-line Implant 3.3	20	1.28 mm hex screwdriver
	Screw-line / Root-line Implant 3.8, 4.3, 5.0, 6.0	20	
Dentsply Implants	ANKYLOS® C/X C/ 3.5, 4.5, 5.5, 7.0 (non-indexed)	15	1.0 mm hex screwdriver
	ANKYLOS® C/X /X 3.5, 4.5, 5.5, 7.0 Indexed)	15	
	OsseoSpeed EV3.0 Green. EV 3.6 Purple. EV 4.2 Yellow. EV 4.8 Blue, EV 5.4 Brown, Profile EV 4.2 Yellow, Profile EV 4.8 Blue	25	0.050 hex screwdriver
	OsseoSpeed /OsseoSpeed TX3.0 Yellow	15	
	OsseoSpeed / OssooSpcod TX 3.5, 4.0 Aqua	20	
	OsseoSpeed / OsseoSpeed TX 4.5, 5.0 Lilac	25	
	OsseoSpeed TX Profile 4.5, 5.0	25	
	XIVE® S 3.0, 3.4, 3.8, 4.5, 5.5	24	1.22 mm hex screwdriver
	FRIALIT 3.4, 3.8, 4.5, 5.5	24	
Implant Direct	Implant Direct	35	0.050 (1.25 mm) hex screwdriver
MIS	MIS® Biocom & Seven	30	0.050 (1.25 mm) hex screwdriver
Neoss	Neoss	32	Neoss Unigrip
Nobel Biocare	NobelActive 3.0	15	Nobel Biocare Unigrip
	NobelActive/NobelReplace Conical Connection NP 3.5, RP 4.3, 5.0	35	
	NobelReplace NP 3.5, RP4.3, WP 5.0, 6.0	35	
	Brånemark System NP 3.3, RP 3.75, 4.0, WP 5.0, 5.5	35	
	Nobel Biocare Multi-unit Abutment Angled	15	
	Nobel Biocare Multi-unit Abutment Straight	35	
Southern Implant	Southern Implant External	32	0.048 hex
	Southern Implant Tri Nex	32	Unigrip
	Southern Implant Octa	32	Star/Torx

(Continued)

Table 29.2 (Continued)

Manufacturer	Implant	Torque Ncm	Screwdriver
Straumann	Bone Level 3.3 NC (Narrow CrossFit)	35	SCS screwdriver
	Bone Level 4.1, 4.8 RC (Regular CrossFit)	35	
	Standard/Standard Plus 4.8 RN (Regular Neck)	35	
	Standard/Standard Plus 4.8 WN (Wide Neck)	35	
	Standard Plus 3.3 NN (Narrow Neck)	35	
	Screw Retained Abutment (Straight and Angled)	35	
Thommen	Thommen SPI® 3.5	15	Four lobe
	Thommon SPI® 4.0, 4.5, 5.0, 6.0	25	
	Thommen SPI® zirconia abutment	20	
Zimmer Dental	Tapered Screw-Vent 3.5, 4.5, 5.7/Tapered Screw-Vent 3.5, 4.5, 5.7 Friction Fit	30	1.25 mm hex screwdriver
	Screw-Vent 3.3, 3.7, 4.5/Screw-Vent 3.3, 3.7, 4.5 Friction Fit	30	
	SwissPlus 4.8	35	

Table 29.3 Examples of permanent and temporary luting agents.

Permanent luting agent	Temporary luting agent
• Zinc phosphate	• Zinc oxide
• Zinc polycarboxylate	• Eugenol cement
• Glass ionomer	
• Self-adhesive resin cement	
• Resin cement	

much cement should be placed within the restoration, but that it should be approximately 3% of its total volume. Excess cement increases the difficulty of cleaning up excess material and increases the chance of damage to surrounding tissue and altering occlusion due to the hydraulic pressure that builds during seating. Too little cement increases the risk of leakage and loss of retention.

29.1.6 Screw Access Channel Management – Screw-Retained Crowns

The screw access channel should be restored with a material that is functional, aesthetic (particularly if on a buccal or occlusal surface), and, most importantly, easily removed. To ensure retrievability, a barrier material such as polytetrafluoroethylene (PTFE), Teflon tape, cotton, or gutta percha is used to cover the abutment screw, and then a restorative material such as composite resin is placed on top. The screw access should be dried, barrier material placed over the abutment screw, and finally a composite restorative material placed.

29.1.7 Pink Porcelain

Pink porcelain may be used to simulate gingiva and is particularly useful where there are soft tissue defects (Figure 29.1). Re-establishing hard and soft tissues with surgery can be complex, unpredictable, and costly. As Papaspyridakos et al. [11] discuss, use of pink porcelain is limited in cases of moderate to high smile lines (i.e. where the transition is more difficult to mask).

Hygiene is critical to long-term maintenance of dental implants, and while pink porcelain is a useful tool in replacing missing soft tissue, it must not hinder access for oral hygiene practices (Figure 29.2).

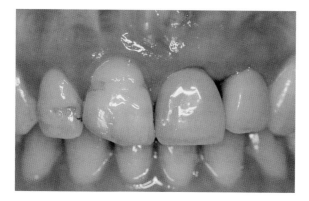

Figure 29.1 Implants in upper left central and incisor positions demonstrating presence of large embrasure space or 'black hole'. This is aesthetically displeasing.

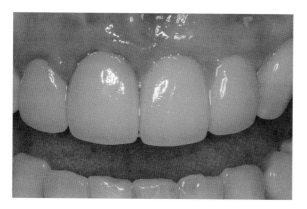

Figure 29.2 Note the gingival embrasure space has been closed with pink porcelain. It is important to assess the ability to cleanse this interdental area easily for long-term peri-implant health.

29.2 Procedures

The healing abutment or provisional restoration is unscrewed, and the clinician should ensure that the peri-implant soft tissue is healthy and ready for delivery of the definitive prosthesis. A description of procedures is given in Chapter 26 on 'Screw versus Cemented Implant-Supported Restorations'.

29.2.1 Delivering a Cement-Retained Crown – Chairside Copy Abutment Technique

This technique allows a copy abutment to be made so that the crown can be cemented onto the copy abutment, removing all the excess cement and leaving a thin film thickness within the crown, which is then seated onto the actual abutment *in situ*. This allows the correct amount of cement to adhere within the crown, minimising any overflow excess.

29.2.1.1 Creating a Polyvinyl Siloxane Copy Abutment
1) Take PTFE (Teflon) tape and line the intaglio of the crown, this will act as a spacer (Figure 29.3a). You may use a hand instrument and then manually seat the crown onto the abutment to aid in the fit.
2) Inject polyvinyl siloxane (PVS) material into the intaglio of the crown and over fill so you have a handle to hold (Figure 29.3b).
3) Remove this PVS copy abutment from the crown and discard the PTFE tape. You now have a copy of the abutment.

29.2.1.2 Delivering a Cement-Retained Crown Using a Copy Abutment Technique
1) Soak the abutment and restoration in a chlorhexidine liquid or disinfectant.
2) After removal of the healing abutment or provisional restoration insert the abutment without delay to prevent the soft tissue collapsing and making it more difficult to insert.
3) Ensure the abutment is inserted in the correct orientation and hand tightened with a manual driver.
4) Take a parallel peri-apical radiograph to confirm seating. The use of a film holder is encouraged.
5) Fit the crown either dry or with an appropriate try-in paste.
6) Confirm passive fit, marginal adaptation, proximal contacts, aesthetics, and occlusion.
7) Sit the patient up and show the restoration using a hand mirror with the correct lighting. Confirm and record the patient's consent to cement the restoration.
8) Use a torque wrench and tighten the abutment screw to the manufacturer's torque recommendation. Dry and clean the screw access of the abutment. Place PTFE (Teflon) tape over the screw. Leave most of the screw channel open as it can aid in collecting excess cement.

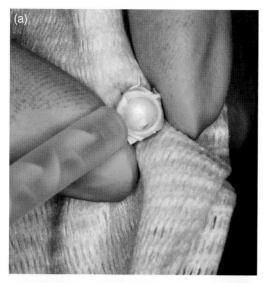

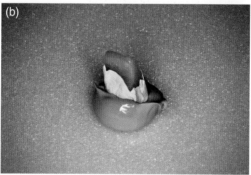

Figure 29.3 (a) Fabricating a copy abutment by lining the intaglio of the crown with PTFE tape. (b) A quick-setting silicone material such as bite registration material is then injected into the crown with enough to form a base. Once the silicone material has set, the replica of the abutment has been constructed. Prior to final cementation *in situ* the crown loaded with cement is seated onto the copy abutment, removing the majority of cement and rendering a simpler clean up with minimal cement excess.

9) Using the luting agent of your choice, load the crown and then place it onto the PVS copy abutment and wipe off the excess cement. Ensure this is done swiftly within the working time of the restoration. Inspect the intaglio of the crown to see if there are any areas without cement. Conservatively add to these areas only if needed.
10) Seat the crown and if the luting material is light-cured then 'tack cure' for three seconds per side of the crown. Then proceed to remove excess with an instrument such as a curved sickle scaler. Alternatively, prior to tack curing you may use a cross-over floss technique to remove excess cement.
11) Take a post-cementation radiograph to confirm marginal fit and the absence of residual cement.

29.3 Tips

- When torquing an implant restoration to seat, tissue blanching may be observed, as a result of pressure from the restoration. This is transient ischaemia and may last five minutes. If vascularity does not return there will be a need to adjust the contours of the restoration. Note that if a provisional restoration has been used then this may not occur due to the idealised contours developed, which allows the contours to be copied in the final restoration.
- Use a periapical film holder to ensure the radiograph is parallel ensuring the threads are sharp and visible on the radiograph.
- When using a cement-retained prosthesis ensure that supragingival margins (or at least equigingival margins) are adopted, especially on the palatal of the restoration which allows cement to escape because supragingival margins allow for straightforward and complete removal of cement.

References

1 Wittneben, J.G., Millen, C., and Brägger, U. (2014). Clinical performance of screw-versus cement-retained fixed implant-supported reconstructions – a systematic review. *Int. J. Oral Maxillofac. Implants* 29 (Suppl): 84–98.

2 Alani, A. and Corson, M. (2011). Soft tissue manipulation for single implant restorations. *Br. Dent. J. Lond.* 211 (9): 411–416.

3 Monaco, C., Evangelisti, E., Scotti, R. et al. (2016). A fully digital approach to replicate peri-implant soft tissue contours and emergence profile in the esthetic zone. *Clin. Oral Implants Res.* 27 (12): 1511–1514.

4 Alani, A. and Corson, M. (2011). Soft tissue manipulation for single implant restorations. *Br. Dent. J.* 211 (9).

5 Mihram, W.L. (1997). Dynamic biologic transformation of the periodontium: a clinical report. *J. Prosthet. Dent.* 78: 337–340.

6 Carlssen, G. (2009). Dental occlusion: modern concepts and their application in implant prosthodontics. *Odontology* 97: 8.

7 Koyano, K. and Esaki, D. (2015). Occlusion on oral implants: current clinical guidelines. *J. Oral Rehabil.* 42 (2): 153–161.

8 Lewis, M.B. and Klineberg, I. (2011). Prosthodontic considerations designed to optimize outcomes for single-tooth implants. A review of the literature. *Aust. Dent. J.* 56: 181–192.

9 Gultekin, P., Alper Gultekin, B., Aydin, M., and Yalcin, S. (2013). Cement selection for implant-supported crowns fabricated with different luting space settings. *J. Prosthodont.* 22: 112–119.

10 Nematollahi, F., Beyabanaki, E., and Alikhasi, M. (2016). Cement selection for cement-retained implant-supported prostheses. *J. Prosthodont.* 25: 599–606.

11 Papaspyridakos, P., Amin, S., El-Rafie, K., and Weber, H.P. (2018). Technique to match gingival shade when using pink ceramics for anterior fixed implant prostheses. *J. Prosthodont.* 27: 311–313.

30

Occlusion and Implants

Christopher C.K. Ho and Subir Banerji

30.1 Principles

A comprehensive understanding of occlusal principles is fundamental to long-term stability of implants and the overlying superstructure prosthesis. Incorrect loading and parafunctional forces may negatively influence the long-term survival, with the possibility of crestal bone loss, as well as mechanical complications such as screw loosening, screw fractures, damage to veneering porcelain, or abutment fracture. Implants may remain integrated, yet suffer from prosthetic complications that may be financially costly to repair or rectify. A clinician's objective is to provide successful implant therapy with optimal health and little to minimal requirements for maintenance and repair.

Osseointegrated implants are effectively ankylosed in bone, thus possess minimal to no movement in function, while natural teeth possess a periodontal apparatus and may move within their respective bony housing, providing a shock absorbing function. The mean values of axial displacement of teeth in the socket are 25–100 μm, whereas the range of motion of osseointegrated dental implants has been reported to be approximately 3–5 μm [1, 2]. Upon a lateral load the natural tooth moves rapidly 56–108 μm and rotates at the apical third of the root [3]; consequently the lateral force on the tooth is diminished immediately along the root. Lateral load to an implant occurs gradually, reaching about 10–50 μm under a similar lateral load. In addition, there is concentration of greater forces at the crest of surrounding bone with no rotation of the implant [2], which results in the highest stress in the crestal bone. The crestal bone around dental implants may act as a lever fulcrum when a force is applied, leading to increased risk of crestal bone loss.

Natural teeth possess peripheral afferent feedback due to the pulpo-dentinal complex, as well as periodontal mechanoreceptors providing reflex control to the central nervous system [4]. This allows a uniquely discriminating sense of feel and directional specificity for mastication, allowing the texture and hardness of food to be sensed, as well as control of the muscles of mastication and swallowing.

In contrast, the peripheral feedback system is different for implants because they lack the pulpo-dentinal complex and periodontal apparatus. However, studies of

Practical Procedures in Implant Dentistry, First Edition. Edited by Christopher C.K. Ho.
© 2022 John Wiley & Sons Ltd. Published 2022 by John Wiley & Sons Ltd.
Companion website: www.wiley.com/go/ho/implant-dentistry

dental implants have shown there is an alternative peripheral mechanism along with central neural plasticity. The term 'osseoperception' is used to describe the concept that the patient's occlusal perception may originate from the nerve fibres innervating the TMJ, skin, and oral musculature, and that this is associated with neuroplasticity of the neural system, allowing adaptation to these changes.

It has been suggested that osseointegrated implants without periodontal mechanoreceptors may be more susceptible to occlusal overloading because the ability to adapt to occlusal force and mechanoperception are significantly reduced in dental implants. Implants exhibit low tactile sensitivity and low proprioceptive motion feedback. Overloading refers to stress around the implant components and bone–implant interface that is not biologically acceptable. Dental implants may suffer from occlusal overload because they lack the suspensory periodontal ligaments that provide a shock absorption function in natural teeth.

Edentulous patients rehabilitated with fixed implant-supported bridges in both arches behave as though anesthetised [5, 6]. Svensson and Trulsson [5] report that patients with fixed dental prostheses on natural teeth showed a similar change in motor control and that, as a result, higher biting forces were developed with food holding and biting, as with implant prostheses. Furthermore, during chewing on foods with different hardnesses, people with dental implants showed impaired adaptation of jaw muscle activity to food hardness [7]. Hammerle et al. [8] report the mean threshold value of tactile perception for implants (100.6 g) was 8.75 times higher than that of natural teeth (11.5 g), demonstrating the less sensitive feedback experienced with implant restorations.

These properties of dental implants mean that careful planning of the occlusion must be performed. Adverse loading may be due to poor occlusal planning, parafunction, excessive cantilever forces, improper occlusal designs, premature contacts, as well as inaccuracy of fit of a prosthesis leading to poor distribution of forces applied. It is important, therefore, to control implant occlusion within physiological limits and to provide optimal implant loading for long-term implant success.

Studies have suggested that occlusal overload may contribute to implant bone loss and/or loss of osseointegration in successfully integrated implants [9–13]. In contrast, other authors believe that peri-implant bone loss and failure are primarily associated with biological complications such as peri-implant infection [14, 15]. They question the causality of occlusal overloading for peri-implant tissue loss due to insufficient scientific evidence. However, it is agreed that occlusal overload may cause mechanical complications on dental implants and prostheses such as screw loosening and/or fracture, prosthesis fracture, and implant fracture, eventually leading to compromised implant longevity [16].

Cantilever forces may introduce a larger force on the implant prosthesis because it acts as a force magnifier; depending on the position and direction of force, this may result in overloading on supporting implants. Shackleton et al. [17] found that long cantilevers (>15 mm) induced more implant–prosthesis failures than shorter cantilevers (<15 mm).

In summary, it appears that heavy occlusal forces and poor distribution of occlusal contacts may be factors in overloading, and may lead to higher susceptibility to implant bone loss, implant fractures/loss, and prosthesis failures (Table 30.1).

Table 30.1 Possible overloading factors involved in implantology.

Parafunctional habits – sleep and awake bruxism

Excessive cantilevers

Excessive occlusal prematurity

Large occlusal tables – bucco-lingual width and mesiodistal dimensions

Steep cuspal inclinations

Insufficient numbers of supporting implants for fixed dental prosthesis

Poor occlusion

Insufficient occluding units

30.1.1 Excessive Forces on Dental Implants

Loss of osseointegration and excessive marginal bone loss from excessive lateral load provided with premature occlusal contacts were demonstrated in several animal studies [10–12]. In non-human primate studies, it was observed that five out of eight implants lost osseointegration due to excessive occlusal overloading after 4.5–15.5 months of loading [10, 11]. Among the three remaining implants, one showed severe crestal bone loss and the other two showed the highest bone–implant contact and density. The results suggested that implant loading might have significantly affected the responses of peri-implant osseous structures. However, it should be noted that the loss of osseointegration observed could be attributed to the unrealistically high occlusal overload used in the study. Similar studies were performed in monkeys with different heights of hyperocclusion of 100, 180, and 250 μm [12, 18]. After four weeks of loading, bone loss was observed in the 180 and 250 μm groups, but not in the 100 μm group.

30.1.2 Bruxism and Implants

Wolff's law states that 'Every change in the function of a bone is followed by certain definite changes in its internal architecture and its external conformation.' This means that bone in a healthy person/animal will adapt to loads so that if loading increased to a particular bone then the bone will remodel itself over time to become stronger to resist the load. Frost [19] proposed a 'mechanostat' mechanism that transformed mechanical usage into appropriate signals that then directed bone to different biological activities. These thresholds of bone strain would then allow either bone apposition or resorption, along with normal levels that would allow remodelling.

Parafunctional activity has been proposed to cause overloading of implants [10–12], but there are few controlled trials showing an association in humans, with no causative relationship has been found. Manfredini et al. [20] in their systematic review report that bruxism is unlikely to be a risk factor for biological complications around dental implants, although there are suggestions that it is a risk factor for mechanical complications. Lobbezoo et al. [21] recommend a careful approach for management that is 'experience based and not evidence based'. There are a few practical guidelines as listed in Table 30.2. Besides the recommendation to reduce

Table 30.2 Practical suggestions for reducing the risk of implant failure in bruxers [20].

Use as many implants as possible
Make sure that implants are as large as possible
Splint implants together for more even distribution of loads
Regard the presence of low-density bone tissue as a risk factor for failure
Respect the normal timing of implant loading
Do not perform occlusal rehabilitation with cantilevers
Allow adequate freedom of movement at the occlusal contact areas in maximum intercuspation
Create flatter cuspid planes to allow better transmission of lateral forces
Make a hard resin protective occlusal splint

Source: Manfredini, D., Bucci, M.B., Sabattini, V.B., and Lobbezoo, F. (2011). Bruxism: overview of current knowledge and suggestions for dental implants planning. *Cranio* 29(4): 304–312.

or eliminate bruxism itself, these guidelines concern the number and dimensions of the implants, the design of the occlusion and articulation patterns, and the protection of the final result with a hard occlusal stabilisation splint (night guard).

30.2 Procedures

Many guidelines and theories have been proposed regarding the optimal occlusal schemes required for implant prosthodontics, but evidence is scarce on specific occlusal designs [22].

Koyano and Esaki [23] report there is insufficient evidence to establish clinical guidelines for implant occlusion and recommend that conventional occlusal concepts should be applied for occlusion on implants.

Three occlusal concepts – balanced, group function, and mutually protected occlusion – have been established. All three have maximum intercuspation (MIP) during habitual and/or centric occlusion.

- *Balanced occlusion*: The teeth are contacting bilaterally during all excursions. A balanced approach is used primarily with complete dentures.
- *Group function occlusion*: The posterior teeth contact on the working side during lateral movements, without any balancing side occlusal contacts.
- *Mutually protected occlusion*: The posterior teeth contact in MIP with light contacts on the anterior teeth. In excursive movements there is anterior guidance. This occlusal scheme is based on the concept that the canine is a key element of occlusion avoiding heavy lateral shearing forces on the posterior teeth. Gibbs et al. [24] found that anterior or canine guidance decreased chewing force compared with posterior guidance.

Various different occlusal philosophies have been prescribed for implant prostheses with success, although the scientific literature does not support any one particular approach. Misch and Bidez [25] proposed an implant-protected occlusion for implant restorations that was designed to minimise occlusal forces on implant. Several modifications to conventional occlusal concepts were recommended, including narrowing the occlusal table and reducing the cuspal inclination, correcting the load direction by providing axial loading, providing

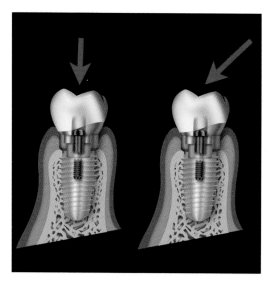

Figure 30.1 Directing occlusal loads axially rather than allowing lateral loads minimises bending moments within implants, reducing the risk of overloading.

load-sharing contacts, reducing cantilevers, and elimination or reduction of occlusal contacts in implants with unfavourable biomechanics and increasing implant surface areas.

The basic principles of implant occlusion include the following [26]:

- Bilateral stability in centric (habitual) occlusion
- Evenly distributed occlusal contacts and force (Figure 30.1)
- No interferences between retruded position and centric (habitual) position
- Wide freedom in centric (habitual) occlusion
- Anterior guidance whenever possible
- Smooth lateral excursive movements without working/non-working interferences.

30.2.1 Clinical Occlusal Applications

The following occlusal considerations for different clinical situations with implant rehabilitation have been suggested (Kim et al. 2005).

Full Arch Implant-Fixed Dental Prosthesis (FAIFDP)
- Bilateral balanced occlusion has been successfully used for an opposing complete denture, while group function occlusion has been used for opposing natural dentitions. Alternatively, a mutually protected occlusion with a shallow anterior guidance can also be recommended for opposing natural dentition.
- Bilateral antero-posterior simultaneous contacts in centric relation and MIP should be obtained to evenly distribute occlusal force during excursions.
- Smooth lateral excursive movements should be attained without any working/non-working occlusal contacts on cantilevers.
- For occlusal contacts, wide freedom (1–1.5 mm) in centric relation and MIP allows axial loading of the implants.
- Cantilevers should not exceed 15 mm in the mandible and 10–12 mm in the maxilla.

Occlusion on Overdentures
- Kim et al. [26] suggest bilateral balanced occlusion with lingualised occlusion on a normal ridge. On the other hand, mono-plane occlusion was recommended for a severely resorbed ridge [27].
- Peroz et al. [28] reported on a randomised clinical trial comparing two occlusal schemes, balanced occlusion and canine guidance, in 22 patients with conventional complete dentures and found that canine guidance was comparable to balanced occlusion in denture retention, aesthetics, and masticatory ability.

Occlusion on Posterior Fixed Prostheses
- An implant-protected occlusion should be prescribed with anterior guidance in excursions, and initial occlusal contact made on natural dentition before contact on implant prostheses. Group function occlusion may need to be used if the anterior teeth are periodontally compromised. During laterotrusion, working and non-working interferences should be avoided in posterior restorations [29].
- Moreover, a narrowed occlusal table is recommended with reduced inclination of cusps, centrally oriented contacts with a 1–1.5 mm flat area, and minimisation of cantilever pontics.

Occlusion on Single-Tooth Implant Restorations
- A single-tooth implant is designed to minimise occlusal force on the implant with the adjacent natural dentition supporting and distributing the forces.
- Excursive movements in laterotrusion and protrusion is obtained by the natural dentition, while any working and non-working contacts are avoided.
- It is recommended that light contacts are made when the patient is biting with a heavy bite while with light occlusion these would have no contact in MIP.
- Other prosthodontic concepts should be adopted to minimise forces such as reduced inclination of cusps, centrally oriented contacts with a 1–1.5 mm flat area, and a narrowed occlusal table (Figure 30.2).

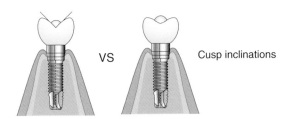

VS   Cusp inclinations

Figure 30.2 Steep cuspal inclinations may produce a bending moment allowing lateral load to the implants. A flat area around centric contacts may direct occlusal force in an apical direction. The reduction of cusp inclination can decrease the resultant bending moment with a lever-arm reduction and improvement of axial loading force. It is recommended that implant restorations should have a reduced cusp inclination, shallow occlusal anatomy, and wide grooves and fossae.

30.3 Tips

- Rangert et al. [30] recommend regular re-evaluation and periodic occlusal adjustments are necessary to prevent potential overload that occurs with the positional changes of natural teeth. Often occlusion may alter due to positional changes, and further restorative dentistry performed over a patient's lifetime. In addition, enamel on teeth wears more rapidly than porcelain on implant restorations, which may result in supra-contact of the implant restoration, possibly overloading the restoration. Regular review and possible adjustment of occlusion should be performed.
- In the restoration of implant-supported fixed dental prostheses, the maintenance of free-standing teeth not rigidly supported as part of a fixed prosthesis may improve the feedback system and jaw muscle control, allowing periodontal mechanoreceptor feedback to be independently activated from those remaining teeth. For example, in a failing dentition it may be feasible to maintain a posterior molar which would not be part of the overall reconstruction yet act as an important feedback mechanism, providing better overall function.
- When assessing occlusion, it is advisable to raise the patient from a supine position to check the chewing cycle to ensure that in the masticatory cycle there are no supra-contacts on the anterior teeth in the patient's envelope of function.

References

1 Schulte, W. (1995). Implants and the periodontium. *Int. Dent. J.* 45: 16–26.
2 Sekine, H., Komiyama, Y., Hotta, H., and Yoshida, K. (1986). Mobility characteristics and tactile sensitivity of osseointegrated fixture-supporting systems. In: *Tissue Integration in Oral Maxillofacial Reconstruction* (ed. D. van Steenberghe), 326–332. Amsterdam: Excerpta Medica.
3 Parfitt, G.J. (1960). Measurement of the physiological mobility of individual teeth in an axial direction. *J. Dental Res.* 39 (3): 608–618.
4 Klineberg, I.J., Trulsson, M., and Murray, G.M. (2012). Occlusion on implants – is there a problem? *J. Oral Rehabil.* 39 (7): 522–537.
5 Svensson, K.G. and Trulsson, M. (2011). Force control during food holding and biting in subjects with tooth-or implant – supported fixed prosthesis. *J. Clin. Periodontol.* 38: 1137–1147.
6 Trulsson, M. and Gunne, H.S. (1998). Food-holding and –biting behaviour in human subjects lacking periodontal receptors. *J. Dent. Res.* 77: 574–582.
7 Grigoriadis, A., Johansson, R.S., and Trulsson, M. (2011). Adaptability of mastication in subjects with implant-supported bridges. *J. Clin. Periodontol.* 38: 395–404.
8 Hämmerle, C.H., Wagner, D., Brägger, U. et al. (1995). Threshold of tactile sensitivity perceived with dental endosseous implants and natural teeth. *Clin. Oral Implants Res.* 6 (2): 83–90.
9 Adell, R., Lekholm, U., Rockler, B., and Branemark, P.I. (1981). A 15-year study of osseointegrated implants in the treatment of the edentulous jaw. *Int. J. Oral Surg.* 10: 387–416.
10 Isidor, F. (1996). Loss of osseointegration caused by occlusal load of oral implants. A clinical and radiographic study in monkeys. *Clin. Oral Implants Res.* 7: 143–152.

11 Isidor, F. (1997). Histological evaluation of peri-implant bone at implants subjected to occlusal overload or plaque accumulation. *Clin. Oral Implants Res.* 8: 1–9.

12 Miyata, T., Kobayashi, Y., Araki, H. et al. (2000). The influence of controlled occlusal overload on peri-implant tissue. Part 3: a histologic study in monkeys. *Int. J. Oral Maxillofac. Implants* 15: 425–431.

13 Rangert, B., Krogh, P.H., Langer, B., and Van Roekel, N. (1995). Bending overload and implant fracture: a retrospective clinical analysis. *Int. J. Oral Maxillofac. Implants* 10: 326–334.

14 Lang, N., Wilson, T.G., and Corbet, E.F. (2000). Biological complications with dental implants: their prevention, diagnosis and treatment. *Clin. Oral Implants Res.* 11 (Suppl): 146–155.

15 Tonetti, M. and Schmid, J. (1994). Pathogenesis of implant failures. *Periodontology* 2000 (4): 127–138.

16 Schwarz, M.S. (2000). Mechanical complications of dental implants. *Clin. Oral Implants Res.* 11 (Suppl 1): 156–158.

17 Shackleton, J.L., Carr, L., Slabbert, J.C., and Becker, P.J. (1994). Survival of fixed implant-supported prostheses related to cantilever lengths. *J. Prosthet. Dent.* 71: 23–26.

18 Miyata, T., Kobayashi, Y., Araki, H. et al. (1998). The influence of controlled occlusal overload on peri-implant tissue: a histologic study in monkeys. *Int. J. Oral Maxillofac. Implants* 13 (5): 677–683.

19 Frost, H.M. (1987). Bone "mass" and the "mechanostat": a proposal. *Anat Rec.* 219 (1): 1–9.

20 Manfredini, D., Bucci, M.B., Sabattini, V.B., and Lobbezoo, F. (2011). Bruxism: overview of current knowledge and suggestions for dental implants planning. *Cranio* 29 (4): 304–312.

21 Lobbezoo, F., Brouwers, J.E., Cune, M.S., and Naeije, M. (2006). Dental implants in patients with bruxing habits. *J. Oral Rehabil.* 33 (2): 152–159.

22 Carlsson, G.E. (2009). Dental occlusion: modern concepts and their application in implant prosthodontics. *Odontologia* 97 (1): 8–17.

23 Koyano, K. and Esaki, D. (2015). Occlusion on oral implants: current clinical guidelines. *J. Oral Rehabil.* 42 (2): 153–161.

24 Gibbs, C.H., Mahan, P., Lundeen, H. et al. (1981). Occlusal forces during chewing – influences of biting strength and food consistency. *J. Prosthet. Dent.* 46: 561–567.

25 Misch, C.E. and Bidez, M.W. (1994). Implant-protected occlusion: a biomechanical rationale. *Compendium (Newtown, Pa.).* 15 (11): 1330–1332.

26 Kim, Y., Oh, T.J., Misch, C.E., and Wang, H.L. (2005). Occlusal considerations in implant therapy: clinical guidelines with biomechanical rationale. *Clin. Oral Implants Res.* 16 (1): 26–35.

27 Mericske-Stern, R.D., Taylor, T.D., and Belser, U. (2000). Management of the edentulous patient. *Clin. Oral Implants Res.* 11 (Suppl 1): 108–125.

28 Peroz, I., Leuenberg, A., Haustein, I., and Lange, K.P. (2003). Comparison between balanced occlusion and canine guidance in complete denture wearers – a clinical, randomized trial. *Quintessence Int.* 34 (8): 607–612.

29 Lundgren, D. and Laurell, L. (1994). Biomechanical aspects of fixed bridgework supported by natural teeth and endosseous implants. *Periodontology* 2000: 23–40.

30 Rangert, B.R., Sullivan, R.M., and Jemt, T.M. (1997). Load factor control for implants in the posterior partially edentulous segment. *Int. J. Oral Maxillofac. Implants* 12: 360–370.

31

Dental Implant Screw Mechanics

Christopher C.K. Ho and Louis Kei

31.1   Principles

An implant screw joint consists of two parts – the implant fixture and the abutment, tightened together by a screw. The screw is tightened by a rotational force (torque), allowing the screw when tightened to elongate, producing a tensile force. This tensile force is commonly referred to as the 'preload'. The preload allows a clamping force between the screw head and the seat within an implant connection. The preload produced within an implant screw joint is generally directly proportional to the tightening torque. The manufacturer usually recommends a specific torque for each screw/abutment assembly, which is dictated by the material and design of the specific screw joint.

The implant screw joint is constantly subjected to external joint-separating forces and factors within the oral cavity that may include the following:

- Excursive contacts
- Off-axis centric contacts
- Interproximal contacts
- Cantilever contacts
- Non-passive framework of a dental prosthesis
- Parafunctional activity
- Long crown height:implant ratio.

A screw may loosen if forces trying to separate the parts are greater than the preload within the screw joint. Excessive joint-separating forces cause slippage between threads of the screw and threads, resulting in a loss of preload. When preload is lost, micromotions within the screw joint increase during function. The anti-rotational features of the abutment–implant interface cease to engage properly and the protection it offers to the screw against excessive external forces is lost. When the external forces exceed the yield strength of the screw, the screw plastically deforms and it may fracture as a result (Figure 31.1).

Practical Procedures in Implant Dentistry, First Edition. Edited by Christopher C.K. Ho.
© 2022 John Wiley & Sons Ltd. Published 2022 by John Wiley & Sons Ltd.
Companion website: www.wiley.com/go/ho/implant-dentistry

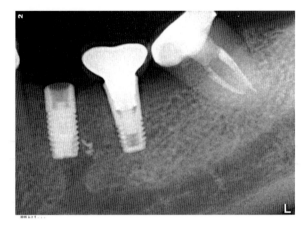

Figure 31.1 Radiograph of fractured abutment screw within an internal connection implant. Careful use of ultrasonics was able to gently dislodge this fractured screw.

31.1.1 Factors Affecting Implant Screw Joint Stability

31.1.1.1 Preload

In order to maximise screw joint stability, McGlumphy et al. [1] recommend 'maximum' clamping forces (preload) should be generated. The ideal preload for a particular screw was recommended at 75% of the yield strength of the screw material.

The more torque applied to an abutment screw, more preload is achieved within the screw joint assembly [2].

31.1.1.2 Embedment Relaxation (Settling Effect)

Embedment relaxation, or the settling effect of screw joints, describes the phenomenon whereby a significant loss of preload is observed after the screw is initially tightened into place within the joint assembly. This occurs because no surface is completely smooth, and because of this micro-roughness no two surfaces are completely in contact with one another. When the screw joint assembly is subjected to external loads, wear of the contact areas occurs, bringing the two surfaces closer to each other. As a result of this, a loss of preload follows.

It has been reported in the literature that 2–10% of the initial preload is lost due to embedment relaxation of the screw joint assembly [3–5]. The magnitude of settling depends on the initial surface roughness, surface hardness, and the magnitude of loading forces. Siamos et al. [5] observed a decrease of up to 29% of torque in implant joint assemblies three hours after the initial tightening. However, when the abutment screws were re-tightened 10 minutes after the initial tightening, the torque loss after three hours reduced to only 19%.

31.1.1.3 Screw Material and Coating

The material from which the prosthetic screw is fabricated directly influences the amount of preload generated within the screw joint assembly. A screw with a high yield strength can tolerate higher insertion torque and is therefore able to generate a higher preload. Jorneus et al. [4] compared the torque generated from three screws fabricated from different metal alloys and concluded that the gold alloy screw produced the highest preload (compared to two titanium alloy screws).

More recently, implant manufacturers have experimented by adding a solid lubricant on abutment screw surfaces to decrease the coefficient of friction [6]. It is thought that a reduction in the surface friction may reduce the embedment relaxation of the screw joint, leading to higher preloads and better joint stability. Examples of solid lubricants include:

- Gold-Tite® – gold alloy screw (80% Pd, 10% Ga, 10% Cu/Au/Zn) coated with 0.76 μm of pure gold (3i Implant Innovations, Inc.)
- TorqTite® – titanium alloy screw coated with amorphous carbon (Nobel Biocare)
- Teflon coating.

Martin et al. [2] evaluated the materials and surfaces of four commercially available abutment screws on preload generation and found the greatest preload values at 20 and 32 Ncm were by the Gold-Tite and TorqTite abutment screws (compared with non-coated gold alloy and titanium alloy screws).

31.1.1.4 Screw Design

Jorneus et al. [4] compared the preload generated by two abutment screw head designs (flat head and conical head) and found a significantly lower preload was generated with abutment screws having a conical head design. The authors speculated that the conical screw lost a major part of the torque as friction between the conical screw head and the abutment, thereby allowing less preload generated within the screw joint assembly.

31.1.1.5 Abutment/Implant Interface Misfit

Abutment/implant interface misfit has been considered a significant factor in screw joint failure. In a laboratory study by Binon [7], a series of 10 incrementally larger UCLA abutments were loaded off-axis with 133 N and cycled at 1150 vertical strokes per minute. Rotational misfit between internal and external hexagons ranged from 1.94 degrees for the smallest abutment to 14.87 degrees for the largest. It was found that there was a strong direct correlation between the amount of hexagonal misfit and screw loosening. The authors concluded the greater the rotational freedom, the greater the probability of screw loosening.

31.1.1.6 Abutment/Implant Interface Design

The anti-rotational element offered by the abutment/implant interface design is crucial in the preservation of the abutment screw preload during function. A correctly fitting prosthetic interface can significantly reduce the amount of joint-separating forces transferred onto the abutment screw, reducing the chances of abutment screw loosening or fracture. Historically, the prosthetic connection was an external hex, but more recent connections have been developed with a Morse-like taper connection, which provides more even distribution of forces and reduced screw loosening.

Binon [7] removed the external hex from the implant fixture and subjected the implant/abutment assembly to simulated functional loading. It was found the absence of the external implant hex extension significantly increased the likelihood to screw loosening. Weiss et al. [8] recorded repeated opening torque values of seven commercially available implant/abutment assemblies and found that systems with Morse taper and spline connections consistently maintained higher preload values than the external hex connections.

31.1.1.7 Functional Forces
McGlumphy and colleagues proposed the following strategies to minimise joint-separating forces on the implant/abutment assembly:

- Minimise prosthesis cantelever
- Minimise contacts in lateral excursion
- Minimise off-axis centric contacts
- Reduce cuspal angles.

Bakaeen et al. [9] investigated the influence of the bucco-lingual width of the occlusal table on the torque required to loosen gold prosthetic screws after subjecting implants and implant-supported restorations to simulated occlusal loads. The authors discovered a significant reduction in screw untightening torque (proxy for a higher loss of preload) in the restorations with a wide occlusal table compared to restorations with a narrow occlusal table.

31.1.1.8 Number of Implants
Bakaeen et al. [9] compared the incidence of screw loosening and values of untightening torque of the screws among crowns supported by one wide-diameter implant or two standard implants after loading *in vitro*. The crowns were subjected to a 6 kg load for 16 660 cycles over 5.5 hours and were loaded at the outer and inner inclines and cusp tips. The authors found missing molars restored with one wide-diameter implant had a greater incidence of screw loosening than those with two implants.

31.1.1.9 Torque Wrench
An appropriate amount of torque applied to the screw by a clinician is crucial to the long-term implant joint stability. Inadequate tightening may cause premature loosening of the screw while in function, yet excessive torque that exceeds the yield strength of the screw will create permanent deformation in the screw shank, leading to screw fracture.

Gutierrez et al. [10] tested the accuracy of torque delivery of 35 implant torque wrenches that has been in clinical service between one month and three years. These torque wrenches were engineered to be accurate within a margin of error of ±3%. The authors discovered that of the 35 torque wrenches tested, 25 produced a torque that was high, 5 low, and only 6 wrenches were within the 3% limit. The biggest error recorded was 455% greater than the 10 Ncm the torque wrench was intended to deliver. Severe corrosion of the spring was discovered when the offending torque wrench was disassembled.

31.2 Procedures

Table 31.1 provides practical recommendations to limit implant screw loosening or fracture.

31.2.1 Techniques for Retrieving a Fractured Screw

31.2.1.1 The Ultrasonic Scaler Technique [11]
1) Make an access hole occlusally through the crown to access the screw head.
2) Retrieve the crown along with the abutment.
3) Once the crown and abutment are removed, take a radiograph to reconfirm the fractured part of the abutment screw inside the implant.

Table 31.1 Practical measures to limit implant screw loosening and or fracture.

Screw selection	Use genuine manufacturer-supplied abutment and prosthetic screws to ensure quality and consistency
	Use gold-coated abutment screw if high preload is required
	Avoid using conically shaped head abutment screws
	Select internal hexagon prosthetic screws where possible over slotted prosthetic screws
	Use a brand new screw for the delivery of a new prosthesis (avoid allowing the lab to use the new screw for the fabrication of the restoration)
Screw tightening	Apply the manufacturer's recommended torque values
	Retorque the abutment/prosthetic screw after 10 minutes from the initial tightening to minimise preload loss due to embedment relaxation
	Minimise unnecessary opening and closing of abutment/prosthetic screws, especially when a gold-coated screw is selected
Abutment/implant connection selection	Use reputable implant manufacturers to ensure high quality and precisely machined fit
	In cases with expected high occlusal loads, select an interface that offers superior anti-rotational features for better abutment screw protection
Prosthesis design	Minimise cantilever
	Ensure passive framework fit
Occlusal design	Minimise excursive contacts
	Minimise off-axis centric contacts
	Reduce cusp height and angles
	Reduce width of occlusal table
Torque wrench	Annual calibration to ensure accurate torque output of the torque wrench
	Inspection for any corrosion in the spring component in detent joint wrenches

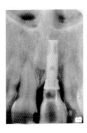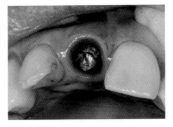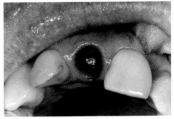

Figure 31.2 Stripped screw head. The top of the screw is carefully removed allowing the release of the clamping force with the remaining screw loose within the screw channel. An ultrasonic is used to gently vibrate the screw until sufficient amount can be grasped and unscrewed.

4) Use a fine tapered carbide bur to make a notch on the occlusal surface of abutment screw between the centre of the screw and its periphery. Take care not to touch the internal threads of the implant with the bur, but ensuring that the notch is made off-centre (Figure 31.2).
5) Insert an ultrasonic scaler tip into the implant and to engage the notch created.
6) Start the ultrasonic scaler at a very low speed, and move the tip of the scaler mechanically counterclockwise to remove the fractured screw.

31.2.1.2 Screwdriver Technique

A diamond flame-shaped or thin tapered carbide bur can be modified to prepare a groove on the fractured screw. The diamond particles of the upper part of the flame-shaped bur can be removed and polished in order not to damage the internal screw thread of the implant.

1) Create a thin groove on the screw.
2) Position a flat screwdriver into the groove prepared in the fractured screw in the implant and slowly rotate counterclockwise.

31.2.1.3 Manufacturer Rescue Kits

Implant manufacturers produce rescue kits–drills that work in reverse. They are carefully drilled in a counterclockwise direction into the fractured screw. These are guided through specific mounts made to fit within implant connections so that drilling is down the long axis of the screw.

1) Use a rescue kit to drill a hole.
2) Once a hole is made within the screw, a reverse-thread screwdriver can be inserted into the fractured screw and the offending screw removed.
3) The internal channel should be carefully flushed of any metal shavings and a screw tap can be used to ensure the internal threads are clean and precise prior to replacing the screw.

31.3 Tips

- In cases of repeated screw loosening it is prudent to assess the occlusion and possible overload as well as passivity of fit. Consider replacing the screw as this may be weakened and susceptible to fracture.

- Broken screw removal is often difficult and should be undertaken with the use of magnification and good illumination. If there is difficulty in removal, then it would be best to refer to an experienced practitioner to remove rather than attempting removal with inadvertent damage to the internal thread.
- Screws can sometimes accidentally fall out of a prosthesis. The author inserts chlorhexidine gel within the screw channels so that the screws are maintained by the sticky nature of the gel to remain in the screw channels.
- Always protect the screw head from damage by using PTFE tape/gutta percha or cotton wool over the screw head before restoration.

References

1 McGlumphy, E.A., Mendel, D.A., and Holloway, J.A. (1998). Implant screw mechanics. *Dent. Clin. N. Am.* 42: 71–89.

2 Martin, W.C., Woody, R.D., Miller, B.H., and Miller, A.W. (2001). Implant abutment screw rotations and preloads for four different screw materials and surfaces. *J. Prosthet. Dent.* 86: 24–32.

3 Winkler, S., Ring, K., Ring, J.D., and Boberick, K.G. (2003). Implant screw mechanics and the settling effect: an overview. *J. Oral Implantol.* 29: 242–245.

4 Jorneus, L., Jemt, T., and Carlsson, L. (1992). Loads and designs of screw joints for single crowns supported by osseointegrated implants. *Int. J. Oral Maxillofac. Implants* 7: 353–359.

5 Siamos, G., Winkler, S., and Boberick, K.G. (2002). The relationship between implant preload and screw loosening on implant-supported prostheses. *J. Oral Implantol.* 28: 67–73.

6 Elias, C.N., Figueira, D.C., and Rios, P.R. (2006). Influence of the coating material on the loosing of dental implant abutment screw joints. *Mater. Sci. Eng. A* 26: 1361–1366.

7 Binon, P.P. (1996). The effect of implant/abutment hexagonal misfit on screw joint stability. *Int. J. Prosthodont.* 9: 149–160.

8 Weiss, E.I., Kozak, D., and Gross, M.D. (2000). Effect of repeated closures on opening torque values in seven abutment-implant systems. *J. Prosthet. Dent.* 84: 194–199.

9 Bakaeen, L.G., Winkler, S., and Neff, P.A. (2001). The effect of implant diameter, restoration design, and occlusal table variations on screw loosening of posterior single-tooth implant restorations. *J. Oral Implantol.* 27: 63–72.

10 Gutierrez, J., Nicholls, J.I., Libman, W.J., and Butson, T.J. (1997). Accuracy of the implant torque wrench following time in clinical service. *Int. J. Prosthodont.* 17: 562–567.

11 Walia, M.S., Arora, S., Luthra, R., and Walia, P.K. (2012). Removal of fractured dental implant screw using a new technique: a case report. *J. Oral Implantol.* 38: 747–750.

32

Prosthodontic Rehabilitation for the Fully Edentulous Patient
Christopher C.K. Ho

32.1   Principles

The emotional and behavioural effects of tooth loss in edentulous patients encompass grief, lowered self-confidence, altered self-image, dislike of appearance, inability to discuss taboo subject, privacy, behaving in a way to keep tooth loss secret, altered behaviour when socialising and forming close relationships, sense of premature ageing, and lack of preparation [1]. Combined with the poorer function and continuing ridge resorption that occurs with tooth loss, this may make removable prostheses more difficult for some patients. Although there has been a decline in edentulism over the last 30 years, the overall increase in the adult population means the numbers of edentulous patients are increasing [2].

The treatment options for the fully edentulous patient include the following:

- Conventional removable dental prosthesis
- Implant-retained overdenture
- Implant-supported overdenture
- Implant-supported bridgework
- Zygomatic implant reconstructions.

Clinical assessment should include the usual protocols required for planning implant treatment, but there are additional specific factors that should be carefully assessed including the following:

- *Restorative space*: This is the interocclusal space from the soft tissue to the antagonist occlusal plane and must be sufficient to be able to incorporate the prosthetic componentry (Figure 32.1). Insufficient space may lead to technical complications with fracture of either componentry or veneering materials. In the fully edentulous patient, it may be necessary to carry out an alveolectomy to attain sufficient restorative space, adjustment of opposing dentition or alternatively, opening of the occlusal vertical dimension (OVD) to create the desired space.

Practical Procedures in Implant Dentistry, First Edition. Edited by Christopher C.K. Ho.
© 2022 John Wiley & Sons Ltd. Published 2022 by John Wiley & Sons Ltd.
Companion website: www.wiley.com/go/ho/implant-dentistry

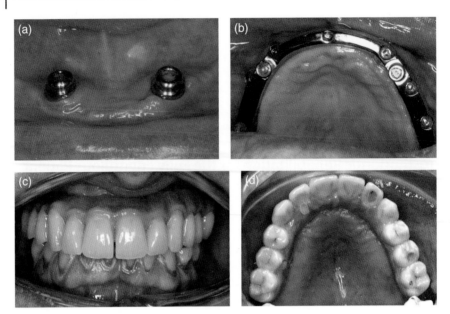

Figure 32.1 Interocclusal space requirements with different restorative options. (a) Locator-retained implant overdenture: 8–9 mm. (b) Milled bar implant overdenture: 11 mm. (c) Implant-fixed complete denture: 11–12 mm. (d) Full arch implant-supported metal ceramic bridgework: 7 mm.

- *Transition line and lip support*: The 'prosthesis–tissue junction' in full arch implant rehabilitation may need to be hidden under the maxillary lip line for optimal aesthetics. It is difficult to achieve perfect soft tissue aesthetics around multiple dental implants without considerable surgical expertise and skill. Assessing the smile line is important, as patients with high smile line may reveal excessive amounts of soft tissue and may not be able to hide the transition line between the soft tissue and the final bridge (Figure 32.2). Adequate lip support may need to be provided by the flange of the removable prosthesis. A fixed prosthesis in this instance may make it impossible for effective peri-implant cleaning. Lip and facial support are often deciding factors when the clinician must choose between fixed or removable prostheses.
- *Dentofacial aesthetics and OVD*: It is important to utilise facially generated treatment planning protocols to develop optimal dentofacial aesthetics. This is staged into four steps including:
  1) *Setting the maxillary incisal edge*: It is important to have an initial starting point, and this starts with the maxillary incisal edge position. The average 30-year-old woman displays 3.4 mm of tooth structure, whereas males display 1.9 mm [3]. The clinician may modify this depending on the patient's aesthetic requirements. When restoring a dentate appearance, Waliszewski [4] found that 55% of patients preferred a normal setup of teeth, 19% preferred supernormal (enhanced display of maxillary teeth), and 26% preferred a denture look. Determining patient's wants and desires to assess their individual requirements is important and requires input from the patient.

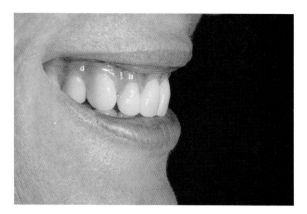

Figure 32.2 The transition line or prosthesis tissue junction is visible in this high smile line patient. In some cases, this would not be aesthetic and a need to carry out a removable prosthesis with a flange would be necessary so that the junction is hidden. An alternative option would have been to carry out more alveolectomy so that the junction is hidden behind the upper lip. Correct diagnostics and assessment of the dentofacial aesthetics is important to provide the optimal aesthetic result for the patient.

2) *Positioning the maxillary occlusal plane*: The posterior maxillary teeth are set with the cusp tips positioned parallel to the camper plane (ala-tragal line).
3) *Setting the mandibular incisal edge*: This provides the OVD, and there are several different procedures that clinicians may use to determine the correct OVD. The most used protocols include an assessment of the facial appearance, the use of phonetic sounds (sibilant 's', fricative 'f' sounds, 'm' sounds), and swallowing. The use of the 's' sound is particularly useful for assessing the freeway space and determining whether the patient has sufficient physiological space for phonetics and function. The pronunciation of the 's' sound provides the closest speaking distance, so when a patient pronounces 's' the edges of the anterior teeth come close to touching.
4) *Positioning the mandibular occlusal plane*: The mandibular posterior teeth are positioned to fit to the maxillary teeth, and another important landmark is the mandibular occlusal plane, which is situated normally at a height half to two-thirds of the retromolar pad.

32.1.1 Number of Implants for Full Arch Implant Rehabilitation

32.1.1.1 Removable Overdenture

The literature reports that for a removable overdenture prosthesis in the mandible two implants are very successful (Figure 32.3). Two expert opinion statements have been made on the standard of care to support two implant overdentures for the edentulous mandible: the McGIll consensus statement [5] and the York statement [6]. However, in the maxilla, long-term prospective studies are needed. There have been no randomised controlled trials in the maxilla, although there are clinical reports on the higher numbers of failures and complications for maxillary

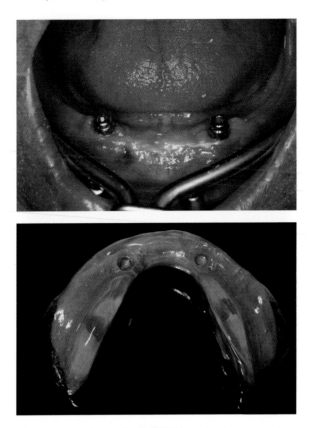

Figure 32.3 Completely removable mandibular dental prosthesis using two locator attachments.

implant overdentures. Nonetheless, the design and planning of removable implant-retained overdentures requires full extension of the denture-fitting surface to maximise support of sthe denture.

In the edentulous mandible, the wearing of a fully removable prosthesis is considered to be extremely difficult with poor comfort and function. The aim has been to minimise financial costs to allow a larger proportion of this cohort of patients to improve their quality of life. The use of one implant placed in the mandibular symphysis area to support an overdenture has been reported to have no statistical difference on overall survival and success [7]. However, it is reported they have a tendency to need more prosthetic maintenance, with fractures through the acrylic in the attachment area.

The use of more than two implants to support a removable implant over-denture is sometimes advised; in these cases due to the larger number of implants (normally four or more) the support can actually be achieved from the implants without having to have full extensions and tissue support. This means the support is very similar to that of a fixed implant-supported bridge, but it allows the overdenture to be removed and makes maintenance simpler (Figure 32.4).

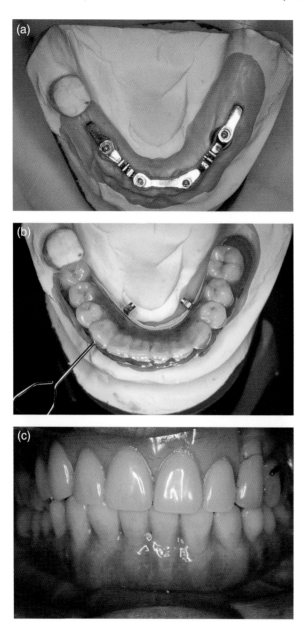

Figure 32.4 Fixed/removable implant-supported bridgework. (a) Titanium bar. (b) The use of a MK1 attachment on a bar with lateral cross-pins to retain the removable superstructure. This prosthesis provides excellent stability while having the ability to be removed. (c) Removable overdenture *in situ*.

32.1.2 Fixed Implant-Supported Bridgework

There is a lack of evidence on the optimum number of implants for a fixed implant supported bridge, but there is well-documented literature on the use of four to six implants as a treatment option for full arch implant-supported

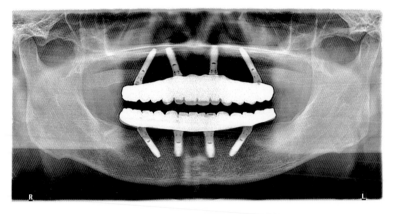

Figure 32.5 All on 4® implant-supported bridgework with angled posterior implants to avoid the maxillary sinus for the maxilla and to avoid the mental foramen in the mandible. The increase in antero-posterior spread of the implants allow a reduction in distal cantilever length.

bridgework. There has also been the use of three implants to support a fixed bridge in the edentulous mandible with the historical Brånemark Novum™ (Nobel Biocare), and more recently Trefoil™ (Nobel Biocare).

The use of a minimum of four implants have been recommended for full arch implant rehabilitation, but clinicians should perform a comprehensive assessment and treatment planning to determine if there may be a need to add more implants to support a fixed reconstruction. Such indications for more implants may include those with higher risk factors for complications or failure such as smokers, bruxers, patients with poor quality and quantity of bone or diabetes, etc.

The All-on-4® treatment concept (Nobel Biocare) is a graft-less solution utilising four implants, with the posterior implants tilted to avoid anatomical regions such as the maxillary sinus or the mental foramen (Figure 32.5). The objective at placement is to ensure sufficient antero-posterior spread of the implants, minimising cantilever forces. Cantilever forces are a force magnifier, and there is a higher incidence of technical complications (20.3 versus 9.7% for non-cantilever fixed partial denture prostheses, while the peri-implant marginal bone loss has been shown to be similar [8]. By tilting implants, the posterior implants are placed in a more posterior location, minimising the distal cantilever forces.

32.2 Procedures

32.2.1 Occlusal Vertical Dimension

OVD is the distance measured between two points when the occluding teeth are in contact. In the fully edentulous patient, because there is a loss of all occlusal contacts, prosthodontic management requires the subjective determination of the OVD (Table 32.1). This provides the height of the lower third of the face, and will provide satisfactory dentofacial aesthetics as well as providing adequate freeway space for correct masticatory function and speech. Altering the vertical dimension may also change occlusal relationships and will provide prosthetic convenience or sufficient room to house the prosthetic componentry required

Table 32.1 Methods of assessing occlusal vertical dimension.

Pretreatment records – old models and previous photographs

Incisor height measurement – 18 mm distance between gingival margins in occlusion

Phonetics – sibilant 's', fricative 'f' sounds, 'm' sounds

Patient relaxation – swallowing

Assessment of facial appearance

Radiographic – cephalometric

Neuromuscular – EMG of muscles in rest position

for dental implants. Abduo [9] reported that a permanent increase in OVD up to 5 mm is a safe and predictable procedure, with associated signs and symptoms being self-limiting, with a tendency to resolve within two weeks. Increasing the OVD may result in a reduction in masticatory muscle activity; with adaptation muscles will lengthen and relax, leading to a resolution of symptoms within one to two weeks and adaptation within a month.

32.2.2 Phonetics

The use of phonetics is an important step to ensure that tooth position is correct. Pound [10, 11] describes how speech can be used in planning removable prostheses, and this can also be applied in full arch implant prosthodontics.

- **'F' – *fricative sounds***: To create the 'f' sound the jaw is held nearly closed. The upper back side of the bottom lip is pressed very lightly into the bottom of the top teeth. Air is pushed out the mouth between the top teeth and the upper back side of the bottom lip. Asking the patient to say 'fifty-five' will locate the incisal edges of the maxillary anterior teeth. The maxillary teeth will contact the vermillion border or wet–dry line of the lower lip, providing a guide to adequate length as well as labio-palatal position. Increased length may start to impact on speech and the patient may complain that they are hitting their lip or feel that their teeth are too long.
- **'S' – *sibilant sounds***: To create the 's', the front of the tongue is placed close to the tooth ridge. The tip of the tongue should be close to the upper back side of the top front teeth. The tongue is kept tense as air is pushed between a small groove along the centre of the tip of the tongue and the front of the tooth ridge. The front sides of the tongue touch the side teeth toward the front of the mouth. The lips are held slightly tense during the sound. Asking the patient to say 'sixty-six' or 'She sells sea shells on the sea shore' will demonstrate the closest speaking distance. Excessive opening of the vertical dimension will create difficulty in annunciating the 's' sounds with the patient finding insufficient room for pronouncing the sound or that their teeth are clicking together on speech.
- **'M' *sound***: To create the 'm sound', the lips are pressed together, causing the air to be blocked from leaving the mouth. The soft palate drops, allowing air to pass out through the nose. Asking the patient to say 'Emma' will demonstrate the rest position and repose position of the maxillary teeth. This will allow determination of maxillary tooth length when lips are at rest (repose position).

Additionally, this will give the postural rest position of the mandible. This position is where the muscles that close the jaws and those that open them are in a state of minimal contraction so as to maintain the posture of the mandible. This space that exists between the maxilla and mandible is called the 'freeway space', and the allowance of at least 2 mm of freeway space is necessary for correct function.

32.2.3 Swallowing

During the function of swallowing saliva, the mandible leaves its rest position and rises to the natural vertical dimension of occlusion; then, as the saliva is forced backward into the pharynx by the tongue, the mandible is retruded along with the tongue to its natural centric relation [12].

32.2.4 Facial Appearance

An important outcome is satisfactory masticatory function and speech, but also improved dentofacial aesthetics. Having suffered loss of teeth, fully edentulous patients will experience continual ridge resorption atrophy. Because of this, they may experience a loss of lip support, a loss of facial height, and suffer from being 'over-closed'. The lower face height and accompanying smile may be significantly improved by opening the vertical dimension, as well as the correct placement of teeth. Furthermore, this may assist in improving the occlusal relationship. The improved quality-of-life measures result not only from the return of function but also from the improvement in appearance and self-image.

32.2.5 Impression Taking

The aim of multiple unit impression taking is passive fit of the final prosthesis, to create as accurate a fit as possible to avoid bone strain resulting from uncontrolled loading of the implants through the superstructure. Poor fit may lead to mechanical strain and load on the prosthesis, resulting in possible screw loosening, as well as mechanical fracture of componentry. To increase the accuracy of multiple unit impressions it is recommended that impression copings are splinted prior to taking the impression. In a systematic review, Papaspyridakos et al. [13] found the splinted impression technique is more accurate for both partially and completely edentulous patients. The open tray technique is more accurate for completely edentulous patients, and is recommended in full arch cases.

32.2.6 Abutment Selection

The prosthodontic rehabilitation of full arch cases may involve the use of a transmucosal abutment called a 'multi-unit abutment'. These are intermediary metal abutments that allow correction of angulation and issues around divergent implant insertion paths. Because of the anatomy of the alveolar ridge it may not be possible to place implants parallel to each other and hence attempts to connect internally with screws may encounter insertion path issues. Multi-unit abutments have a tapered wide-angle cone with different heights; they are also available in angulated versions allowing for correction of angulated implants such as in 'all-on-4' protocols, as well as in cases of the need to angulate the screws in aesthetic regions so that access holes are not visible.

32.2.7 Prosthodontic Options for Fixed Bridgework

A decision on the final choice of material will depend on restorative space, aesthetic requirements, clinician preference, and financial budget. Options include the following:

- All acrylic bridgework
- Acrylic titanium hybrid bridge
- Ceramo-metal hybrid bridge (precious metal and layered feldspathic porcelain)
- Zirconia/titanium/cobalt-chrome bridge – layered feldspathic porcelain
- Zirconia/titanium/cobalt-chrome bridge – individual all-ceramic crowns
- Monolithic zirconia on titanium/cobalt-chrome bar (Figure 32.6).

32.2.8 Occlusion

There are many different occlusal schemes available and insufficient evidence to establish clinical guidelines for implant occlusion [14]; however, it has been reported that conventional occlusal concepts should be adopted and these include the following:

- Reduce force on implant prostheses
- Narrow occlusal table
- Reduce cusp inclination
- Reduce non-axial loading
- Reduce length of cantilever.

Further information can be read in Chapter 30.

32.3   Tips

- An implant-retained overdenture gains tissue support from the denture base, and it is imperative to ensure correct impression of all the denture borders to capture the peripheral extensions and primary support areas.
- In full arch fixed implant-supported bridgework it is often advantageous for a patient to be provided with a provisional prosthesis to ensure they are comfortable with its desired function, occlusion, and aesthetics prior to fabrication of the definitive prosthesis.
- A verification jig can be used to check that the initial master impression is correct and a simple procedure used to ensure passive fit for the final prosthesis. This jig is essentially a second impression splinting impression coping and resin together, which is then verified on the master cast to ensure accuracy.

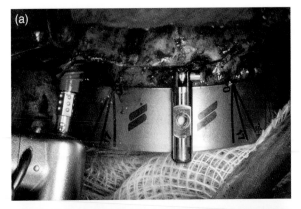

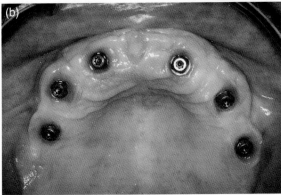

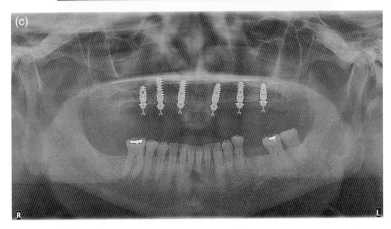

Figure 32.6 (a) Placement of six implants in the maxilla for full arch implant-supported bridgework. (b) Implants with excellent soft tissue health. (c) Orthopantomogram.

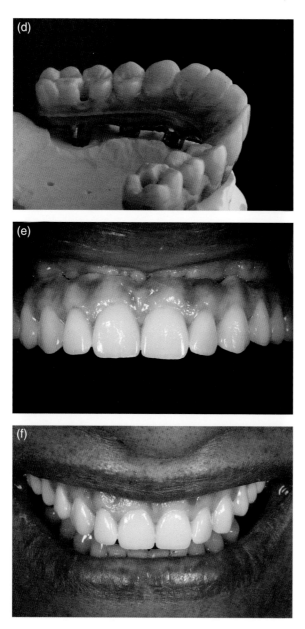

Figure 32.6 (Cont'd) (d) Definitive prosthetic restoration: zirconia (monolithic) on titanium bar. (e) Implant restoration *in situ* demonstrating access for hygiene and easily cleanable contours. (f) Final aesthetic smile. Note that the transition line of the final prosthesis is hidden under the lip line.

- It is important to correctly design a fixed bridge to allow access for oral hygiene, as well as ensuring the fitting surface is not concave, which would trap food and microorganisms. The use of acrylic in contact with the tissues should also be discouraged, because acrylic is a porous material that can harbour microorganisms, leading to a 'denture-stomatitis' type reaction. The use of metal or zirconia may be better suited in contact with the tissues.
- The cantilever length on full arch implant-supported bridgework should not extend past 15 mm in the mandible and 10 mm in the maxilla [15]. Maintain light occlusion on cantilevers and ensure clearance in lateral excursions.

References

1 Fiske, J., Davis, D.M., Frances, C., and Gelbier, S. (1998). The emotional effects of tooth loss in edentulous people. *Br. Dent. J.* 184 (2): 90–93.

2 Douglas, C.W., Shih, A., and Ostry, L. (2002). Will there be a need for complete dentures in the United States in 2020? *J. Prosthet. Dent.* 87: 5–8.

3 Vig, R.G. and Brundo, G.C. (1978). The kinetics of anterior tooth display. *J. Prosthet. Dent.* 39 (5): 502–504.

4 Waliszewski, M. (2005). Restoring dentate appearance: a literature review for modern complete denture esthetics. *J. Prosthet. Dent.* 93 (4): 386–394.

5 Feine, J.S., Carlsson, G.E., Awad, M.A. et al. (2002). The McGill consensus statement on overdentures. Mandibular two-implant overdentures as first choice standard of care for edentulous patients. *Gerodontology* 19 (1): 3–4.

6 British Society for the Study of Prosthetic Dentistry (2009). The York consensus statement on implant-supported overdentures. *Eur. J. Prosthodont. Restor. Dent.* 17 (4): 164–165. Erratum in: Eur. J. Prosthodont. Restor. Dent. 2010; 18(1): 42.

7 Bryant, S.R., Walton, J.N., and MacEntee, M.I. (2015 Jan). A 5-year randomized trial to compare 1 or 2 implants for implant overdentures. *J Dent Res.* 94 (1): 36–43.

8 Zurdo, J., Romão, C., and Wennström, J.L. (2009 Sep). Survival and complication rates of implant-supported fixed partial dentures with cantilevers: a systematic review. *Clin Oral Implants Res.* 20 (Suppl 4): 59–66.

9 Abduo, J. (2012). Clinical considerations for increasing occlusal vertical dimension: a review. *Aust. Dent. J.* 57: 2–10.

10 Pound, E. (1970). Utilizing speech to simplify a personalized denture service. *J. Prosthet. Dent.* 24 (6): 586–600.

11 Pound, E. (1977). Let /S/ be your guide. *J. Prosthet. Dent.* 38 (5): 482–489.

12 Shanahan, T.E. (1955). Physiologic jaw relations and occlusion of complete dentures. *J. Prosthet. Dent.* 5: 319–324.

13 Papaspyridakos, P., Chen, C.J., Gallucci, G.O. et al. (2014). Chronopoulos accuracy of implant impressions for partially and completely edentulous patients: a systematic review. *Int. J. Oral Maxillofac. Implants* 29 (4): 836–845.

14 Koyano, K. and Esaki, D. (2015 Feb). Occlusion on oral implants: current clinical guidelines. *J Oral Rehabil.* 42 (2): 153–161.

15 Kim, Y., Oh, T., Misch, C.E., and Wang, H.L. (2005). Occlusal considerations in implant therapy: clinical guidelines with biomechanical rationale. *Clin. Oral Implant. Res.* 16: 26–35.

33

Implant Maintenance

Kyle D. Hogg and Christopher C.K. Ho

33.1 Principles

Dental implants can be an aesthetic and predictable method of replacing missing teeth. While dental implants are not subject to caries or endodontic pathology like natural teeth, they can develop peri-implant mucositis and peri-implantitis, similar to the natural dentition exhibiting gingivitis and periodontitis. Long-term studies show that both biological and technical complications can arise for both implants and implant-supported restorations [1]. Despite high survival rates over long periods of time, the need for maintenance and revision procedures related to dental implants and their restorations does exist. This can result in significant resources in terms of time and finances allocated to keep the implants healthy and functioning appropriately. The need for continual maintenance, a defined individualised maintenance plan consisting of both at home and professional care, and counselling on the cost of ownership of the implant rehabilitation should be discussed and documented as part of the process of achieving informed consent prior to treatment. Additionally, surgical and prosthetic planning should be conducted in such a way as to minimise avoidable biological and technical complications, with special consideration given to delivering prostheses with contours permitting use of appropriate cleansing devices [2].

The most common biological complications that occur with dental implant treatment are peri-implant mucositis and peri-implantitis (Figure 33.1). Peri-implant mucositis is the plaque-induced reversible inflammatory response of the marginal peri-implant soft tissues. It does not present with appreciable bone loss. While it is also plaque-induced, peri-implantitis features progressive marginal bone loss and clinical signs of infection of the peri-implant soft tissues. Central to the disease process of both conditions is the accumulation or presence of bacterial plaque. A causative relationship between plaque accumulation and inflammatory changes in the peri-implant soft tissues has been shown [3]. A comparison of peri-implant mucositis and peri-implant health can be seen in Figure 33.1. It is generally thought that untreated peri-implant mucositis can progress into peri-implantitis, which can lead to implant failure. This is of

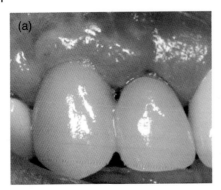
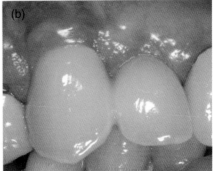

Figure 33.1 Comparison of peri-implant mucositis and healthy peri-implant tissues. (a) Presence of gingival inflammation, soft tissue swelling, and tissue that bleeds easily upon gentle probing. The patient was reluctant to perform basic hygiene around the cantilevered provisional fixed partial denture (FPD) UR 2–3 on the implant in the UR 3 position. (b) Restoration of a healthy peri-implant environment on the same individual around the final cantilevered FPD UR 2–3 after non-surgical supportive therapy and patient education. Note the lack of swelling, inflammation, and bleeding.

Table 33.1 Treatment strategies for maintaining peri-implant tissue health.

Individualised patient education on how to effectively clean and maintain prosthesis and implants
At-home mechanical debridement
Professional in-office mechanical debridement
Chlorhexidine mouthwash/gel
Antiseptic mouthwash
Subgingival irrigation (WaterPik)

importance because the incidence of peri-implant mucositis is fairly common and likely underdiagnosed.

Different maintenance regimens as well as surgical and non-surgical interventions have been proposed for treatment of peri-implant diseases (Table 33.1). Prevention strategies should be aimed at preventing and eliminating the accumulation of bacterial plaque on restorations, abutments, and any susceptible surface of the implant itself via patient education on home care and hygiene instruction, professional in-office supportive therapy on a recall interval that matches the individual's risk assessment, and provision of restorations that facilitate cleaning. As peri-implant diseases have high rates of recurrence, repeated interventions and close monitoring of patients of patients with a past history of the conditions should be considered.

33.1.1 Radiographic Analysis

Implant success is generally evaluated on the basis of clinical findings such as bleeding on probing, pocket depth, and implant mobility; along with radiographic follow-up examinations which provide evidence of changes in peri-implant bone over time. Detection of adverse changes may allow for necessary treatment or improved oral hygiene practices. To monitor marginal bone loss, conventional imaging techniques such as (intra-oral) dental films and (extra-oral) panoramic radiographs have been recommended post-operatively. These have traditionally been taken with either peri-apical radiographs using the long cone technique and a film holder or panoramic radiography [4].

Radiographic interpretation to assess crestal bone has limitations, as a two-dimensional radiograph only displays mesial and distal levels of bone. Bone loss may occur on the facial/buccal aspect of an implant. The absence of radiolucency around an implant does not mean that bone is present at the interface. Bone may be superimposed on an implant. The literature proposes that as much as 40% decrease in density is necessary to be visible on a radiograph due to dense crestal bone [5]. Diagnostic periapical radiographs aim to capture a clear depiction of sharp threads on the radiograph, with the abutment–implant connection as a clear line between the two components. Thus, the radiographs need to be parallel to the implant, and this can be difficult. The apex is often apical to the adjacent natural teeth, and below muscle attachments. This can result in a foreshortened, non-diagnostic image. Often, baseline radiographs are obtained when the prosthesis is delivered, and subsequent radiographs are obtained one-year post insertion, and the images compared. If no changes are apparent the radiographic examinations may be scheduled every two to three years unless other clinical signs warrant more frequent examinations. If there are bony changes noted, then radiographs might be taken more frequently to monitor for deterioration.

Some authors advocate the precision of periapical radiographs in the evaluation of the marginal bone crest changes and its superiority to panoramic radiographs [6]; however, orthopantomograms may be well suited for measurements because of standardised projections [7]. Modern orthopantomograms have complex rotational scanning mechanisms, and the inherent symmetrical imaging error in the vertical plane can be corrected by the magnification factor. Panoramic radiographs produce readable images of the maxilla and mandible, and can be used in patients with limited mouth opening and those who gag. The downside is that they provide 2D views, which may be out of focus because of the superimposition of the vertebral column on the anterior region, are distorted geometrically, and magnify the structures imaged. Batenburg et al. [8] reported that intra-oral radiography may be difficult to near impossible due to the atrophy-related elevation of the floor of the mouth, which can raise the floor of mouth making the film hard to position. In such situations, extra-oral imaging was found to be superior to intra-oral small-format radiography, which was not applicable in all patients (59% in this study) because of atrophy-related elevation of the floor of the mouth.

There are additional problems in assessing bony changes with radiographs, such as the following:

- Intra-examiner and inter-examiner variability.
- Non-standardised image taking. For example, if a radiographic jig is not used to take reproducible radiographs each image may be taken in a different alignment, making accurate comparison impossible.

- Different methods used to assess bone height from the counting of implant threads to using a computer-based interactive image analysis system.
- Different implant geometries and connections, making comparison difficult.
- Diagnostic bias.
- Diagnostic clarity and resolution of comparative radiographs.

Because of this the influence of radiographic imaging factors should be taken into consideration when assessing bony changes around dental implants. These comparative difficulties must be understood so that bony changes are diagnosed correctly and managed appropriately to deal with further bone loss.

33.2 Procedures

Developing an individualised maintenance programme for patients receiving a dental implant restoration with a structured schedule of review will help to prevent biological and technical complications from occurring and allows the clinician to recognise any need for intervention and potentially limit the extent of the complication. To be effective, the maintenance programme must collect clinical and, when appropriate, radiographic data in an organised and repeatable fashion. The plan must be evaluated frequently to determine its effectiveness, and altered as conditions change. A good maintenance programme allows the patient, dental auxiliaries, and clinician to work together to maintain the health, function, and aesthetics of the implant restoration. The following discussion of clinical procedures will commence with delivery of the definitive implant restoration.

With the patient comfortably seated in the dental chair, prepare to deliver the definitive implant restoration. It is good practice to show the patient the component restorative parts prior to delivery to help them better understand how to adequately clean around the restoration. A trial fitting of the restoration should then be conducted to permit the clinician to evaluate, among other things, the contours, proximal contacts, gingival embrasures, and both static and dynamic occlusion. The contours of the restoration should allow for cleansing and prevent stagnation or plaque accumulation. The proximal contacts should be sufficiently loose to allow floss to access but not so open as to allow food to impact. The gingival embrasure design should permit the insertion of cleaning aids or floss threaders. In general, the static occlusion of a single-implant restoration should be light enough such that a ribbon of shim stock is not held by the implant restoration and the antagonistic tooth under light to moderate pressure, but under increasing occlusal force the shim stock is held. Additionally, excursive contacts on the implant restorations should be eliminated or kept to a minimum when possible.

After the trial fitting has been completed to the satisfaction of the clinician the implant restoration may be definitively delivered. When providing implant abutments with cemented crowns, great care must be taken not to introduce excess cement into the peri-implant sulcus. Excess cement in this area is often hard to detect, can be even more challenging to remove, and can lead to peri-implant pathology (see Figure 33.2). Upon delivery of the restoration a baseline radiograph should be taken. The film or sensor should be oriented parallel to the long

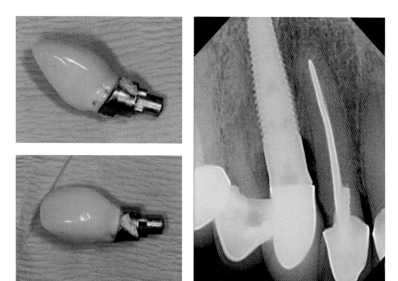

Figure 33.2 Excess cement on buccal and lingual of restoration. The clinical images depict excess cement retained on the abutment and crown of the implant in the UR 3 site. The radiograph shows recurrent decay of the UR 2 and peri-implant bone loss. The patient presented with pain, swelling, and suppuration from the implant sulcus consistent with peri-implantitis.

axis of the implant. The baseline radiograph establishes a reference point of where the hard tissue contours were in relation to the implant at time of restoration. It is important to note that while the radiograph may pick up excess radiopaque cement present on the image, it is poorly sensitive and not a reliable means of establishing that all cement has been removed from the peri-implant sulcus. Steps taken to minimise excess cement being loaded in the crown and a thorough tactile and visual examination of the sulcus are more appropriate means to avoid cementation-related complications.

Time should be taken to instruct and demonstrate to the patient how to adequately clean around the delivered restoration. The patient should then repeat back and perform the cleaning exercise, allowing for remediation of the hygiene techniques and establishing that the patient is equipped to proficiently perform the at-home care required.

A recall interval of between three and six months should be established based upon the individual risk factors of the patient. Factors to be considered in determination of the recall interval include oral hygiene and effectiveness of plaque control, previous history of peri-implant disease, peri-implant bleeding or suppuration, tobacco use, and the needs of the remaining dentition. When examined by the clinician or dental hygienist at a recall visit, the patient should be asked if they are having any trouble with the implant rehabilitation, along with the rest of the dentition. Prior to any instrumentation of the implant the site should be inspected visually, noting the appearance of the peri-implant soft tissues and checking for any signs of oedema or tissue recession. The soft tissues around the implant should be gently compressed to check for any signs of

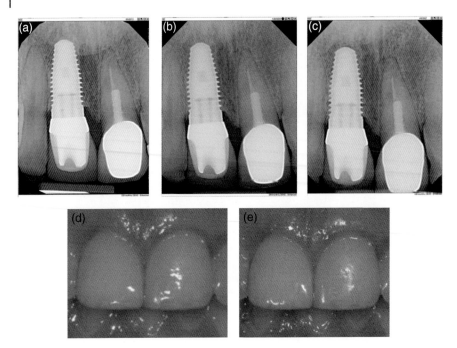

Figure 33.3 Series of radiographs and photographs permitting evaluation of peri-implant hard and soft tissues. High-quality repeatable radiographs (a)–(c) demonstrate the stability of the crestal bone relative to the implant over time. (a) Baseline radiograph. (b) One-year follow-up. (c) Six-year follow-up. Clinical images (d) and (e) depict the stability and health of the peri-implant soft tissues over the same six-year interval, with (d) being the baseline and (e) the six-year follow-up.

suppuration from the sulcus, which would indicate pathology. Following this, gentle periodontal probing can be conducted. Because of the differences in the attachment of natural teeth and implants and the prosthetic transition from implant to clinical crown, the absolute probing depth around implants is not comparable to teeth. What is more important is the presence or absence of bleeding upon probing and the relative changes in probing depths over time associated with the implant. The implant can be percussed to check for mobility or pain. The static and dynamic occlusion should also be re-evaluated with thin articulating paper and a ribbon of shim stock to ensure its stability and fidelity to the prescribed occlusal scheme. The patient should also be screened for parafunctional activity.

Professional mechanical debridement with gold or titanium scalers, and/or ultrasonic or piezoelectric scalers with plastic or carbon tips are suitable for debridement of the restored implant. Although some standard metal scalers may be too hard or abrasive for the debridement of the implant, many plastic hand scalers are not sufficiently rigid to remove plaque or calculus effectively.

A second pre-scripted radiograph, taken in the same fashion as the baseline radiograph (as seen in Figure 33.3), should be conducted one year following the restoration of the implant. The capture of a similar high-quality image allows the clinician to evaluate the stability of the bone levels visible on the radiograph when compared to the baseline. In the absence of clinical and radiographic signs of peri-implantitis, the radiographic interval can be extended to match that of the remaining dentition. If those conditions are not met then an interventive treatment should be initiated promptly or the patient referred to a specialist colleague for further management.

33.3 Tips

1) Discuss with the patient the expectations for maintenance and review prior to initiating treatment. Be sure the patient understands the potential for biological and technical complications associated with the implant rehabilitation, the importance of at-home and professional debridement, and the responsibility for the cost of future maintenance.
2) Develop an individualised maintenance plan for the patient focussing on disease prevention via plaque control and review the effectiveness of and compliance with the plan frequently.
3) Recognise the clinical and radiographic signs and symptoms of peri-implant mucositis or peri-implantitis early and intervene or refer to a specialist colleague for further care.
4) Reassess occlusion on implant restorations frequently, particularly if there have been changes to the dentition.

References

1 Jung, R.E., Zembic, A., Pjetursson, B.E. et al. (2012). Systematic review of the survival rate and the incidence of biological, technical, and aesthetic complications of single crowns on implants reported in longitudinal studies with a mean follow-up of 5 years. *Clin. Oral Implants Res.* 23 (Suppl. 6): 2–21.
2 Lang, N., Wilson, T., and Corbet, E. (2000). Biological complications with dental implants: their prevention, diagnosis, and treatment. *Clin. Oral Implants Res.* 11 (Suppl): 146–155.
3 Pontoriero, R., Tonelli, M.P., Carnevale, G. et al. (1994). Experimentally induced peri-implant mucositis: a clinical study in humans. *Clin. Oral Implants Res.* 5: 254–259.
4 Updegrave, W.J. (1951). The paralleling extension-cone technique in intraoral dental radiography. *Oral Surg. Oral Med. Oral Pathol.* 4 (10): 1250–1261.
5 White, S. and Pharoah, M. (2014). Oral Radiology: Principles and Interpretation, 248–250. St. Louis, MO: Elsevier Health Sciences.
6 de Almeida, F.D., Carvalho, A.C.P., Fontes, M. et al. (2011). Radiographic evaluation of marginal bone level around internal-hex implants with switched platform: a clinical case report series. *Int. J. Oral Maxillofac. Implants* 26 (3): 587–592.

7 Tal, H. and Moses, O. (1991). A comparison of panoramic radiography with computed tomography in the planning of implant surgery. *Dentomaxillofac. Radiol.* 20 (1): 40–42.

8 Batenburg, R.H., Meijer, H.J., Geraets, W.G., and van der Stelt, P.F. (1998). Radiographic assessment of changes in marginal bone around endosseous implants supporting mandibular overdentures. *Dentomaxillofac. Radiol.* 27 (4): 221–224.

34

The Digital Workflow in Implant Dentistry

Andrew Chio and Anthony Mak

There are two types of dental implant treatment workflows: the traditional analogue treatment modality and the digital implant workflow.

Full and proper treatment planning protocols are the foundation of any fixed restorations of the arch that are supported by dental implants. They generally include the following protocols:

- Articulated study models from diagnostic impressions.
- Diagnostic wax-ups, intra-oral wax-ups or diagnostic appliance fabricated to evaluate aesthetics and phonetics.
- Radiographs, including peri-apicals and cone beam computed tomography (CBCT) scan to evaluate osseous support for dental implants.
- Fabrication of a radiographic guide and the secondary adaptation to a surgical guide.

Analogue systems have traditionally relied on conventional impression techniques used to create a plaster model from which all subsequent procedures from the diagnostic wax-up to the prosthesis fabrication are manually completed by the ceramist.

The use of a full digital workflow eliminates the disadvantages and difficulties commonly associated with conventional analogue techniques. Some of these common limitations include:

- The discomfort commonly associated with the impression procedure.
- The potential for distortion of the impression material and inaccuracies of subsequent steps in the manufacturing process.
- Potential of damage to the dental cast.
- Delay due to logistics of sending lab work between the dental practice and the laboratory.

These disadvantages of the analogue system do not occur in the full digital workflow where the impression is taken with an intra-oral scanner and the design of the prosthesis is done on computer-aided design (CAD) software. The data from the digital impression is also simply sent over the Internet, significantly reducing the time needed to manufacture the wax-ups and prosthesis.

Practical Procedures in Implant Dentistry, First Edition. Edited by Christopher C.K. Ho.
© 2022 John Wiley & Sons Ltd. Published 2022 by John Wiley & Sons Ltd.
Companion website: www.wiley.com/go/ho/implant-dentistry

One of the main advantages of the full digital workflow is the simplicity in accurately diagnosing and virtually planning the implant position using the digital intra-oral scan and CBCT data. This in turn allows the fabrication of an accurate surgical implant guide that enables the placement of the implant fixtures in a simplified and predictable manner.

Full digital workflows in implant treatment planning and surgical workflows in short have the following benefits:

- They reduce the number of patient visits for the procedure.
- They provides for a simplified and predictable workflow in implant treatment planning and guided surgery.
- Better angulation and accuracy of placement of single and multiple implants is possible.
- The prosthetic design process is much simpler and easier.

34.1 Components and Steps of the Digital Implant Workflow

34.1.1 Digital Diagnostic Impression

The digital implant workflow begins with the intra-oral scanning of the pre-surgical area (Figure 34.1). Current digital scanners have been shown in the literature to be quite accurate, with an accuracy range of 6.9–45.2 μm [1, 2]. These scanners also acquire and render three-dimensional (3D) models easily and rapidly [3] and are able to generate digital models that are as reliable as plaster cast models [4].

Evidence in the literature is mixed regarding the accuracy and practicality of complete arch digital impressions, particularly in relation to edentulous cases where implant fixtures are placed in a cross-arch configuration. However, it

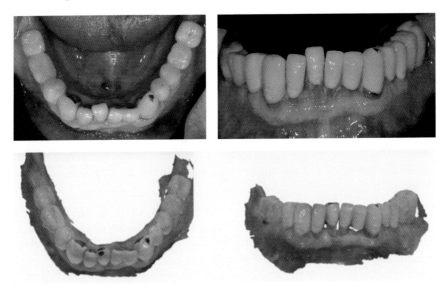

Figure 34.1 Digital surface scans acquired from the intra-oral scan of the lower arch.

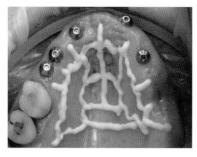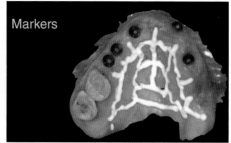

Figure 34.2 Incorporated resin or silicone-based markers to increase the number of reference points on large edentulous spans.

should be noted that the current generation of digital impression systems are more accurate for full arches and faster than previous systems [1]. The development of novel techniques such as the author's full arch scan protocol, which incorporates the use of resin or silicone-based markers to increase the number of reference points on large edentulous spans, can aid in improving the accuracy of the surface acquisition procedure (Figure 34.2).

In addition to being more efficient and convenient than conventional impression technique, studies have also indicated that patients often prefer the intraoral scanning approach over the traditional impression [5, 6].

34.1.2   Cone Beam Computed Tomography

CBCT scans allow the production of ultra high-resolution 3D rendering of the patient's oral anatomy (Figure 34.3). CBCT today can be seen as the standard of care for implant placement because it brings the following factors:

- Low-dosage optimisation, bringing CBCT radiation dosages in line with conventional panographs [7].
- Short scan times [7].
- Accurate data that has been verified in the literature [8, 9].

34.1.3   Digital Implant Treatment Planning

The patient's scanned image (STL file) and the CBCT scans (DICOM) are then compiled and matched together using a diagnostic 3D modelling software (Figures 34.4 and 34.5).

The data compiled by the diagnostic 3D modelling software allows the following to be accomplished:

- Accurate assessment of the bone volume and bone density.
- Illustration of the anatomical structures of the teeth, gums, and teeth in the image.
- Identification of critical anatomic landmarks such as nerves, sinuses, and proximal teeth so they can be avoided through safety zones in the planning software.

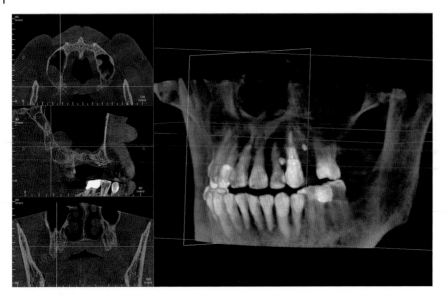

Figure 34.3 Cone beam computed tomography (CBCT) scan.

Prosthetically driven implant treatment planning is also simplified and easily visualised with the use of the diagnostic software as it allows for the following to be accomplished:

- Merging of the location of the planned prosthesis from a digital wax-up to the preoperative scans.
- Visualisation of the prosthetic plan to aid pre-surgical planning.
- Accurate determination of implant width, depth, and size prior to surgery.
- Planning for multiple implants that can be instantly paralleled using the software to simplify the restoration of cases involving multiple fixtures.

Correct implant positioning has the advantage of favourable aesthetic and prosthetic outcome and the potential to ensure optimal occlusal and implant loading [10–14].

34.1.4 The Digital Surgical Guide

Once the placement position of the virtual implant has been determined to ensure they are at the ideal angulation, location, and depth to support optimal prosthetic results, a surgical guide can be designed (Figures 34.6 and 34.7).

The surgical guide 'transfers' all the information from the planning software to allow the reproduction of the virtual plan on the patient during the implant surgical procedure. Tooth-supported surgical guides tend to be more stable and lead to better precision than other types of guides (bone-supported, mucosa-supported) [15–19].

There are two methods of manufacturing the computer-generated surgical guide: an additive stereolithographic 3D printing process or a subtractive milling process. Certain software platforms allow for in-office 3D printing while others require the fabrication of the guide at an off-site facility. In addition, many software platforms also deliver an individual drilling protocol with sequenced instrumentation and depth stops incorporated into the surgical guide for safe 3D implant placement.

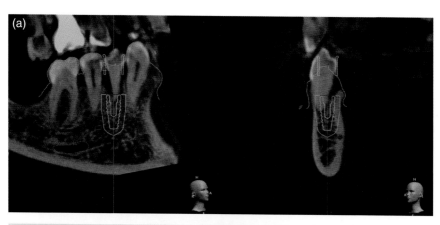

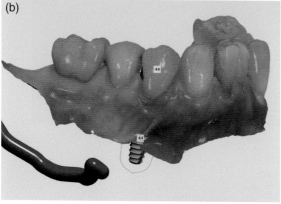

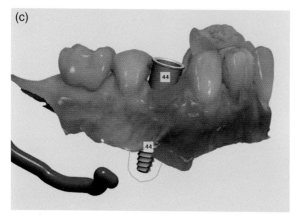

Figure 34.4 (a–d) Digital planning of implant placement based from a restorative perspective.

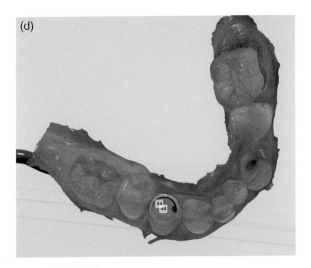

(d)

Figure 34.4 (Continued)

(a)

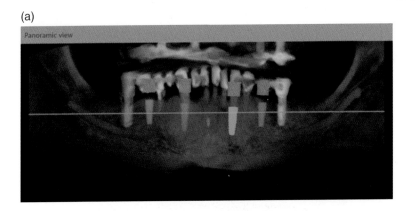

(b)

(c)

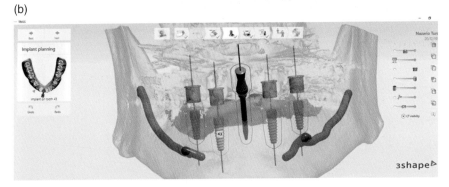

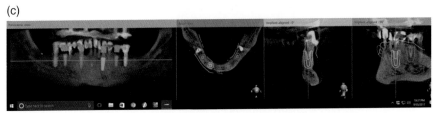

Figure 34.5 (a–c) Digital planning of implant placement based from a restorative perspective. (complex case). *Source:* (b) 3Shape A/S. (c) Used with permission from Microsoft Corporation.

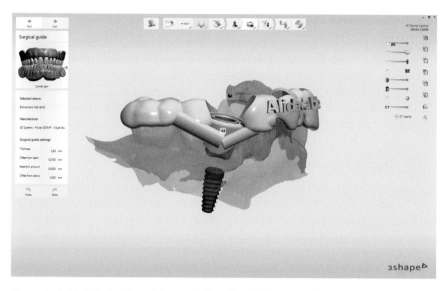

Figure 34.6 Digital planning of the surgical guide with the optimal 3D implant positioning. *Source:* 3Shape A/S.

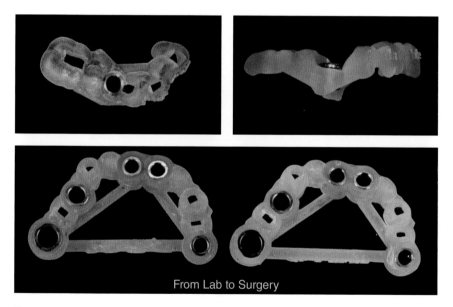

Figure 34.7 The digitally planned surgical guide.

It should be noted that some drawbacks do present with the use of the digital manufactured surgical guide. The lack of space has been referred to in the literature, affecting especially the lower posterior regions [20, 21]. Shortcomings including surgical guide shape, length of the metal sleeve/surgical drill, and template supporting problems have been reported by authors in several studies [20, 22–25].

34.1.5 Pre-surgical Fabricated Temporary Prosthesis

Digitally designed and fabricated provisional restorations in a full arch configuration can be manufactured and milled before the surgical procedure for immediate temporisation. It should be noted that slight deviations can occur during guided implant surgery compared to what had been digitally planned. The choice of material for the abutment and temporary prosthesis should ideally be adjustable to allow for these potential deviations.

34.1.6 Guided Implant Surgery

In comparison to freehand surgery, the implementation of a computer-generated surgical guide (Figure 34.8) significantly reduces the chance of positional error at the time of fixture placement [26, 27]. As a result, the implementation of the digital implant-guided surgery, with the use of a guided surgery kit (Figure 34.9), allows for greater accuracy in fixture placement and simplification of the subsequent restorative process [28].

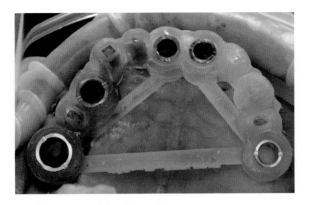

Figure 34.8 The surgical guide seated intra-orally.

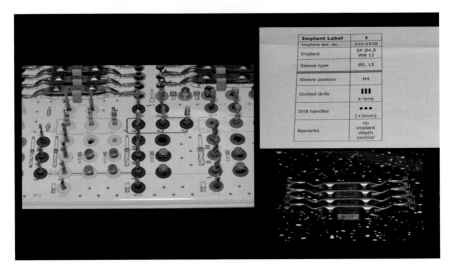

Figure 34.9 Straumann BLX Guided Surgery kit.

The benefits of guided implant surgery also extend to tangible patient benefits including significantly less intra-operative and post-operative complications, including pain [29]. Increased patient comfort has partially been linked to the ability to execute the guided implant surgery using a flapless approach. Some studies have indicated that the flapless approach may be the preferable method for executing guided surgery [30, 31]. Reduced post-operative pain and swelling, reduced intra-operative bleeding, preservation of soft and hard tissue, and maintenance of periosteal blood supply are advantages commonly associated with implant surgery using a flapless approach [32]. Some studies have also shown that the flapless technique has the potential to enhance aesthetics through the preservation of the papillae [33].

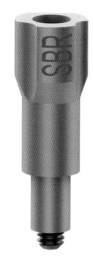

Figure 34.10 Intra-oral scan marker.

34.1.7 Implant Digital Impressions

Digital impressions with an intra-oral scanner can also be utilised in the restorative phase of the implant workflow. Intra-oral scan bodies have been developed for most major implant brands and facilitate the transfer of the implant brand, position, and alignment to be scanned and transferred to a digital model (Figures 34.10–34.13). This information is then utilised to develop the abutment and subsequent restoration. All other prosthodontic records, including the bite registration and the opposing arch, are also captured with the intra-oral scanners.

34.1.8 Manufacturing of the Customised Prosthesis

The digital implant records can either be used for in-office fabrication of the final abutment and prosthesis or delivered via the Internet to a dental laboratory. For more complicated cases, digital laboratory technologies may be better suited for the design and manufacturing of the corresponding restorative components. These laboratory-based systems have been shown to offer more scope and prosthetic options compared to in-office systems [34].

Digital design and manufacturing methods have simplified and streamlined the complex process of fabricating restorations [35] and also provide for greater efficiency compared to the conventional approach when it comes to the restoration of the implant-supported prosthesis (Figure 34.14) [36].

Technological developments in digital dentistry from both hardware and software perspectives continue to improve simplicity, while maintaining the predictability and accuracy, in the provision of implant restorative procedures. Some recent developments are photogrammetry and dynamic navigation.

Photogrammetry is a technique that collects 3D coordinate measurements to record the geometric properties of objects and their spatial position from photographic images by an extra-oral receiver [37–40]. Introduced in dentistry by Lie and Jemt [41] in 1994 to study the distortion of implant frameworks, this technique

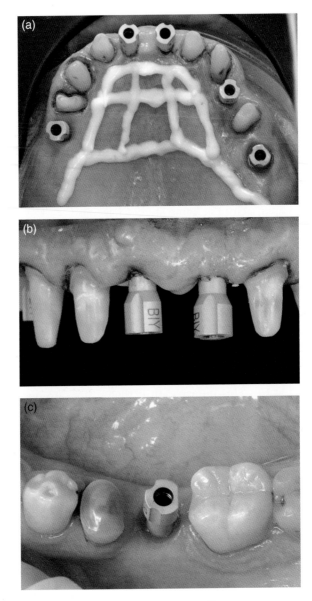

Figure 34.11 (a–c) Intra-oral scan markers *in situ* intra-orally.

has been reported in the literature as a potentially viable alternative to record the positions and angulations of multiple dental implants [37–42].

Dynamic navigation for surgical implant placement enables the tracking of the tip of the implant drill and mapping it to a pre-acquired CBCT scan. This provides for real-time and live drilling and placement guidance during implant surgery. The available literature demonstrates the accuracy of the system;

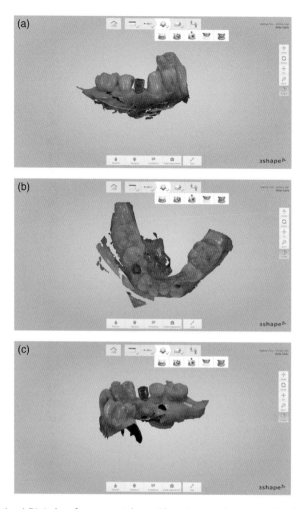

Figure 34.12 (a–c) Digital surface scans taken with an intra-oral scanner with the scan marker capturing the position and orientation of the implant fixture for a single-unit implant case. *Source:* 3Shape A/S.

however, the complex workflow and the cost of such systems have currently prevented the broader adoption of this technology [10, 43, 44].

In concluding this chapter, it should be noted that the body of this chapter has described the contemporary protocols in the digital implant workflow, also known as the single-scan protocol. There is also a double-scan protocol where the patient wearing a radiographic guide and the radiographic guide alone are scanned separately. Fiduciary markers incorporated in the radiographic guide allow for the matching of the two scans. This protocol allows for the digitisation of the surgical guide and the creation of a surgical guide using the appropriate planning software.

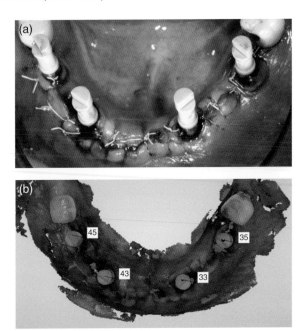

Figure 34.13 (a, b) Scan bodies inserted with an intra-oral digital scanner digitally capturing the position and orientation of the implant fixture for a multiple-unit implant case.

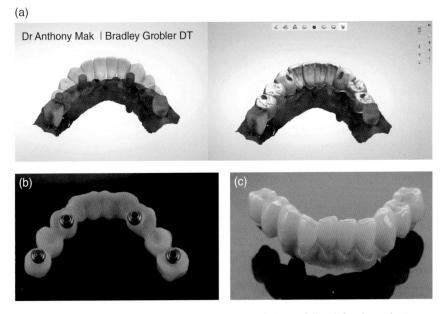

Figure 34.14 (a–c) Digital design and manufacturing of a lower full arch fixed prosthesis. *Source:* (a) Dr. Anthony Mak | Bradley Grobler DT. (b) 3Shape A/S.

References

1 Renne, W., Ludlow, M., Fryml, J. et al. (2016). Evaluation of the accuracy of 7 digital scanners: an in vitro analysis based on 3dimensional comparisons. *J. Prosthet. Dent.* 16: 30514–30515.

2 Hack, G. and Patzelt, S. (2015). Evaluation of the accuracy of six intraoral scanning devices: an invitro investigation. *J. Am. Dent. Assoc.* 10: 1–5.

3 Schepke, U., Meijer, H.J., Kerdijk, W., and Cune, M.S. (2015). Digital versus analog completearch impressions for singleunit premolar implant crowns: operating time and patient preference. *J. Prosthet. Dent.* 114 (3): 403–406.

4 Rossini, G., Parrini, S., Castroflorio, T. et al. (2016). Diagnostic accuracy and measurement sensitivity of digital models for orthodontic purposes: a systematic review. *Am. J. Orthod. Dentofacial Orthop.* 149: 161–170.

5 Gjelvold, B., Chrcanovic, B.R., Korduner, E.K. et al. (2016). Intraoral digital impression technique compared to conventional impression technique. A randomized clinical trial. *J. Prosthodont.* 25 (4): 282–287.

6 Wismeijer, D., Mans, R., Genuchten, M., and Reijers, H.A. (2014). Patients preferences when comparing analogue implant impressions using a polyether impression material versus digital impressions (intraoral scan) of dental implants. *Clin. Oral Implants Res.* 25 (10): 1113–1118.

7 EzEldeen, M., Stratis, A., Coucke, W. et al. (2017). As low dose as sufficient quality: optimization of conebeam computed tomographic scanning protocol for tooth autotransplantation planning and followup in children. *J. Endod.* 43: 210–217.

8 Lund, H., Gröndahl, K., and Gröndahl, H.G. (2009). Accuracy and precision of linear measurements in cone beam tomography Accuitomo tomograms obtained with different reconstruction techniques. *Dentomaxillofac. Radiol.* 38: 379–386.

9 Agbaje, J.O., Jacobs, R., Maes, F. et al. (2007). Volumetric analysis of extraction sockets using cone beam computed tomography: a pilot study on ex vivo jaw bone. *J. Clin. Periodontol.* 34: 985–990.

10 Tahmaseb, A., Wismeijer, D., Coucke, W., and Derksen, W. (2014). Computer technology applications in surgical implant dentistry: a systematic review. *Int. J. Oral Maxillofac. Implants* 29 (Supplement): 25–42.

11 Baggi, L., Pastore, S., Di Girolamo, M., and Vairo, G. (2013). Implantbone load transfer mechanisms in complete-arch prostheses supported by four implants: a three-dimensional finite element approach. *J. Prosthet. Dent.* 109 (1): 9–21.

12 Cecchetti, F., Germano, F., Bartuli, F.N. et al. (2014). Simplified type 3 implant placement, after alveolar ridge preservation: a case study. *Oral Implantol. (Rome)* 7 (3): 80–85.

13 Gargari, M., Comuzzi, L., Bazzato, M.F. et al. (2015). Treatment of peri-implantitis: description of a technique of surgical 2 detoxification of the implant. A prospective clinical case series with 3-year follow-up. *Oral Implantol.* 8 (1): 1–11.

14 Spinelli, D., Ottria, L., De Vico, G.D. et al. (2013). Full rehabilitation with nobel clinician® and procera implant bridge®: case report. *Oral Implantol.* 6 (2): 25–36.

15 Cassetta, M., Stefanelli, L.V., Giansanti, M., and Calasso, S. (2012). Accuracy of implant placement with a stereolithographic surgical template. *Int. J. Oral Maxillofac. Implants* 27: 655–663.

16 Geng, W., Liu, C., Su, Y. et al. (2015). Accuracy of different types of computer-aided design/computer-aided manufacturing surgical guides for dental implant placement. *Int. J. Clin. Exp. Med.* 8: 8442–8449.

17 Nokar, S., Moslehifard, E., Bahman, T. et al. (2011). Accuracy of implant placement using a CAD/CAM surgical guide: an in vitro study. *Int. J. Oral Maxillofac. Implants* 26: 520–526.

18 Dandekeri, S.S.L., Sowmya, M.K., and Bhandary, S. (2013). Stereolithographic surgical template: a review. *J. Clin. Diagn. Res.* 7: 2093–2095.

19 Moon, S.Y., Lee, K.R., Kim, S.G., and Son, M.K. (2016). Clinical problems of computer-guided implant surgery. *Maxillofac. Plast. Reconstr. Surg.* 38: 15.

20 Lin, Y.K., Yau, H.T., Wang, I.C. et al. (2015). A novel dental implant guided surgery based on integration of surgical template and augmented reality. *Clin. Implant Dent. Relat. Res.* 17: 543–553.

21 Cushen, S.E. and Turkyilmaz, I. (2013). Impact of operator experience on the accuracy of implant placement with stereolithographic surgical templates: an in vitro study. *J. Prosthet. Dent.* 109: 248–254.

22 Valente, F., Schiroli, G., and Sbrenna, A. (2009). Accuracy of computer-aided oral implant surgery: a clinical and radiographic study. *Int. J. Oral Maxillofac. Implants* 24: 234–242.

23 Papaspyridakos, P. and Lal, K. (2008). Flapless implant placement: a technique to eliminate the need for a removable interim prosthesis. *J. Prosthet. Dent.* 100: 232–235.

24 Beretta, M., Poli, P.P., and Maiorana, C. (2014). Accuracy of computer- aided template-guided oral implant placement: a prospective clinical study. *J. Periodontal. Implant. Sci.* 44: 184–193.

25 Koshy, E., Surathu, N., and Raj, F.S. (2009). Computer guided implant surgery: a clinical report. *Int. J. Clin. Implant. Dent.* 1: 23–29.

26 Di Giacomo, G., Cury, P.R., de Araujo, N.S. et al. (2005). Clinical application of stereolithographic surgical guides for implant placement: preliminary results. *J. Periodontol.* 76: 503–507.

27 Arisan, V., Karabuda, C.Z., Mumcu, E., and Özdemir, T. (2013). Implant positioning errors in freehand and computeraided placement methods: a singleblind clinical comparative study. *Int. J. Oral Maxillofac. Implants* 28: 190–204.

28 Van Assche, N., Vercruyssen, M., Coucke, W. et al. (2012). Accuracy of computeraided implant placement. *Clin. Oral Implants Res.* (Suppl 6): 112–123.

29 Nkenke, E., Eitner, S., Radespiel-Tröger, M. et al. (2007). Patient-centred outcomes comparing transmucosal implant placement with an open approach in the maxilla: a prospective, nonrandomized pilot study. *Clin. Oral Implants Res.* 18 (2): 197–203.

30 Fortin, T., Bosson, J.L., Isidori, M., and Blanchet, E. (2006). Effecct of flapless surgery on pain experienced in implant placement using an imageguided system. *Int. J. Oral Maxillofac. Implants* 21: 298–304.

31 Arisan, V., Karabuda, C.Z., and Ozdemir, T. (2010). Implant surgery using boneand mucosasupported steriolithographic guides in totally edentulous jaws; surgical and postoperative outcomes of computeraided vs. standard techniques. *Clin. Oral Implants Res.* 21: 980–988.

32 Hockl, K., Stoll, P., Stoll, V. et al. (2001). Flapless implant surgery and its effect on periimplant soft tissue. *Int. J. Oral Maxillofac. Surg.* 40 (10): e24.

33 Cosyn, J., Hooghe, N., and De Bruyn, H. (2012). A systematic review on the frequency of advanced recession following single immediate implant treatment. *J. Clin. Periodontol.* 39: 582–589.

34 Abduo, J., Bennamoun, M., Tennant, M., and McGeachie, J. (2016). Impact of digital prosthodontics planning on dental esthetics: biometric analysis of esthetic parameters. *J. Prosthet. Dent.* 115: 57–64.

35 Joda, T. and Brägger, U. (2014). Complete digital workflow for the production of implantsupported singleunit monolithic crowns. *Clin. Oral Implants Res.* 25: 1304–1306.

36 Joda, T., Katsoulis, J., and Brägger, U. (2016). Clinical fitting and adjustment time for implantsupported crowns comparing digital and conventional workflows. *Clin. Implant Dent. Relat. Res.* 18: 946–954.

37 Suarez, M.J., Paisal, I., Rodriguez-Alonso, V., and Lopez-Suarez, C. (2018). Combined stereophotogrammetry and laser-sintered, computer-aided milling framework for an implant-supported mandibular prosthesis: a case history report. *Int. J. Prosthodont.* 31 (1): 60–62.

38 Agustín-Panadero, R., Peñarrocha-Oltra, D., Gomar-Vercher, S., and Peñarrocha-Diago, M. (2015). Stereophotogrammetry for recording the position of multiple implants: technical description. *Int. J. Prosthodont.* 28 (6): 631–636.

39 Sánchez-Monescillo, A., Sánchez-Turrión, A., Vellon-Domarco, E. et al. (2016). Photogrammetry impression technique: a case history report. *Int. J. Prosthodont.* 29 (1): 71–73.

40 Pradíes, G., Ferreiroa, A., Özcan, M. et al. (2014). Using stereophotogrammetric technology for obtaining intraoral digital impressions of implants. *J. Am. Dent. Assoc.* 145 (4): 338–344.

41 Jemt, T., Bäck, T., and Petersson, A. (1999). Photogrammetry – an alternative to conventional impressions in implant dentistry? A clinical pilot study. *Int. J. Prosthodont.* 12 (4): 363–368.

42 Pradíes, G., Gomar-Vercher, S., and Peñarrocha-Diago, M. (2017). Maxillary full-arch immediately loaded implant-supported fixed prosthesis designed and produced by photogrammetry and digital printing: a clinical report. *J. Prosthodont.* 26 (1): 75–81.

43 Jung, R.E., Schneider, D., Ganeles, J. et al. (2009). Computer technology applications in surgical implant dentistry: a systematic review. *Int. J. Oral Maxillofac. Implants* 24 (Suppl): 92–109.

44 Brief, J., Edinger, D., Hassfeld, S., and Eggers, G. (2005). Accuracy of image-guided implantology. *Clin. Oral Implants Res.* 16 (4): 495–501.

35

Biological Complications

Christopher C.K. Ho

35.1 Principles

The literature suggests that the use of dental implants after appropriate treatment planning can result in high survival and success rates with longstanding predictability. However, implants are also susceptible to a range of technical and biological complications. As the numbers of patients with dental implants increase, it is inevitable the incidence of biological complications will increase, which may pose a significant future healthcare problem.

Biological implant complications include implant loss and inflammation of the peri-implant tissue. Loss of osseointegration with loss of implant can be further divided into 'early' or 'late' implant failure based on the timing of implant removal or lack of osseointegration. Histologically, an implant with loss of osseointegration has a predominantly fibrous tissue capsule, preventing direct contact between implant and bone, resulting in impaired implant function. Other biological implant complications, which occur more commonly, are peri-implant diseases. Peri-implant diseases include peri-implantitis and peri-implant mucositis, characterised by the presence or absence of bone loss, respectively.

Albrektsson et al. [1] proposed criteria for success of annual bone loss of 1.0 mm in the first year and 0.1 mm in the years thereafter, or annual bone changes of 0.2 mm at the contact zone between the implant and surrounding bone, as natural biological process. This was described as a 'steady state'. An increased level of bone loss is commonly seen in the first year after loading, followed by a phase of lower bone loss with almost stable levels of crestal bone. As a consequence, after 10 years, bone resorption of 2.8 mm was accepted as 'normal'.

These criteria were reviewed by Smith and Zarb [2], and they suggested the following new criteria:

1) The individual unattached implant is immobile when tested clinically.
2) No evidence of peri-implant radiolucency is present as assessed on an undistorted radiograph (Figure 35.1).

Practical Procedures in Implant Dentistry, First Edition. Edited by Christopher C.K. Ho.
© 2022 John Wiley & Sons Ltd. Published 2022 by John Wiley & Sons Ltd.
Companion website: www.wiley.com/go/ho/implant-dentistry

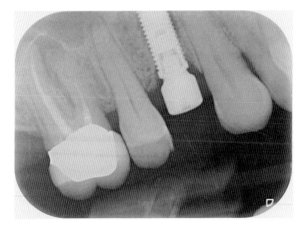

Figure 35.1 Peri-implant radiolucency noted around failing implant.

3) The mean vertical bone loss is less than 0.2 mm annually after the first year of service.
4) No persistent pain, discomfort, or infection is attributable to the implant.
5) The implant design does not preclude placement of a crown or prosthesis with an appearance that is satisfactory to the patient and dentist.

By these criteria, a success rate of 85% at the end of a five-year observation period and 80% at the end of a ten-year period are minimum levels for success.

35.1.1 Attachment Differences

Natural teeth and dental implants present subtle anatomical and biological differences, which may contribute to the pathogenesis of bone loss. Epithelium attaches to dental implants in a mechanically fragile surface adhesion rather than a direct structural attachment with hemi-desmosomal and internal basal lamina attachment. In comparison, teeth have connective tissue attachment to cementum with Sharpey fibres. The fibres in the connective tissue around implants are oriented running parallel to implants in a circular manner and is merely a result of abutting soft scar-like connective tissue against the implant surface (Figure 35.2). Teeth also possess a periodontal ligament allowing slight transient movement in response to load. The ability of peri-implant mucosa to regenerate is limited as loss of a tooth leads to the loss of the periodontal ligament, an important source of vascular supply.

The progression of peri-implant diseases is more rapid and destructive than that seen in natural teeth due to combination of a weaker mechanical attachment of the supracrestal parallel collagen fibres, along with the poorer vascularity compared to natural teeth. Hence, the early detection and treatment of peri-implant diseases is crucial for long-term success.

The ability of peri-implant mucosa to regenerate is limited by compromised number of cells and poor vascularity because of the loss of the periodontal ligament with its inherent blood supply.

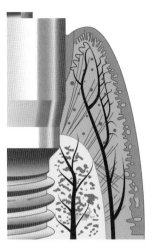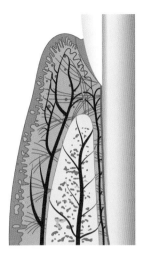

Figure 35.2 Periodontal and peri-implant interface. The implant interface consists of supracrestal collagen fibres oriented in a parallel rather than a perpendicular configuration, and has a weaker mechanical attachment compared to natural teeth.

35.1.2 Crestal Bone Loss

It appears from the literature that accepted bone loss after the first year should be less than 0.2 mm annually. Many studies have reported on bone loss that occurs in the first year of placing an abutment and found it to be from 1 to 1.5 mm. It is suggested that this is due to the microgap within a restoration, which leads to the formation of a biological width around implants. Prevention of late implant bone loss is a critical component in long-term implant success. Continuing bone loss at a rate greater than 0.2 mm annually requires scrutiny and may require intervention.

The incidence of crestal bone loss has been a controversial issue, with much written on the magnitude and consequences. The reason for crestal bone loss is poorly understood with infection or overload being the main factors thought to be responsible. The infection theory suggests that implants behave like teeth and are susceptible to a similar type of disease as teeth [3], while overload [4] has been presented as an alternative reason with stresses within bone leading to bone loss. A further theory is centred on compromised healing/adaptation, where different local and systemic factors may influence the biology of osseointegration or influence the maintenance of osseointegration once implants are subjected to the demands of supporting a prosthesis [5].

35.1.3 Peri-implant Disease

Peri-implantitis was introduced as a term for infectious pathological conditions of peri-implant tissues more than five decades ago. Most literature sources report this as an infectious condition of the tissues around osseointegrated implants with loss of supporting bone and clinical signs of inflammation (bleeding and/or suppuration on probing).

In 1994, the First European Workshop on Periodontology developed a consensus report to more clearly define peri-implant disease [6]. Peri-implant mucositis was defined as a reversible inflammation of the soft tissues surrounding an implant in function with no loss of supporting bone. Clinical signs of this process included bleeding and/or suppuration on probing and increased periodontal probing depths (PD) between 4 and 5 mm. Peri-implantitis was defined as an inflammatory process not only affecting soft tissues around a dental implant in function, but also including evidence of loss of supporting bone. Clinical signs included periodontal PD of greater than 5 mm, bleeding and/or suppuration on probing, while evidence of bone loss is most often determined radiographically. Typically, the pattern of bone loss around affected dental implants presents as a crater-type defect. The Sixth European Workshop on Periodontology in 2008 revised the definition of peri-implant diseases: *peri-implant mucositis* is the presence of inflammation in the mucosa at an implant with no signs of loss of supporting bone; *peri-implantitis*, in addition to the mucosal inflammation, is characterised by the loss of supporting bone [7].

Recently, a further theory on bone loss has been proposed relating to a provoked foreign body reaction [8]. Albrektsson et al. [9] postulated that osseointegration is a foreign body response to an implant. A chronic inflammatory response results with embedding or separation of bone (osseo-separation) around an implant. This bone loss may be an imbalance in the foreign body response, influenced by various factors including the implant, clinician experience and skill, as well as patient characteristics, which may sustain or aggravate the response. Once severe marginal bone loss has occurred a secondary biofilm-mediated infection may ensue.

35.1.3.1 Prevalence of Peri-implant Diseases

Numbers of patients with peri-implant disease have increased as a result of more implants being inserted, as well patients now having had implants over multiple decades. Peri-implantitis has been reported to occur at a prevalence in the order of 10% of implants and 20% of patients, 5–10 years after implant placement [10].

Derks et al. [11] assessed 2765 patient files in a national register of Swedish social insurance and found that 22% of patients experienced peri-implantitis and 43% had peri-implant mucositis. Early implant loss occurred in 4.4% of patients (1.4% of implants), while 4.2% of the patients who were examined nine years after therapy presented with late implant loss (2.0% of implants). Multi-level analysis revealed higher odds ratios for early implant loss among smokers and patients with an initial diagnosis of periodontitis. Renvert et al. [12] in a 21–26 year follow-up study of occurrence of peri-implant mucositis and peri-implantitis started with 294 patients and after 20–26 years analysed 86 of those patients, finding a diagnosis of peri-implant mucositis of 54.7% and peri-implantitis of 22.1%. They also found that individuals with three or more implants were at higher risk.

35.1.3.2 Risk Factors in Peri-implant Disease

A difficult challenge in implant therapy is detecting individuals at higher risk for implant loss. A risk factor may be defined as 'an environmental, behavioural, or biological factor that, if present directly increases the probability of a disease (or adverse event) occurring and, if absent or removed, reduces that probability' (Table 35.1).

Table 35.1 Possible factors that may influence crestal bone loss.

Patient specific	**General**
	• Medical, e.g. diabetes
	• Social, e.g. smoking
	• Dental, e.g. history of periodontitis
	• Genetic
	Local
	• Biomechanics – overload
	• Prosthetic procedures and design of prosthesis
	• Soft tissue biotype and keratinisation
	• Oral hygiene
Non-patient specific	**Implant risk factors**
	• Macroscopic design
	• Surface characteristics
	• Implant connection
	Clinician risk factors
	• Lack of knowledge of procedure
	• Inexperience in carrying out the procedure
	• Not using appropriate protocol
	Time

Several risk factors have been identified for peri-implant disease including:

• History of periodontitis
• Smoking
• Poor oral hygiene
• Excess cement
• Exposed threads and surface coatings (roughened surfaces)
• No plaque removal access (ridge lap crown, connected prostheses)
• Incorrect restoration contour
• Poor marginal fit of implant restoration
• Lacking keratinised gingiva and insufficient bone volume
• Lack of preventive maintenance
• Inadequately performed surgical procedures.

35.1.3.2.1 *Cement versus Screw Retention* An implant prosthesis can be secured to an implant via cementation (using a provisional or definitive cement) on an implant abutment that is screw retained to the implant. The clinical decision as to which retention system depends on several factors including the implant alignment, retrievability, and passivity of fit.

A major disadvantage with cemented implant restorations is that complete removal of any excess cement can be difficult. It has been demonstrated that in attempting complete removal of cement, remnants are often left, in addition to scratches and gouges made onto titanium abutments [13].

Wilson et al. [14] in a prospective study found a positive relationship between excess cement and peri-implant disease. Linkevicius et al. [15] reported in a retrospective case analysis that implants with cement remnants in patients with history of periodontitis are more likely to lead to peri-implant disease. In a cement-retained restoration the deeper position of the margin the greater amount of undetected cement was found [16].

A randomised controlled trial by Crespi et al. [17] compared the bone loss between cement-retained and screw-retained crowns. The study included 28 patients with 272 implants. They reported that in the cement-retained group (CRG) mean bone levels were -1.23 ± 0.45 mm, while the screw-retained group (SRG) showed mean bone levels of -1.01 ± 0.33 mm. At three-year follow-up, a slight increase was found (0.30 ± 0.25 mm in CRG and 0.45 ± 0.29 mm in SRG). After that point, marginal bone levels remained stable over time, up to the eight-year follow-up.

Sailer et al. [18] report in a systematic review that cemented reconstructions exhibited more serious biological complications (implant loss, bone loss >2 mm), whereas screw-retained reconstructions exhibited more technical problems. Screw-retained reconstructions are more easily retrievable than cemented reconstructions and, therefore, technical and eventually biological complications can be treated more easily.

35.1.3.2.2 Prosthodontic Contour Katafuchi et al. [19] reported on whether prosthodontic contour in implants (bone and tissue level), specifically restoration emergence angle, was associated with peri-implantitis. They found the prevalence of peri-implantitis was significantly greater in the bone-level group when the emergence angle was >30 degrees compared to an angle ≤30 degrees (Figure 35.3). In the tissue-level group, no such correlation was found. For bone-level implants, when a convex profile was combined with an angle of >30 degrees, the prevalence of peri-implantitis was 37.8% with a statistically significant interaction between emergence angle and profile. Furthermore, Yi et al. [20] reported on the association between prosthetic features and peri-implantitis. This retrospective

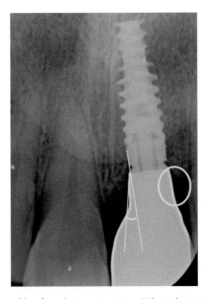

Figure 35.3 Emergence profile of implant restorations. When the emergence angle of an implant restoration is ≥30 degrees there may be an association with peri-implantitis. Furthermore, when the emergence profile is convex this is an additional risk factor.

study on 169 patients (n = implants: 349) found the emergence angle showed a significant correlation with marginal bone loss. They found a statistically greater prevalence of peri-implantitis if emergence angle was ≥30 degrees, when the emergence profile is convex, and in middle implants splinted together with adjacent implants. A similar correlation was not observed in tissue-level implants. They found that crown:implant ratio had no significant effect on the prevalence of peri-implantitis.

Over-contoured implant prostheses, in particular with an emergence angle of ≥30 degrees, is a critical local confounder for peri-implantitis.

35.1.3.2.3 *Prosthodontic Design (Accessibility for Hygiene)*

Serino and Ström [21] in a cross-sectional study on 23 patients found that in partially edentulous patients local factors such as accessibility for oral hygiene at the implant sites were related to the presence or absence of peri-implantitis. Peri-implantitis was a frequent finding in subjects with signs of minimal loss of supporting bone around the remaining natural dentition and no signs of presence of periodontitis (i.e. presence of periodontal pockets of 6 mm at natural teeth). A high proportion (74%) of implants with peri-implantitis were found to have inadequate plaque control and 48% of the implants presenting with peri-implantitis were those with no accessibility/capability for proper oral hygiene. The study's conclusions suggest that bone loss around implants was associated with inadequate plaque control at implant sites, while peri-implantitis was a rare finding around implants that had proper plaque control.

35.1.3.2.4 *Implant Surface*

The majority of implant manufacturers produce implants in the modern age with a moderately rough implant surface. This provides a surface that provides quicker osteointegration with enhanced bone-to-implant contact. The modified surfaces provide higher surface energy, higher adsorption, with stronger and faster osseointegration. Although this may be advantageous for osteointegration this microstructure may be disadvantageous in the management of peri-implant disease because the roughened surfaces increase the surface area for bacterial colonisation. Along with macro-geometry design of implants with larger, more aggressive thread pitch patterns this may lead to more difficulty in cleaning between each thread.

35.2 Procedures

35.2.1 Treatment of Peri-implant Disease

Peri-implant disease is caused by bacterial infection from dental biofilms, and the microbiota is similar to the subgingival bacterial flora associated with chronic periodontitis, being composed of mixed anaerobic species. These pathogens lead to a host response with local inflammatory changes. The primary objective of treatment is to alter the microbiota in the peri-implant region, allowing the host immune system to successfully eliminate the pathogens. This is usually performed with efficient mechanical debridement similar to that used in periodontal disease treatment [22]. In implant rehabilitations this may be made more difficult due to the prosthetic superstructure, with the design precluding the ability to clean effectively. If there has been crestal bone loss, with exposure of threads and roughened surfaces, the ability to effectively decontaminate between threads and within irregularities of the surface is questionable.

Several treatment modalities have been proposed to manage biological complications, including non-surgical mechanical debridement, antiseptics, local and/or systemic antibiotics, lasers, resection with or without implantoplasty, and regenerative approaches. It is suggested that the treatment modalities should be chosen based on the severity of peri-implant diseases, amount of bone loss, and the morphology of peri-implant bony defects. For peri-implant mucositis or peri-implant defects with less than 2 mm destruction, non-surgical treatments are recommended. For peri-implant defects with more than 2 mm destruction, surgical treatments (e.g. resection with or without implantoplasty, guided bone regeneration) are suggested, but also removal of the implant if the bone loss is beyond repair.

35.2.1.1 Methods of Decontamination

Decontamination methods for peri-implantitis aim to remove bacterial biofilm in the peri-implant site, including the pocket and implant surface, and to allow re-osseointegration or at least to minimise bacterial adhesion. Various methods have been advocated for the decontamination of implant surfaces following exposure. Mechanical, chemical, or photodynamic measures along with laser therapy have been used in attempts to eliminate infection, resolve inflammation, and render the surface conducive to re-osseointegration.

35.2.1.1.1 Mechanical Decontamination Mechanical methods involve supragingival and subgingival debridement of the implant with the aim of removing the biofilm without damaging the implant surface.

- *Curettes*: These are specially designed hand instruments for mechanical debridement around implants. Many are made from pure titanium to prevent damage to the surface. Steel is not normally recommended because it is harder than titanium, while carbon fibre and plastic curettes are softer than implant surfaces and do not damage the surface but may break. Clinicians should proceed with caution using softer implant instruments as remnants of the material may remain stuck within the peri-implant tissues, leading to a foreign body reaction and impairing healing. Titanium-coated curettes have a similar hardness to the implant surface and thus do not scratch the surface (Figure 35.4).
- *Ultrasonic devices*: The use of ultrasonic instruments with polyether ether ketone (PEEK)-coated tips can safely be used. They are made of plastic material with a stainless-steel core which can be used on implant surfaces.
- *Air powder abrasive systems*: Standard air powder abrasive systems with sodium bicarbonate are contraindicated due to their higher abrasiveness, but recently developed low abrasive glycine powder and erythritol powder systems

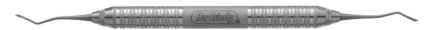

Figure 35.4 Titanium curettes designed for use around dental implants to prevent damage to the surface. *Source:* Courtesy of HuFriedy Group.

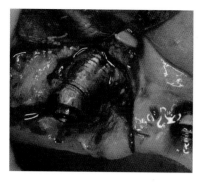 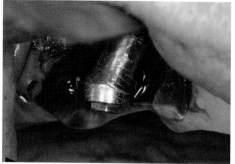

Figure 35.5 Implantoplasty to remove exposed threads and render the surface smooth and highly polished.

have been recommended for effective biofilm removal around implants. They have specially designed plastic nozzles which are directed so that the powder exits laterally with less pressure, preventing the formation of air emphysema in the adjacent tissues.

- *Implantoplasty*: This more aggressive approach smooths the implant surface, leaving a polished surface amenable to oral hygiene (Figure 35.5). It is performed with burs or stones under irrigation, but caution should be exercised not to increase the temperature of the implant. It is easy to contaminate the local area with titanium shavings and this may lead to tattooing of the region.
- *Mechanical plaque control (at-home care)*: The use of manual or powered toothbrushes and interdental aids must be advised as poor oral hygiene is a risk factor for peri-implantitis.

35.2.1.1.2 Chemical Decontamination

- *Antiseptics*: Substances used in the past included citric acid, chlorhexidine, cloramines, tetracyclines, hydrogen peroxide, and sodium chloride. No single method of surface decontamination was found to be superior to another [23]. Antimicrobial agents such as chlorhexidine are often recommended as adjuncts supporting oral hygiene practices. This can be applied as either a mouth rinse or used as a gel applied by toothbrushing. Other antiseptics include essential oil rinses such as that in Listerine®, and triclosan toothpastes.
- *Locally delivered antibiotics*: The use of monolithic ethylene vinyl acetate fibres containing tetracycline placed into the peri-implant sulcus has been advocated and has shown a positive effect on clinical and microbiological parameters around implants [24].

35.2.1.1.3 Lasers and Photodynamic Therapy
Recent studies have demonstrated that the use of lasers can assist in decontamination of titanium implants. Various lasers including erbium-doped yttrium-aluminium-garnet (Er:YAG) and CO2 lasers have been used for implant surface decontamination [25, 26]. Laser decontamination is based on its thermal effect, which denatures proteins and causes cellular necrosis. The lasers possess haemostatic properties, selective calculus ablation, and bactericidal effects. The Er:YAG laser has been

shown to be effective in removing the oral biofilm from implant surfaces without damaging the implant surface. The CO2 laser has also been reported to be safe and not hinder osteoblastic attachment to implant surfaces. However, a major risk while using both types of laser is the temperature increase above the critical threshold (10°C) after 10 seconds of continuous use. Another disadvantage is the high cost of equipment.

Schwarz et al. [27] compared surface decontamination with an Er:YAG laser device with that using plastic scalers with cotton pellets and sterile saline, and found no significant difference in the clinical outcomes following combined surgical therapy of advanced peri-implantitis.

There is a lack of consensus in the literature on the type and settings of lasers that are most favourable for bacterial decontamination of titanium implant surfaces.

Photodynamic therapy is a technique that uses a photosensitising substance that fixes itself to the bacteria of the biofilm. When irradiated with laser, cytotoxic singlet oxygen is produced which is able to destroy the bacterial cells on an implant surface [28].

35.2.2 Treatment of Peri-implant Mucositis

Assessing the aetiology is an important first step, and removing impediments to oral hygiene such as ridge laps, plaque traps as well as encouraging proper oral hygiene practice is integral to treatment. Like gingivitis around natural teeth, aetiology is related to biofilm accumulation in the soft tissues surrounding the implant, combined with a susceptible host response. Anti-infective therapy is thus fundamental to the management of peri-implant mucositis. This should be non-surgical in nature with mechanical debridement of the implant surface using curettes, ultrasonic devices, air-abrasive devices or lasers, with or without the adjunctive use of local antibiotics or antiseptics. The efficacy of these therapies has been demonstrated for mucositis, with controlled clinical trials showing an improvement in clinical parameters, especially in bleeding on probing [29]. When mechanical debridement alone was compared with mechanical debridement plus the adjunctive use of different protocols of chlorhexidine [30–32] or locally delivered tetracycline [33], reductions in bleeding on probing were significant in both test and control groups. They found no clear benefit derived from the use of chlorhexidine or locally delivered tetracycline.

In a study where the oral hygiene was suspended, Salvi et al. [34] looked at experimentally induced mucositis around implants treated through non-surgical mechanical debridement. Their research demonstrated that, compared to gingiva around teeth, the bacterial challenge presented by the cessation of oral hygiene elicited a greater inflammatory response in the peri-implant mucosa. Schierano et al. [35] showed that reversibility of tissue inflammation to pre-experimental levels was possible after oral hygiene care was suspended and reinstituted, but it took three times as long as that with natural teeth (69 versus 21 days). In summary, multiple studies examining peri-implant mucositis have shown that compared to treating gingivitis in natural teeth, the degree and severity of inflammation is greater, and reversibility takes longer and is harder to establish in implant patients.

It is recommended that peri-implant mucositis is treated with mechanical debridement of biofilm and calculus. This is with professional debridement and at-home care with or without adjunctive use of antimicrobials. The oral hygiene at-home care should encourage mechanical plaque control, combined with the use of antiseptic antimicrobials.

35.2.3 Treatment of Peri-implantitis

Treatment of peri-implantitis can be divided into non-surgical and surgical management, based on the severity of the disease and the type of peri-implant defect.

35.2.3.1 Non-surgical Therapy for Peri-implantitis

The management involves thorough debridement of the implant, disrupting the biofilm and reducing the bacterial load. A similar procedural decontamination to that used for mucositis is applied, the main difference being that this is aimed more subgingivally to decontaminate the surface. The available literature seems to suggest non-surgical therapy is not effective, giving only limited improvement, with a clear tendency for disease recurrence [29]. This is most likely because of insufficient decontamination of the implant surface exposed to biofilm, and hence there may be a need to consider surgical intervention.

35.2.3.2 Surgical Therapy for Peri-implantitis

Surgical therapy of peri-implantitis is indicated when non-surgical therapy fails to control the inflammatory changes (Figure 35.6).

Surgical intervention allows:

- Access for cleaning and decontamination
- Access for cleaning and decontamination plus exposure of the affected surfaces for cleaning (apically repositioned flaps)
- Access for cleaning and regenerative techniques.

There are three different surgical approaches:

- *Access flap surgery*: This technique gains access to decontaminate the implant surface, with the intention of maintaining the soft tissue around the implant. An intra-crevicular incision is made with full-thickness mucoperiosteal flaps to allow access with degranulation of the inflamed tissues and surface decontamination. The flaps are then repositioned and sutured. The aim is to eliminate inflammatory changes without altering the soft tissue margin around the implant neck. This technique is often only possible if bone loss is shallow.
- *Apically positioned flap surgery*: This approach is used to apically position tissues around implants, reducing pockets and enhancing oral hygiene procedures. A reverse bevel incision is made depending on the PD and thickness of the peri-implant mucosa. Buccal and palatal/lingual flaps are raised, with the affected tissues removed and the implant surface decontaminated. Vertical releasing incisions may be needed to position the flap apically. Osteoplasty is performed by recontouring the bone, and the flap is then sutured apically, leaving the previously affected areas of the implant exposed. This technique is suitable for non-aesthetic areas for the surgical management of peri-implantitis with one-wall intra-bony or supra-bony defects.
- *Regenerative surgical techniques*: This reconstructive surgery aims to decontaminate the implant surface and support the tissues during the healing of the

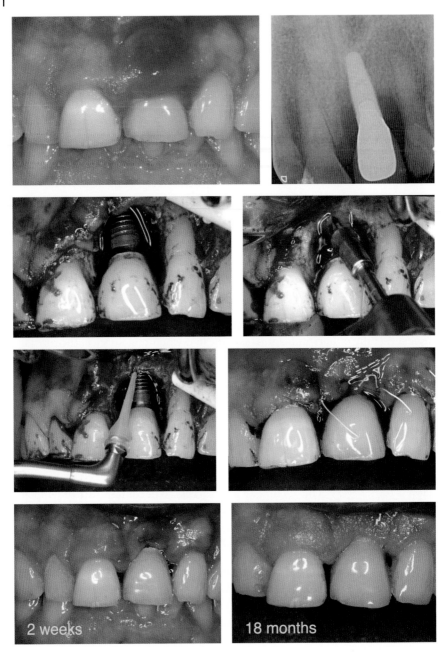

Figure 35.6 Patient with peri-implantitis treated surgically with full-thickness flap elevation with removal of granulation tissue and decontamination with curettes, titanium brushes, and glycine powder with apical positioning. This can be performed in non-aesthetic regions or situations where aesthetics is not important, as in this low smile line patient. Note the resolution of the inflammation and return of gingival health and stippling.

tissues to avoid the recession of the mucosa, while enhancing the possibility of re-osseointegration with regenerative techniques (Figure 35.7). It is suitable for crater-shaped lesions with intra-bony defects. Intra-sulcular incisions are made to maintain the soft tissue margin, and flap elevation on both the buccal and lingual/palatal are made to decontaminate the surface. Graft materials are then placed around the implant, filling the intra-bony defect, and may be covered with a resorbable or non-resorbable membrane. The tissues are coronally positioned and sutured. Animal studies have shown that re-osseointegration may occur on previously contaminated implant surfaces [36].

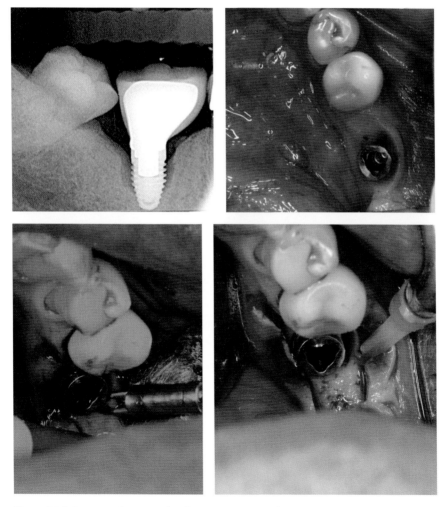

Figure 35.7 Regenerative surgical technique in a case with crater-like intra-bony defects.

(Continued)

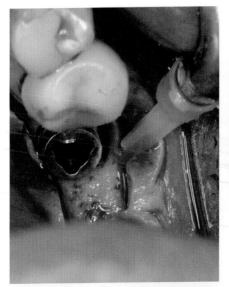
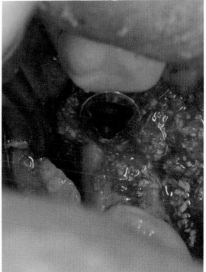
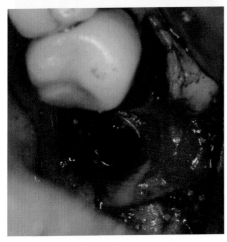

Figure 35.7 (Continued)

35.2.4 Recommendations

- Selection of surgical technique should be based on the characteristics of the peri-implant lesion. In the presence of deep circumferential and intra-bony defects, surgical interventions should aim to provide thorough debridement, implant surface decontamination, and defect reconstruction/regeneration. In the presence of defects without clear bony walls or with a predominant supra-bony component, the aim of the surgical intervention should be the thorough debridement and repositioning of the marginal mucosa to enable the patient to perform effective oral hygiene practices, although this may compromise the aesthetic result of the implant-supported restoration.

- The literature has not revealed the optimal method of surface decontamination of an implant, with lasers not showing any additional advantages over traditional systems; even simply rinsing with saline has shown successful outcomes [23, 27].
- The evidence is limited supporting the use of access flaps but they may be selected for shallow defects or in aesthetic areas after unsuccessful non-surgical treatment.
- When defects are supra-bony or one-wall defects then an apically repositioned flap should be used in a non-aesthetic region.
- A regenerative approach is indicated for peri-implantitis with circumferential and intra-bony defects. Schwarz et al. [37] demonstrated improved outcomes in the presence of circumferential bony defects with bony walls with regenerative surgical approach. There is no evidence to recommend the use of a specific regenerative surgical technique, such as grafting with autogenous or xenograft or bone substitutes [29].

35.2.5 Supportive Care

Supportive periodontal/peri-implant therapy involves regular monitoring using a periodontal probe, removal of supra- and subgingival/mucosal plaque and calculus deposits and provision of individualised oral hygiene instructions.

Heitz-Mayfield et al. [38] evaluated clinical outcomes of supportive peri-implant therapy (SPIT) following surgical treatment of peri-implantitis. Twenty-four partially dentate patients with 36 dental implants diagnosed with peri-implantitis were treated by an anti-infective surgical protocol followed by regular supportive therapy. SPIT included removal of supra- and submucosal biofilm at the treated implants using titanium or carbon fibre curettes, or ultrasonic devices. In addition, professional prophylaxis (calculus/biofilm removal) at other implants/teeth and oral hygiene reinforcement was provided. Clinical measurements and radiographs were obtained at one, three, and five years. A successful treatment outcome was defined as implant survival with the absence of peri-implant PD ≥5 mm with concomitant bleeding/suppuration and absence of progression of peri-implant bone loss. Twelve months after treatment, there was 100% survival of the treated implants and 79% of patients (19 of 24) had a successful treatment outcome according to the defined success criteria. At five years 63% of patients (15 of 24) had a successful treatment outcome. Complete resolution of peri-implantitis, defined as absence of bleeding at all sites, was achieved in 42% of implants at five years.

Costa et al. [39] found that the absence of preventive maintenance in individuals with pre-existing peri-implant mucositis was associated with a high incidence of peri-implantitis. They studied 212 partially edentulous individuals, rehabilitated with dental implants that underwent periodontal and peri-implant clinical examinations. Five years later, 80 individuals who had been diagnosed with mucositis in the baseline examination were re-examined. These individuals were divided into two groups: one group with preventive maintenance during the study period ($n = 39$) and another group without preventive maintenance ($n = 41$). The following parameters were clinically evaluated: plaque index, bleeding on periodontal and peri-implant probing, periodontal and peri-implant PD, suppuration, and peri-implant bone loss. The incidence of peri-implantitis was 43.9% in the group without supportive therapy and 18% in the patients with regular supportive therapy. They concluded the absence of preventive maintenance in individuals with pre-existing peri-implant mucositis was associated with a high incidence of peri-implantitis.

35.3 Tips

- Ensure the contours of implant restorations are not over-contoured and are easy to clean. It is important to ensure the emergence angle of the restoration does not exceed 30 degrees, and that the contour is either flat or concave in profile. There should be accessible channels for which interdental aids or floss can be positioned to cleanse effectively around the prosthesis (Figure 35.8).
- The tissue-fitting surface of implant-supported bridgework should be flat or convex in edentulous pontic areas to allow cleaning and not allow any plaque traps present.
- Remove any flanges that prevent proper access for hygiene. If a prosthesis requires a flange, then consider a removable prosthesis to allow proper hygiene procedures (Figure 35.9).
- Because peri-implant mucositis can progress rapidly, and is more difficult to resolve than gingivitis, an aggressive non-surgical approach is warranted.
- The incidence of peri-implant disease is significantly reduced when patients are involved in a supportive periodontal therapy programme.

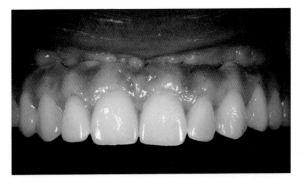

Figure 35.8 Final implant-supported prosthesis demonstrating areas that are accessible for hygiene.

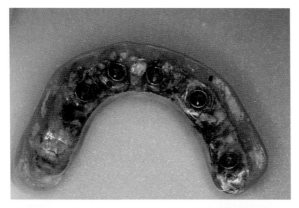

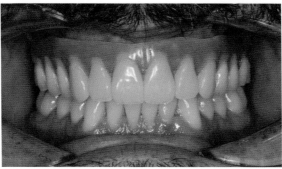

Figure 35.9 Fixed prosthesis with a large flange impeding access for cleaning resulting in a large build-up of food debris and plaque within the prosthesis, predisposing the patient to peri-implantitis.

References

1 Albrektsson, T., Zarb, G., Worthington, P., and Eriksson, A. (1986). The long-term efficacy of currently used dental implants: a review and proposed criteria of success. *Int. J. Oral Maxillofac. Implants* 1 (1): 11–25.
2 Smith, D.E. and Zarb, G.A. (1989). Criteria for success of osseointegrated endosseous implants. *J. Prosthet. Dent.* 62 (5): 567–572.
3 Heitz-Mayfield, L.J. (2008). Peri-implant diseases: diagnosis and risk indicators. *J. Clin. Periodontol.* 35: 292–304.
4 Fu, J.H., Hsu, Y.T., and Wang, H.L. (2012). Identifying occlusal overload and how to deal with it to avoid marginal bone loss around implants. *Eur. J. Oral Implantol.* 5 (Suppl): 91–103.
5 Chvartszaid, D., Koka, S., and Zarb, G. (2008). Osseointegration failure. In: Osseointegration – on Continuing Synergies in Surgery, Prosthodontics, Biomaterials (eds. G. Zarb, T. Albrektsson, G. Baker, et al.), 157–164. Chicago, IL: Quintessence Publishing.
6 Lang, N.P. (1994). Proceedings of the 1st European Workshop on Periodontology. Chicago, IL: Quintessence Publishing.

7 Lindhe, J. and Meyle, J. (2008). Peri-implant diseases: consensus report of the sixth European workshop on periodontology. *J. Clin. Periodontol.* 35: 282–285.

8 Koka, S. and Zarb, G. (2012). On osseointegration: the healing adaptation principle in the context of osseosufficiency, osseoseparation, and dental implant failure. *Int. J. Prosthodont.* 25 (1): 48–52.

9 Albrektsson, T., Dahlin, C., Jemt, T. et al. (2013). Is marginal bone loss around oral implants the result of a provoked foreign body reaction? *Clin. Implant Dent. Relat. Res.* 16 (2): 155–165.

10 Mombelli, A., Müller, N., and Cionca, N. (2012). The epidemiology of peri-implantitis. *Clin. Oral Implants Res.* 23 (s6): 67–76.

11 Derks, J., Håkansson, J., Wennström, J.L. et al. (2015). Effectiveness of implant therapy analyzed in a Swedish population: early and late implant loss. *J. Dent. Res.* 94 (3_suppl): 44S–51S.

12 Renvert, S., Lindahl, C., and Persson, G.R. (2018). Occurrence of cases with peri-implant mucositis or peri-implantitis in a 21–26 years follow-up study. *J. Clin. Periodontol.* 45 (2): 233–240.

13 Agar, J.R., Cameron, S.M., Hughbanks, J.C., and Parker, M.H. (1997). Cement removal from restorations luted to titanium abutments with simulated subgingival margins. *J. Prosthet. Dent.* 78 (1): 43–47.

14 Wilson, T.G. Jr. (2009 Sep). The positive relationship between excess cement and peri-implant disease: a prospective clinical endoscopic study. *Journal of periodontology.* 80 (9): 1388–1392.

15 Linkevicius, T., Puisys, A., Vindasiute, E. et al. (2013). Does residual cement around implant-supported restorations cause peri-implant disease? A retrospective case analysis. *Clin. Oral Implants Res.* 24 (11): 1179–1184.

16 Linkevicius, T., Vindasiute, E., Puisys, A. et al. (2013). The influence of the cementation margin position on the amount of undetected cement. A prospective clinical study. *Clin. Oral Implants Res.* 24 (1): 71–76.

17 Crespi, R., Capparè, P., Gastaldi, G., and Gherlone, E.F. (2014). Immediate occlusal loading of full-arch rehabilitations: screw-retained versus cement-retained prosthesis. An 8-year clinical evaluation. *International Journal of Oral & Maxillofacial Implants.* 29 (6): 1406–1411.

18 Sailer, I., Mühlemann, S., Zwahlen, M. et al. (2012). Cemented and screw-retained implant reconstructions: a systematic review of the survival and complication rates. *Clin. Oral Implants Res.* 23: 163–201.

19 Katafuchi, M., Weinstein, B.F., Leroux, B.G. et al. (2018 Feb). Restoration contour is a risk indicator for peri-implantitis: A cross-sectional radiographic analysis. *Journal of clinical periodontology.* 45 (2): 225–232.

20 Yi, Y., Koo, K.T., Schwarz, F. et al. (2020). Association of prosthetic features and peri-implantitis: a cross-sectional study. *J. Clin. Periodontol.* 47 (3): 392–403.

21 Serino, G. and Ström, C. (2009 Feb). Peri-implantitis in partially edentulous patients: association with inadequate plaque control. *Clinical oral implants research.* 20 (2): 169–174.

22 Renvert, S., Polyzois, I., and Persson, G.R. (2013). Treatment modalities for peri-implant mucositis and peri-implantitis. *Am. J. Dent.* 26 (6): 313–318.

23 Claffey, N., Clarke, E., Polyzois, I., and Renvert, S. (2008). Surgical treatment of peri-impantitis. *J. Clin. Periodontol.* 35: 316–332.

24 Mombelli, A., Feloutzis, A., Brägger, U., and Lang, N.P. (2001). Treatment of peri-implantitis by local delivery of tetracycline: clinical, microbiological and radiological results. *Clin. Oral Implants Res.* 12 (4): 287–294.

25 Bach, G., Neckel, C., Mall, C., and Krekeler, G. (2000 Oct 1). Conventional versus laser-assisted therapy of periimplantitis: a five-year comparative study. *Implant dentistry.* 9 (3): 247–251.

26 Romanos, G.E. and Nentwig, G.H. (2008). Regenerative therapy of deep peri-implant infrabony defects after CO2 laser implant surface decontamination. *International Journal of Periodontics & Restorative Dentistry.* 28 (3): 245–255.

27 Schwarz, F., Sahm, N., Iglhaut, G., and Becker, J. (2011). Impact of the method of surface debridement and decontamination on the clinical outcome following combined surgical therapy of peri-implantitis: a randomized controlled clinical study. *J. Clin. Periodontol.* 38: 276–284.

28 Marotti, J., Tortamano, P., Cai, S. et al. (2013). Decontamination of dental implant surfaces by means of photodynamic therapy. *Lasers Med. Sci.* 28: 303–309.

29 Figuero, E., Graziani, F., Sanz, I. et al. (2014). Management of peri-implant mucositis and peri-implantitis. *Periodontology* 66 (1): 255–273.

30 Heitz-Mayfield, L.J., Salvi, G.E., Botticelli, D. et al. (2011). Anti-infective treatment of peri-implant mucositis: a randomised controlled clinical trial. *Clin. Oral Implants Res.* 22: 237–241.

31 Porras, R., Anderson, G.B., Caffesse, R. et al. (2002). Clinical response to 2 different therapeutic regimens to treat peri-implant mucositis. *J. Periodontol.* 73: 1118–1125.

32 Thone-Muhling, M., Swierkot, K., Nonnenmacher, C. et al. (2010). Comparison of two full-mouth approaches in the treatment of peri-implant mucositis: a pilot study. *Clin. Oral Implants Res.* 21: 504–512.

33 Schenk, G., Flemmig, T.F., Betz, T. et al. (1997). Controlled local delivery of tetracycline HCl in the treatment of periimplant mucosal hyperplasia and mucositis. A controlled case series. *Clin. Oral Implants Res.* 8: 427–433.

34 Salvi, G.E., Agiletta, M., Sculean, A. et al. (2012). Reversibility of experimental peri-implant mucositis compared with experimental gingivitis in humans. *Clin. Oral Implants Res.* 23: 182–190.

35 Schierano, G., Pejrone, G., Brusco, P. et al. (2008). TNF-a, TGF-b2, and IL-1B levels in gingival crevicular fluids before and after de novo plaque accumulation. *J. Clin. Periodontol.* 35: 532–538.

36 Renvert, S., Polyzois, I., and Maguire, R. (2009). Re-osseointegration on previously contaminated surfaces: a systematic review. *Clin. Oral Implants Res.* 20 (Suppl 4): 216–227.

37 Schwarz, F., Sahm, N., Schwarz, K., and Becker, J. (2010). Impact of defect configuration on the clinical outcome following surgical regenerative therapy of peri-implantitis. *J. Clin. Periodontol.* 37: 449–455.

38 Heitz-Mayfield, L.J., Salvi, G.E., Mombelli, A. et al. (2018). Supportive peri-implant therapy following anti-infective surgical peri-implantitis treatment: 5-year survival and success. *Clin. Oral Implants Res.* 29 (1): 1–6.

39 Costa, F.O., Takenaka-Martinez, S., Cota, L.O. et al. (2012). Peri-implant disease in subjects with and without preventive maintenance: a 5-year follow-up. *J. Clin. Periodontol.* 39 (2): 173–181.

36

Implant Prosthetic Complications
Christopher C.K. Ho and Matthew K. Youssef

36.1 Principles

With the increasing placement of dental implants and time in function, the number of late implant failures is growing. This can be a result of either mechanical problems or loss of supporting tissue secondary to infection or peri-implantitis. Understanding potential complications not only aids in management, but also in treatment planning and prevention. The understanding of implant complications is important in patient–clinician communication, informed consent, and post-treatment care. Complications are often bothersome and time consuming for both patient and clinician [1].

The survival of osseointegrated implants has been well documented to be around 95% [2]. Over the past five decades, implant success has been assessed by survival rates, continuous prosthesis stability, minimal radiographic bone loss, and absence of infection in the peri-implant soft tissues. The primary criteria for assessing dental implants are pain, mobility, and bone levels on radiographs.

Key criteria for implant prosthetic success include the following [1–4]:

- Aesthetics – matching the patient's existing dentition with soft tissues matching neighbouring and contralateral dentition
- Soft tissue stability and absence of peri-implant disease
- Implant survival and success
- Occlusal function
- Retrievability
- Passive fit – restorative passivity allows for reduced forces on the dental implant, ensuring maximum abutment to implant contact to allow even stress distribution
- Patient satisfaction.

Possible prosthetic complications [1, 3]:

- Abutment fracture
- Veneering material fracture
- Screw loosening

Practical Procedures in Implant Dentistry, First Edition. Edited by Christopher C.K. Ho.
© 2022 John Wiley & Sons Ltd. Published 2022 by John Wiley & Sons Ltd.
Companion website: www.wiley.com/go/ho/implant-dentistry

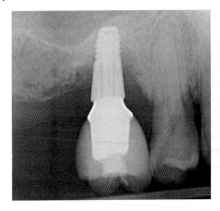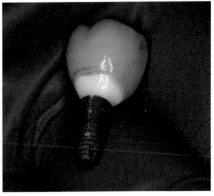

Figure 36.1 Implant fracture. Patient was experiencing unexplained bone loss around their implant and upon removal of the crown it was noted that there was a fracture of the implant.

- Screw fracture
- Acrylic fracture
- Implant fracture
- Framework fracture
- Compromised or poor aesthetic outcome
- Occlusal complications
- Open contacts
- Over-denture mechanical retention complications.

Mechanical problems may result from metal fatigue, material wear, ageing, poor fit, or biomechanical overloading [1, 3]. Furthermore, there may be iatrogenic clinician factors, including operator error, lack of judgement, and inexperience or patient factors, such as parafunction with microtrauma, macrotrauma, or time *in situ*.

Single-unit complications include detachment of prosthetic crown from implant abutment, open contacts, ceramic fracture, poor aesthetics, soft tissue loss, prosthetic screw loosening, fractured abutment, and implant fracture [1, 3]. Full arch complications include the detachment of acrylic teeth, minor acrylic fractures, prosthetic screw loosening, prosthetic screw fractures, and wear of the abutment connection screw thread [3]. Major complications, which are less common, include titanium bar fractures and implant fractures (Figures 36.1 and 36.2).

36.1.1 Incidence of Prosthetic Complications

36.1.1.1 Implant-Supported Single Tooth Crowns and Implant-Fixed Dental Prostheses

Restorative implant success rates vary significantly between papers. Early papers reveal success rates of 80–85% [4]. More recent systematic reviews, with a minimum 10-year review, reveals a success rate of 89% [2]. In a systematic review, Zembic et al. reported prosthetic complication rates over a five-year period, when assessing biological, mechanical, and aesthetic outcomes, to be 12% mechanical and 6% biological [5].

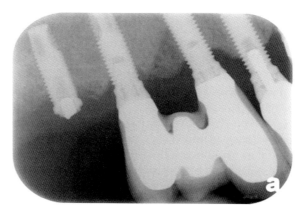

Figure 36.2 Fractured abutment screw (gold screw).

Jung et al. [6] published a systematic review of the survival rate and incidence of technical complications of implant-supported crowns reported in longitudinal studies with a mean follow-up of five years. Technical complications reached a cumulative incidence of 8.8% for screw loosening, 4.1% for loss of retention, and 3.5% for fracture of the veneering material after five years [6]. A 10-year retrospective study on implant-supported single-tooth crowns and implant-fixed dental prostheses (IFDPs) found the most frequent complication was ceramic chipping (20.31%), followed by occlusal screw loosening (2.57%), and loss of retention (2.06%) [7]. Generalised attrition and IFDPs were associated with statistically significantly higher rates of ceramic fractures when compared with single crowns [8]. Moreover, open contacts interproximally has an incidence of 60% after seven years [9, 10].

36.1.1.2 Full Arch Implant-Fixed Dental Prostheses

Full arch prosthetic restoration complications are common. Papaspyridakos et al. [50] specifically investigated biological and technical complications in implant-supported full arch fixed dental hybrid prostheses and found prostheses free of complications after five years 29.3% and 8.6% after ten years. Technical complications involving screws (i.e. loosening or fracture) were reported at a rate of 10.4% after five years and 20.8% after ten years. Chipping or fracture of veneering materials occurred at a rate of 33% and 66.6% at five and ten years, respectively [11]. There were few studies on metal/ceramic full arch prostheses. Bozini et al. in a meta-analysis of prosthetic complications in full arch implant-fixed dental prostheses (FAIFDPs) concluded that there were minimal metal/ceramic studies and that, in metal/acrylic resin studies, veneer fracture and material wear were the most common complication [12].

Irrespective of the exact figures in the literature, a thorough understanding of prosthetic complications, as well as methods of their prevention and management, is a requirement in implant dentistry. Although a full arch implant-supported bridge may be an excellent treatment option for a patient with a completely edentulous ridge(s), the strategic removal of teeth with satisfactory prognosis for the sake of delivering an implant-supported full arch dental hybrid prosthesis should be avoided.

36.1.2   Aetiology of Prosthetic Complications

Understanding the aetiology of implant complications aids in prevention and management. The aetiology of prosthetic implant complications can be largely differentiated into patient and clinician factors. Late implant failures may be multifactorial, and may result from a lack of equilibrium between the biomechanical forces and host factors.

36.1.2.1   Mechanical Overloading
This can occur due to parafunction leading to possible implant overload and metal fatigue/material ageing [8]. Other overload-related factors include inadequate occlusion, the presence of distal cantilevers in IFDPs, or lack of prosthesis passive fit. Misfit at the abutment–implant interface with a lack of passivity may lead to fracture, screw loosening, or abutment/prosthetic screw fracture.

36.1.2.2   Cement Excess
In certain patients there may be the need for cement to retain the restoration due to screw access alignment issues from the underlying bony anatomy. With the introduction of angled screw channels to correct screw access issues this has led to fewer cement-retained restorations. Wilson et al. in a prospective study found a positive relationship between excess cement and peri-implant disease [14]. Linkevicius et al. found implants with cement remnants in patients with history of periodontitis may be more likely to develop peri-implant disease [15]. In a cement-retained restoration the deeper the position of margin, the greater the amount of undetected cement [16]. Dental radiographs should not be considered a reliable method for cement detection as this will only visualise the mesial and distal of the implant fixture.

36.1.2.3   Proximal Contact Loss
The development of an open contact between a natural tooth and a restored implant where there was a firm contact occurs more often than would be expected [9]. This proximal contact loss can result in food trapping, caries, pain, and periodontal issues. It is thought that it occurs as a result of occlusal forces transmitting from the contact areas with a physiological mesial migration of the teeth [10]. This anterior component of force from the occlusion is thought to direct forces to the teeth mesially, and as contact points wear due to friction, the teeth subsequently drift mesially. The ankylosed implant does not shift, however natural teeth may migrate mesially, creating proximal contact loss. An alternative theory is that craniofacial growth beyond adulthood may lead to occlusal alterations. Greenstein et al. [51] in a review found that an interproximal gap developed in 34–66% of cases after an implant restoration was placed. This would happen as early as three months after prosthetic rehabilitation, usually on the mesial of the restoration.

36.2   Procedures

36.2.1   Occlusion

Animal studies on overloaded implants in a split mouth, with one side given regular oral hygiene and the other little hygiene, have shown that marginal bone loss stopped at the implant neck when oral hygiene was well maintained, but

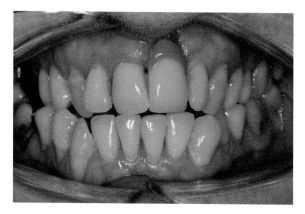

Figure 36.3 Poor implant positioning and attempted prosthetic recovery with pink porcelain. This placement has led to difficulty in cleaning around the prosthesis with subsequent inflammation.

progressed in poorly maintained environments [12]. In cases where peri-implant inflammation was pre-existing, overloading of the implant resulted in significant increase in marginal bone loss [13].

36.2.2 Unfavourable Implant Position

Unfavourable implant position can lead to an aesthetic compromise as well as resulting in unfavourable access for hygiene (Figure 36.3). Innovations in restorative solutions allowed recovery of poor placement with the introduction of pre-fabricated or custom angulated abutments. However, in some cases it may be necessary to use a cement-retained restoration. The aim is to provide forces along the long axis of the implant to prevent unfavourable stress distribution throughout the prosthesis. If an implant is placed in a position that is aesthetically undesirable a decision needs to be made to either remove the implant or restore it. Pre-surgical planning with cone beam computed tomography (CBCT) and appropriate implant planning software allows for accurate pre-surgical assessment of the patient's bone volume and the potential need for bone augmentation [16].

36.2.3 Anterior Implants

Examination of gingival colour at implant sites has shown that irrespective of material choice, when compared to natural dentition, a significant difference in gingival aesthetic outcome is observed (Figure 36.4) [17]. Gold and zirconia abutments showed less aesthetic differences when compared to titanium in the anterior region [17]. Using spectrophotometric analysis, Kim et al. concluded that zirconia abutments demonstrated significantly better colour difference when compared with gold or titanium [18]. However, interestingly, patient aesthetic satisfaction rates do not vary between materials [19].

36.2.4 Implant Fracture

The incidence of implant fracture is between 0.16 and 1.5% [20]. Several factors may contribute, including small-diameter implants, improper occlusal scheme,

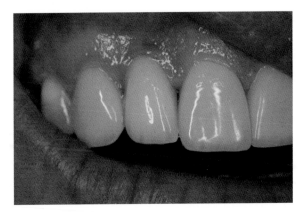

Figure 36.4 Minor gingival discolouration in the anterior region adjacent to healthy tissue.

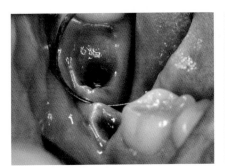 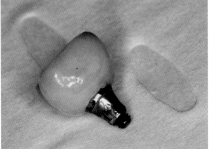

Figure 36.5 Continued screw loosening of the abutment and re-tightening led to a fracture of the implant. Note the poor form of the conical connection/engaging hex within the abutment, which is the most likely reason for misfit and continued loosening.

and parafunction (Figure 36.5). A further predisposing factor is crestal bone loss, which may lead to bending stress of the implants and in particular loss of supporting bone to the structurally weaker zone of the implants at the end of the prosthetic screw.

Management
- If an implant has fractured, it can be explanted with the use of trephines or piezosurgery, and possibly a new larger implant may be inserted if appropriate.
- In certain cases, when an implant fractures superficially leaving sufficient internal thread, it may be possible to use a new prosthetic post cemented into place. However, explantation and replacement would the best long-term option.
- If an implant is not being replaced, it may be possible to leave the remaining apical portion integrated in bone and the edentulous space restored with conventional prosthodontic procedures like a removable dental prosthesis or bridgework.

36.2.5   Screw Loosening

Gold and titanium screws are normally used, and gold screws have a higher modulus of elasticity and show less screw loosening with improved clamping forces. Titanium alloy has better mechanical properties and is stronger than gold, with metal fatigue occurring more frequently with gold screws [5, 6]. A screw is tightened by applying torque which develops a force within the screw called the preload. As the screw is tightened it elongates, producing tension. Elastic recovery of a screw pulls the components together, providing the clamping force. Wittneben et al. [52] in a 10-year restrospective study on complication rates with implant-supported fixed dental prostheses and single crowns found occlusal screw loosening occurred in 2.57%.

Management
- Calibration of torque drivers and motors must be continually checked, and the use of mechanical torque gauges should be used to ensure correct torque is achieved.
- Chronic loosening of gold or abutment screws or fracture of components will need critical assessment of the prosthesis for fit, and also any excessive forces subjected to the prosthesis.
- If a screw is continually loosening this may lead to stretching, with possible damage and weakening. This may require a new replacement screw prior to refitting the prosthesis.

36.2.6   Abutment Screw Fracture

The fracture of an abutment screw within an implant can lead to a complicated procedure to retrieve the broken screw, or may require the explantation and replacement of the implant. When a screw fractures, a loss of clamping force occurs, with the loss of preload; often the fractured screw is loose apically and can be unwound. There are situations where the apical part may be stuck or the threads damaged and impossible to retrieve.

Management
- Artery forceps/haemostats can be used to remove the broken screw when it is fractured above the head of the implant.
- An ultrasonic scaler can be used to disengage the fractured screw. The oscillations from the scaler gradually reverse the screw, if the tip of the scaler is placed directly on top of the screw.
- Use of rescue retrieval kits. The majority of implant manufacturers produce specific kits with instruments designed to fit into their implants with drills, drill guides, and tapping instruments. These kits work by unscrewing the screw. Other kits will drill into the screw, creating splinters of metal that can be removed.
- A small bur running in reverse at low speed may act to turn out the screw.

36.2.7   Stripped Screw Head

A common prosthetic complication encountered is damage to the head of the screw or stripping of the internal head, which renders the implant screwdriver ineffective in removing or tightening a screw.

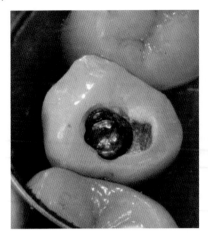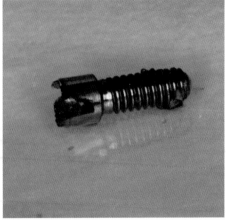

Figure 36.6 Stripped screw head. A fine slot has been cut into the top of the screw so that a flat driver can be used to unwind the screw to remove.

Management

- The first attempt may be to use a brand new driver or to modify the driver slightly by removing the end and shortening it by 0.5 mm. Removing the end makes the driver slightly larger, which may allow it to engage the screw to remove it.
- The second step to try is to cut a slot in the screw with a fine carbide bur (Figure 36.6). This may then allow engagement of a flat screwdriver to remove the screw.
- The final step is to remove the head of the screw, which then removes the preload or clamping force of the screw and allows the restoration to be removed. Because the head of the screw is removed, the remaining screw is loose and can be removed.

36.2.8 Passive Fit

Dental implant superstructure fit is a key component in preventing undesirable biological and mechanical events. The term passive fit in implant prosthetics is defined as 'zero strain on the supporting implant components and the surrounding bone in the absence of an applied external load' [21]. In 1994, Carlsson suggested that passive fit prosthetics was not possible, and a level of misfit was inevitable [22]. Natural teeth may move within bony sockets, but implants are ankylosed. Moreover, due to the machine fit of prostheses, it is crucial to have an accurate fit, as on screwing the restoration to seat there may be internal stresses that may lead to microfractures in the bone, with subsequent crestal bone loss, or mechanical problems such as loosening or fracture.

A passively fitting superstructure enables reduced stress along the implant and surrounding bone [23]. Osseointegrated implants do not possess a periodontal ligament and so have limited or no biological freedom for misfit. Implants are believed to experience approximately 10 μm of movement range [24]. Framework misfit to osseointegrated implants induces stresses on internal components of the prosthesis, the implants, and the surrounding bone [25]. However, some tolerance for misfit is present between the prosthesis and the implants [26]. Clinically establishing a quantifiable amount of misfit that is acceptable is extremely difficult [27]. The exact amount probably depends on a variety of factors including: 'bone quality, length and diameter of implants, and implant surface characteristics' [21].

Clinical measurement of the passive fit of implant framework superstructures is a contentious topic. Multiple fit checking methods have been established with varying degrees of success and are empirical in nature [28]. They include the following:

- *Alternate finger pressure*: Apply alternate pressure on either side of the prosthesis when seating the prosthesis to assess for rocking movements [28]. This technique aims to divulge any fulcruming on the prosthesis. Saliva movement on pressure at the implant–abutment interface may be seen if there is a misfit [29].
- *Radiographic assessment:* This should always be incorporated, irrespective of fit tests undertaken. Radiographs should be taken, juxtaposed with any alternate testing of fit [18, 30, 32]. This is especially relevant when superstructure connection is positioned subgingivally (Figure 36.7).
- *Direct vision and tactile sensation*: Use an explorer around the margins of the restoration framework using tactile sensation and vision to review the fit [30, 31]. Lighting and magnification improve visualisation of margins while using an explorer [30]. A fine explorer can be used to maximise the ability to detect framework fit discrepancies, but it is not a sensitive instrument to detect accurately.

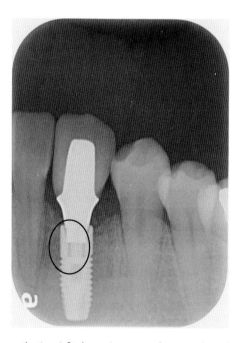

Figure 36.7 Implant prosthetic misfit due to incorrect abutment insertion.

- *One-screw test*: One screw at the terminal aspect of the prosthesis is tightened, while remaining abutment interfaces are examined for discrepancies [25, 28, 33]. This technique is paramount with long-span frameworks, as discrepancies become more apparent further away from the terminally screwed abutment. This test can be used in conjunction with aforementioned techniques.
- *Screw resistance test* [25]: This was designed based on the clinical decision that 150 μm was an acceptable level of misfit. A full rotation equates to 300 μm when using a gold Nobel Biocare screw with a Nobel Biocare implant. Therefore, once resistance is noted, only a half turn (180 degrees) is considered an acceptable amount of superstructure misfit. The prosthesis is tightened from the mesial abutment first and gradually moving to the terminal abutment. A maximum torque of 10–15 Ncm should be used to fully seat the prosthesis within a half turn from the point of resistance [25]. A five-year follow-up using this technique showed no mechanical fatigue fractures, suggesting this test is clinically adequate for fit assessment [25, 28]. Nevertheless, radiographs, direct vision, illumination, finger pressure, floss, and disclosing media should be used in conjunction with the screw resistance test for framework fit verification.

36.2.9 Mechanical and Biological Complications of Framework Misfit

Finite element analysis assessed on levels of misfit under occlusal-like loads show increased stress on surrounding implant bone [37, 38]. The degree of misfit was also found to be correlated to the amount of strain applied on implant and prosthetic components as well as stress transfer to bone [39]. Jimbo et al. hypothesised that vertical fractures of the implant which were commonly found adjacent to regions of bone loss were due to prosthesis misfit [40, 41]. Through finite element analysis, they demonstrated that as the degree of misfit increases, the stress levels on the implant and its surrounding bone increase [41]. They also showed that the stress levels reduced when a multi-unit abutment was used [41]. Adell et al. found an increasing fracture rate over time, introducing the possibility of metal fatigue as a contributing factor [29]. Establishing a relationship between framework misfit and implant failure is extremely difficult. One must consider the implications of occlusal stresses, implant length and diameter, implant surface topography, patient factors, prosthesis design, impression techniques, splinted versus non-splinted prosthesis, and more. Further to this the degree of misfit and the direction will impact potential complications. Vertical, horizontal, and angulation misfits exist. Finite element analysis from several authors has shown that stress patterns due to misfit may result in increased stresses to componentry and underlying bone of 30–40% [42–44].

Animal studies have been used to examine the clinical state that results from implant framework misfit. Tests included clinical evaluation of mobility, radiographic evaluation, histological analysis, microscopic measurements, photogrammetry, and laser scanning. Peri-implant bone response was the key outcome of interest in these studies. Unfortunately, the majority of the studies were completed without loading and assessed response to vertical misfit only. 'None of the studies confirmed any negative effects on peri-implant bone due to framework misfit' alone [42]. Another paper by Jemt et al. showed no statistical correlations between the changes in marginal bone levels to variations in prosthesis misfit using intra-oral radiographs on seven patients [26].

As a result, although finite element analysis shows increased stress application to the bone, the animal studies did not reflect this due to poor-quality research. Nevertheless, we should not ignore the importance of accurately taking an impression and providing a stable passive implant prosthesis.

36.2.10 Impression Technique

Modern technology revolves around digital dentistry and digital impression taking. When assessing digital impression techniques, the Trios® scanner (3Shape) averaged 0.028 mm of inaccuracy when scanning six implants across a single arch [45]. However, a clinical comparative study comparing digital and conventional implant impression techniques showed traditional methods have a statistically relevant advantage in accuracy [46]. Furthermore, splinting impression copings with acrylic resin demonstrated better accuracy than non-splinted impressions [47]. In efforts toward a passively fitting framework it is important to take accurate impressions. Implant impression copings joined together intraorally with acrylic resin show the most consistent results [46, 47].

Possible errors creating prosthetic superstructure misfit may include:

- Impression procedure – mandibular flexure, technique, material, machining tolerance of impression copings – splinting, non-splinting custom tray, angulation of implants, roughening of impression copings, and pickup versus transfer technique.
- Master cast fabrication.
- Framework fabrication – cast, distortion with addition of porcelain.

36.2.11 Gingival Fistula

A gingival fistula may result from a loose implant crown, fractured restorative screw, or fractured crown. Excess cement has also been shown to cause the formation of a fistula (Figure 36.8). Management includes tightening of the abutment screw to the manufacturer's recommended torque level, removal of excess cement, debridement of biofilm and irrigation with saline, and regular review.

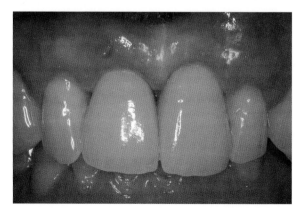

Figure 36.8 Fistula present on the labial gingivae around the maxillary right central incisor. This may present from a loose implant crown, fractured restorative screw, fractured crown, or excess residual cement.

36.2.12 Prevention of Prosthetic Complications

Prevention of implant prosthetic complications requires careful diagnosis, sound treatment planning, atraumatic surgical technique, appropriate alignment and spacing of implants, use of fully or partially guided implant placement systems, fabrication of a passively fitting implant prosthesis, good patient oral hygiene measures, and regular maintenance [48].

- Manage occlusal forces carefully, including sufficient numbers of occlusal units, correct occlusal scheme, and minimisation of occlusal interferences. In patients with parafunction the use of a stabilisation splint is recommended.
- Avoid or minimise posterior cantilevers and bucco-lingual restoration offsets. Cantilevers act as a force magnifier and can be destructive.
- Crown:implant ratio; the use of short implants is well evidenced in the dental literature. However, an unfavourable crown:implant ratio may lead to excessive cantilever forces and loosening or fractures of screws/abutments.
- Chronic loosening of gold or abutment screws or fracture of components will need critical assessment of the prosthesis for fit along with assessment of any overloading factors.
- Patients with multiple implant componentry fractures/failure may require placement of additional implants and splinting of the implant restoration.
- Ensure passive fit with an accurate impression technique with correct technical design and fabrication (Figure 36.9).

Furthermore, preventing implant acrylic superstructure fractures involves aligning implants so they are centred over the ridge, beneath occluding forces, to

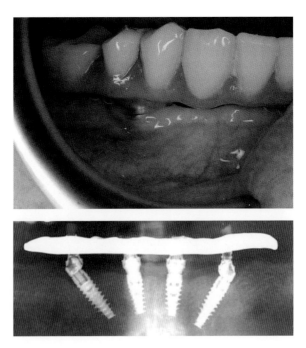

Figure 36.9 Lower 46 implant with prosthesis misfit. The decision was to replace the framework due a noticeable discrepancy.

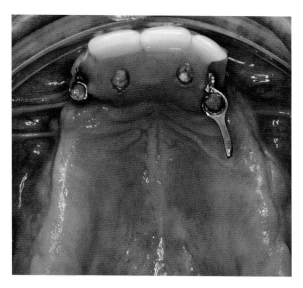

Figure 36.10 Fractured metal framework and acrylic superstructure with poor antero-posterior spread of the implants.

decrease leverage that may be applied to various implant prosthetic components, and the implants themselves [48]. During prosthodontic planning of full arch prosthesis, implant fracture is best avoided by: limiting cantilevers, using an adequate number of implants, well distributed implants, producing a minimum of 10 mm of antero-posterior dimension to the implant distribution, and use of appropriate sized diameter implants in the posterior region (Figure 36.10) [48].

36.3 Tips

- The use of magnification with either loupes or a microscope with illumination is necessary to provide good visual access and ability to assess fit.
- Replace abutment screws if there is chronic loosening or any signs of damage to the screws.
- Refer the patient to a more experienced practitioner if there is difficulty in removal of broken componentry as this may lead to irrecoverable damage.
- Prosthetic complications after the delivery of implant-supported restorations occur continuously over time. It is up to the prudent clinician to minimise possible risk factors but also to inform patients that they may experience possible complications that may need continuing maintenance.

References

1 Goodacre, C.J., Kan, J.Y., and Rungcharassaeng, K. (1999). Clinical complications of osseointegrated implants. *J. Prosthet. Dent.* 81 (5): 537–552.
2 Moraschini, V., Poubel, L.D., Ferreira, V.F., and dos Sp Barboza, E. (2015). Evaluation of survival and success rates of dental implants reported in

longitudinal studies with a follow-up period of at least 10 years: a systematic review. *Int. J. Oral Maxillofac. Surg.* 44 (3): 377–388.

3 (2017). Long-term prosthetic complications in full-arch rehabilitations supported by four implants. *Clin. Oral Implants Res.* 28: 316.

4 Albrektsson, T., Zarb, G., Worthington, P., and Eriksson, A.R. (1986). The long-term efficacy of currently used dental implants: a review and proposed criteria of success. *Int. J. Oral Maxillofac. Implants* 1 (1): 11–25.

5 Zembic A, Kim S, Zwahlen M, Kelly JR. Systematic review of the survival rate and incidence of biologic, technical, and esthetic complications of single implant abutments supporting fixed prostheses. *Int. J. Oral Maxillofac. Implants* 2014;29: 99–116.

6 Jung, R.E., Zembic, A., Pjetursson, B.E. et al. (2012). Systematic review of the survival rate and the incidence of biological, technical, and aesthetic complications of single crowns on implants reported in longitudinal studies with a mean follow-up of 5 years. *Clin. Oral Implants Res.* 23 (Suppl 6): 2–21.

7 Wittneben, J.G., Buser, D., Salvi, G.E. et al. (2014). Complication and failure rates with implant-supported fixed dental prostheses and single crowns: a 10-year retrospective study. *Clin. Implant Dent. Relat. Res.* 16 (3): 356–364.

8 Chrcanovic, B.R., Kisch, J., Albrektsson, T., and Wennerberg, A. (2017). Bruxism and dental implant treatment complications: a retrospective comparative study of 98 bruxer patients and a matched group. *Clin. Oral Implants Res.* 28 (7): e1–e9.

9 Pang, N.S., Suh, C.S., Kim, K.D. et al. (2017). Prevalence of proximal contact loss between implant-supported fixed prostheses and adjacent natural teeth and its associated factors: a 7-year prospective study. *Clin. Oral Implants Res.* 28 (12): 1501–1508.

10 Byun, S.J., Heo, S.M., Ahn, S.G., and Chang, M. (2015). Analysis of proximal contact loss between implant-supported fixed dental prostheses and adjacent teeth in relation to influential factors and effects. A cross-sectional study. *Clin. Oral Implants Res.* 26 (6): 709–714.

11 Esposito, M., Hirsch, J., Lekholm, U., and Thomsen, P. (1999). Differential diagnosis and treatment strategies for biologic complications and failing oral implants: a review of the literature. *Int. J. Oral Maxillofac. Implants* 14 (4): 473–490.

12 Bozini, T., Petridis, H., Garefis, K., and Garefis, P. (2011). A meta-analysis of prosthodontic complication rates of implant-supported fixed dental prostheses in edentulous patients after an observation period of at least 5 years. *Int. J. Oral Maxillofac. Implants* 26 (2): 304–318.

13 Kozlovsky, A., Tal, H., Laufer, B.Z. et al. (2007). Impact of implant overloading on the peri-implant bone in inflamed and non-inflamed peri-implant mucosa. *Clin. Oral Implants Res.* 18 (5): 601–610.

14 Wilson, T.G. Jr. (2009). The positive relationship between excess cement and peri-implant disease: a prospective clinical endoscopic study. *J. Periodontol.* 80 (9): 1388–1392.

15 Linkevicius, T., Puisys, A., Vindasiute, E. et al. (2013). Does residual cement around implant-supported restorations cause peri-implant disease? A retrospective case analysis. *Clin. Oral Implants Res.* 24 (11): 1179–1184.

16 Linkevicius, T., Svediene, O., Vindasiute, E. et al. (2012). The influence of implant placement depth and impression material on the stability of an open tray impression coping. *J. Prosthet. Dent.* 108 (4): 238–243.

17 Bressan, E., Paniz, G., Lops, D. et al. (2011). Influence of abutment material on the gingival color of implant-supported all-ceramic restorations: a prospective multicenter study. *Clin. Oral Implants Res.* 22 (6): 631–637.

18 Kim, A., Campbell, S.D., Viana, M.A., and Knoernschild, K.L. (2016). Abutment material effect on peri-implant soft tissue color and perceived esthetics. *J. Prosthodont.* 25 (8): 634–640.

19 Bidra, A.S. and Rungruanganunt, P. (2013). Clinical outcomes of implant abutments in the anterior region: a systematic review. *J. Esthet. Restor. Dent.* 25 (3): 159–176.

20 Gupta, S., Gupta, H., and Tandan, A. (2015). Technical complications of implant-causes and management: a comprehensive review. *Natl. J. Maxillofac. Surg.* 6 (1): 3.

21 Sahin, S. and Çehreli, M.C. (2001). The significance of passive framework fit in implant prosthodontics: current status. *Implant Dent.* 10 (2): 85–92.

22 Carlsson, L. (1994). Built-in strain and untoward forces are the inevitable companions of prosthetic misfit. *Nobelpharma News* 8: 5.

23 Michalakis KX, Hirayama H, Garefis PD. Cement-retained versus screw-retained implant restorations: a critical review. *Int. J. Oral Maxillofac. Implants* 2003;18(5): 719–728.

24 Assif, D., Marshak, B., and Schmidt, A. (1996). Accuracy of implant impression techniques. *Int. J. Oral Maxillofac. Implants* 11 (2): 216–222.

25 Jemt, T. (1991). Failures and complications in 391 consecutively inserted fixed prostheses supported by Brånemark implants in edentulous jaws: a study of treatment from the time of prosthesis placement to the first annual checkup. *Int. J. Oral Maxillofac. Implants* 6 (3): 270–276.

26 Jemt, T. and Book, K. (1996). Prosthesis misfit and marginal bone loss in edentulous implant patients. *Int. J. Oral Maxillofac. Implants* 11 (5): 620–625.

27 Buzayan, M.M. and Yunus, N.B. (2014). Passive fit in screw retained multi-unit implant prosthesis understanding and achieving: a review of the literature. *J. Indian Prosthod. Soc.* 14 (1): 16–23.

28 Kan, J.Y., Rungcharassaeng, K., Bohsali, K. et al. (1999). Clinical methods for evaluating implant framework fit. *J. Prosthet. Dent.* 81 (1): 7–13.

29 Adell, R., Eriksson, B., Lekholm, U. et al. (1990). A long-term follow-up study of osseointegrated implants in the treatment of totally edentulous jaws. *Int. J. Oral Maxillofac. Implants* 5 (4): 1.

30 Jemt, T. (1994). How do you test a cast framework fit for a full-arch fixed implant-supported prosthesis. *Int. J. Oral Maxillofac. Implants* 9: 471–472.

31 Loos, L.G. (1986). A fixed prosthodontic technique for mandibular osseointegrated titanium implants. *J. Prosthet. Dent.* 55 (2): 232–242.

32 Hollender, L. and Rockler, B. (1980). Radiographic evaluation of osseointegrated implants of the jaws. *Dentomaxillofac. Radiol.* 9 (2): 91–95.

33 Tan, K.B., Rubenstein, J.E., Nicholls, J.I., and Yuodelis, R.A. (1993). Three-dimensional analysis of the casting accuracy of one-piece, osseointegrated implant-retained prostheses. *Int. J. Prosthodont.* 6 (4): 346–363.

34 Natali, A.N., Pavan, P.G., and Ruggero, A.L. (2006). Evaluation of stress induced in peri-implant bone tissue by misfit in multi-implant prosthesis. *Dent. Mater.* 22 (4): 388–395.

35 Hasan, I., Bourauel, C., Keilig, L. et al. (2015). The effect of implant splinting on the load distribution in bone bed around implant-supported fixed prosthesis with different framework materials: a finite element study. *Ann. Anatomy-Anatomischer Anzeiger* 199: 43–51.

36 Abduo, J. and Lyons, K. (2012). Effect of vertical misfit on strain within screw-retained implant titanium and zirconia frameworks. *J. Prosthodont. Res.* 56 (2): 102–109.

37 Zarb, G.A. and Schmitt, A. (1990). The longitudinal clinical effectiveness of osseointegrated dental implants: the Toronto study. Part III: problems and complications encountered. *J Prosthet. Dent.* 64 (2): 185–194.

38 Jimbo, R., Halldin, A., Janda, M. et al. (2013). Vertical fracture and marginal bone loss of internal-connection implants: a finite element analysis. *Int. J. Oral Maxillofac. Implants* 28 (4): e171–e176.

39 Abduo, J. and Judge, R.B. (2014). Implications of implant framework misfit: a systematic review of biomechanical sequelae. *Int. J. Oral Maxillofac. Implants* 29 (3).

40 Kunavisarut, C., Lang, L.A., Stoner, B.R., and Felton, D.A. (2002). Finite element analysis on dental implant–supported prostheses without passive fit. *J. Prosthodont.* 11 (1): 30–40.

41 Natali, A.N., Gasparetto, A., Carniel, E.L. et al. (2007). Interaction phenomena between oral implants and bone tissue in single and multiple implant frames under occlusal loads and misfit conditions: a numerical approach. *J. Biomed. Mater. Res. Pt. B Appl. Biomater.* 83 (2): 332–339.

42 Vandeweghe, S., Vervack, V., Dierens, M., and De Bruyn, H. (2017). Accuracy of digital impressions of multiple dental implants: an in vitro; study. *Clin. Oral Implants Res.* 28 (6): 648–653.

43 Alsharbaty, M.H., Alikhasi, M., Zarrati, S., and Shamshiri, A.R. (2019). A clinical comparative study of 3-dimensional accuracy between digital and conventional implant impression techniques. *J. Prosthodont.* 28 (4): e902–e908.

44 Öngül, D., Gökçen-Röhlig, B., Şermet, B., and Keskin, H. (2012). A comparative analysis of the accuracy of different direct impression techniques for multiple implants. *Aust. Dent. J.* 57 (2): 184–189.

45 Goodacre, C.J. and Kattadiyil, M.T. (2015). Prosthetic-related dental implant complications: etiology, prevention, and treatment. *Dent. Implant Complicat. Etiol. Prevent. Treat.* 16: 233–258.

46 Papaspyridakos, P., Chen, C.J., Chuang, S.K. et al. (2012). A systematic review of biologic and technical complications with fixed implant rehabilitations for edentulous patients. *Int. J. Oral Maxillofac. Implants* 27 (1): 102–110.

47 Greenstein, G., Carpentieri, J., and Cavallaro, J. (2016). Open contacts adjacent to dental implant restorations: etiology, incidence, consequences, and correction. *J. Am. Dental Assoc.* 147 (1): 28–34.

48 Wittneben, J.G., Buser, D., Salvi, G.E. et al. (2014). Complication and failure rates with implant-supported fixed dental prostheses and single crowns: A 10-year retrospective study. Clin. Implant Dent. *Relat Res.* 16 (3): 356–364.

Index

Page locators in **bold** indicate tables. Page locators in *italics* indicate figures. This index uses letter-by-letter alphabetization.

a

absorbable collagen sponge (ACS)   78
absorbable sutures   156
abutments   243–252
  complications   375, *376*, 377, 382
  custom abutments   243–245,
    244–245
  definitive prosthesis   292,
    296–297, *297*
  design   249–250, *249*
  implant materials, designs, and
    surfaces   96–101, *99–100*
  implant screw joint   307–313
  implant treatment in the aesthetic
    zone   234
  impression taking in implant
    dentistry   219, 220, 223
  laboratory perspective on implant
    dentistry   265, *266*, 267–271,
    268–271, *274*, 275
  location jigs   251, *251*
  material selection   247–249, *248*
  prefabricated abutments   243, *244*,
    245–247, *246–247*, 250
  prosthodontic rehabilitation for fully
    edentulous patient   322–323
  screw- versus cement-retained
    restorations   253, 259–264
  surgical protocols for implant
    placement   177
  timing of implant placement   114

access flap surgery   361, *362*
accessory lingual foramina   63, *64*
acellular dermal matrix   201
acellular extrinsic fibre
  cementum   74–75
acrylic superstructure fractures
  382–383, *383*
ACS *see* absorbable collagen sponge
adjacent teeth   120–122, *120*, **121**
adjunctive soft tissue grafting
  112–113
aesthetics
  abutments   248, 250
  anatomic and biological principles for
    implant placement   37, 43
  bone augmentation   211
  clinical management   232–233
  complications   375, *376*
  definitive prosthesis   290–292,
    295, *295*
  diagnostic keys for single-tooth peri-
    implant aesthetics   232, **232**
  extraction ridge management   73
  general considerations in smile
    evaluation   227–230, *228*
  gingival biotype   230, 232–233
  gingival display, gingival zeniths, and
    papillae of maxillary anterior teeth
    228, 229–230
  implant site preparation   118–119,
    118, 122–124, *123*

Practical Procedures in Implant Dentistry, First Edition. Edited by Christopher C.K. Ho.
© 2022 John Wiley & Sons Ltd. Published 2022 by John Wiley & Sons Ltd.
Companion website: www.wiley.com/go/ho/implant-dentistry

aesthetics (*cont'd*)
  implant treatment in the aesthetic
    zone   227–236
  laboratory perspective on implant
    dentistry   268, *269–270*
  lip contour and length   228
  loading protocols in
    implantology   129
  major deficiencies in hard and soft
    tissues   230–232, *231*
  patient assessment and history
    taking   227
  pre-surgical tissue evaluation
    163–171
  prosthodontic rehabilitation for fully
    edentulous patient   316–317,
    322, *325*
  provisionalisation in
    implantology   241, *241*
  screw- versus cement-retained
    restorations   254–255,
    254–255, 261
  smile line   228–229, *228*
  soft tissue augmentation   199, 201
  surgical protocols for implant
    placement   174
  thickness of soft tissues   234
  timing of implant placement   104–
    107, *104–106*, 109, 114, 233–234
  tooth display   228
  tooth length, shape, alignment,
    contour, and colour   229
  tooth loss and implant placement
    32, *33*
  width of edentulous space   230
  see also dentofacial aesthetics
age of patient   7
air powder abrasive systems   358–359
ALARA principle   14, 23
alcohol   133
allergies   6, 92
allografts   73, 201
alloplasts   73
alternate finger pressure   379
alveolar ridge
  bone augmentation   211–212
  implant site preparation   124, *126*
  mandibular anatomical structures   59

surgical protocols for implant
  placement   173, *175*
tooth loss and implant placement
  31–32, 34
see also extraction ridge management
anaesthesia   49–50, 52, 67–68
analogue/traditional template   15, *15*, 18
angiogenesis   212, 217
angle screw correction   262–263,
  262–263, 267–268, *267–268*
angulation
  abutments   247, *247*, 250
  implant site preparation
    122–123, *124*
  laboratory perspective on implant
    dentistry   267–268, *267–268*
  screw- versus cement-retained
    restorations   262–263, *262–263*
anterior implants   375, *376*
anterior superior alveolar nerve
  (ASA)   40
antibiotics   7, 359
anticoagulants   7
antiseptic decontamination   359
apically repositioned flap   188–190,
  188, *190*, 361
apico-coronal position   176
articulated study models   17–18
ASA *see* anterior superior alveolar
  nerve
attached mucosa   118
attachment differences   352, *353*
Audentes technique   274, *274*
augmentation techniques *see* bone
  augmentation; soft tissue
  augmentation
auriculotemporal nerve   41
autogenous bone grafts
  bone augmentation   212, *213*,
    215–216, *216–217*
  extraction ridge management   73
axontmesis   62

b
beams   280–281, *281*
BH *see* buccal bone height
bi-axial screws   262–263, *262–263*
BIC *see* bone-to-implant contact

biomaterials
  extraction ridge management
    74–78, *76–78*, 82
  timing of implant placement
    109–110
bisphosphonate therapy   8–9
blood clots
  bone augmentation   212
  implant surface treatments   92
  peri-implant emergence profile   195
  surgical instrumentation   144
  surgical protocols for implant
    placement   178
  timing of implant placement   110
  tooth loss and implant placement
    29–31, *31*
bone augmentation   211–217
  autogenous bone graft   212, *213,*
    215–216, *216–217*
  bone graft with non-resorbable
    membrane   213–214, *214*
  defect topography classification
    211–212
  flap design and management for
    implant placement   146
  loading protocols in implantology
    130–131, 134
  materials used for augmentation
    212–213, *213*
  objectives of bone grafting   211
  peri-implant emergence profile   182
  pre-surgical tissue evaluation   165–
    166, *165*
  requirements for successful tissue
    grafting   212
  soft tissue augmentation prior
    to bone grafting   202–203,
    205–206
  soft tissue graft to gain keratinised
    tissue   203–207, *206–209*
  surgical instrumentation   143
  surgical protocols for implant
    placement   177
  timing of implant placement   106,
    108, 112
bone loss
  complications   351–354, *352*, 371
  extraction ridge management   73

implant biomechanics   284
implant site preparation   125
loading protocols in
  implantology   131
maintenance of dental implants
  329–330
occlusion   299–301
screw- versus cement-retained
  restorations   256–257
surgical protocols for implant
  placement   174, 179
timing of implant placement   106,
  107–108
bone quantity/quality
  complications   379
  maxillary anatomical structures   54
  surgical protocols for implant
    placement   174, 177, 179
  timing of implant placement   108
bone resorption
  implant biomechanics   283
  implant materials, designs, and
    surfaces   92, 96
  implant treatment in the aesthetic
    zone   232
  maintenance of dental implants
    329–330
  pre-surgical tissue evaluation   169
  timing of implant placement   106,
    107–108, 112
  tooth loss and implant placement
    29–32, *30–31*
bone sounding   168–169, *169*
bone-to-implant contact (BIC)
  implant materials, designs, and
    surfaces   95
  loading protocols in implantology
    130–131
  timing of implant placement   110
bridgework
  impression taking in implant
    dentistry   223
  prosthodontic rehabilitation for fully
    edentulous patient   319–320,
    319–320, 323–326, *324–325*
  see also full arch restorations
bruxism   301–302, **302**
BT *see* buccal wall thickness

buccal attached gingiva of maxillary
    molars   201
buccal bone height (BH)   74–75
buccal bone thickness   165–166, *165*
buccal grafts   121
buccal–lingual position   106–107
buccally repositioned flap   191–193,
    191–192
buccal plate integrity   169, *169*
buccal plate thickness   109, *110*
buccal roll   152, 183–186, *183–185*
buccal veneer grafting   *165*
buccal wall thickness (BT)   74,
    79–81, 82
bucco-lingual/palatal position   174,
    175–176
bulk implant materials   87–92
    other bulk materials   92
    pure titanium   88–90, *88–90*
    titanium alloys   90, *91*
    zirconia   90–92, *91*

c
CAD/CAM *see* computer-aided design/
    manufacturing
cancellous bone   179, 284
cantilevers   282–283, *283–285*, 300,
    310, 374, 382–383
cardiovascular disorders   6–7
CBCT *see* cone beam computed
    tomography
CCARD *see* Cologne Classification of
    Alveolar Ridge Defects
cement-retained restorations   253–264
    aesthetics   254–255, *254–255*
    clinical performance   256–257
    complications   355–356, 374
    definitive prosthesis   289, 292–294,
        294, 296–297, *297*
    health of peri-implant tissue   256
    hygiene/emergence profile   255, *255*
    inter-arch space   256
    lateral set-screw/cross-pinning
        261–262, *261*
    maintenance of dental implants
        330–331, *331*
    occlusion   256

    passivity   254–255, 257
    procedures for cement retention
        260–261
    provisionalisation   256
    reduced occlusal material
        fracture   255
    retrievability   253, 257–259, 261
chairside copy/replica abutments   263,
    296–297, *297*
checklists   27, 28
closed tray impression techniques
    220–222, **221**
Cologne Classification of Alveolar Ridge
    Defects (CCARD)   211–212
complications
    abutment screw failure   377
    acrylic superstructure
        fractures   382–383, *383*
    aetiology of prosthetic
        complications   374
    anterior implants   375, *376*
    attachment differences   352, *353*
    biological complications   351–369,
        380–381
    causes of peri-implant disease
        353–357, **355**, *356*
    cement excess   374
    crestal bone loss   351, 353, **355**
    criteria for bone loss   351–352, *352*
    flap design and management for
        implant placement   145
    framework misfit   380–381
    gingival fistula   381, *381*
    implant fracture   375–376, *376*
    implant materials, designs, and
        surfaces   97
    implant prosthetic complications
        3–4, 371–386
    impression taking   381
    incidence of prosthetic complications
        372–373
    mechanical overloading   374
    occlusion   374–375, 382
    passive fit   378–380, *379*, 382, *382*
    prevalence of peri-implant disease   354
    prevention of prosthetic complications
        382–383, *382–383*

proximal contact loss   374

screw loosening   *376*, 377, 382

screw- versus cement-retained
   restorations   256–257

stripped screw head   377–378, *378*

supportive care   365–366

treatment of peri-implant disease
   357–366, *358–359, 362–364,*
   366–367

types of mechanical
   complications   371–372, *372–373*

unfavourable implant position
   375, *375*

see also peri-implantitis/mucositis

compressive forces   279–280, *279*, 300

computed tomography (CT) *see* cone
   beam computed tomography

computer-aided design/manufacturing
   (CAD/CAM)   1, 3

abutments   243, 245

diagnostic records   17

digital workflow in implant
   dentistry   335

laboratory perspective on implant
   dentistry   268–274, *270–273*

screw- versus cement-retained
   restorations   255, 259

cone beam computed tomography
   (CBCT)   2

complications   375

diagnostic records   14–19, **15**, 23

digital workflow in implant dentistry
   336, 337, *338*, 344

extraction ridge management   *77*, 82

implant site preparation   119–120

implant treatment in the aesthetic
   zone   232

mandibular anatomical structures
   60–63, *61, 63*, 65, *66*, 69

maxillary anatomical structures   50,
   51, 53

peri-implant emergence profile   196

pre-surgical tissue evaluation   169

surgical protocols for implant
   placement   173–174

timing of implant placement   *109–110*

tooth loss and implant placement   34

connection design   *91*, 96–101,
   98–100, **98**

connective tissue   29–31, *31*

connective tissue grafts
   extraction ridge management   73
   maxillary anatomical structures   56
   pre-surgical tissue evaluation
      166, *166*
   soft tissue augmentation   200, 201,
      205–206

continuous/uninterrupted sutures
   159, *159*

contour management
   abutments   249–251, *249*
   complications   356–357, *356*, 366
   maintenance of dental
      implants   330
   provisionalisation in implantology
      239, **239**
   screw- versus cement-retained
      restorations   259

contraindications   5–6, **6**

cortical bone   174, 179, 284

cranial bones   37

cranial nerves   40–41
   see also individual nerves

crestal bone loss
   complications   351, 353, **355**
   maintenance of dental
      implants   329
   occlusion   299

crestal incision   149, *149*, 151–152,
   153, 191–192

cross-pinning   261–262, *261*

crown:implant ratio   382

crown lengthening   122, *123*

curettage   358, *358*

cusp inclinations   304, *304*

customised impression copings
   222, *222*

cutting torque resistance analysis   134

d

DBBM/DBBMC *see* deproteinised
   bovine bone mineral/collagen

decontamination techniques   358–360,
   358–359

definitive prosthesis   289–298
  aesthetic evaluation   290–292
  cement-retained crown   289,
    292–294, **294**, 296–297, *297*
  chairside copy/replica abutments
    296–297, *297*
  maintenance of dental implants   330
  occlusal verification   290
  pink porcelain   295, *295*
  prosthodontic rehabilitation for fully
    edentulous patient   *325*
  screw-retained crown   289, 294–295
  soft tissue support   289–290, **291**
  torque requirement for delivery   292,
    293–294, 298
dental history   9–10
dental records   26–28
denture-stomatitis   326
deproteinised bovine bone mineral/
    collagen (DBBM/DBBMC)
    74–76, *76*, *79*, *81*, 110
diagnostic records   13–23
  articulated study models   17–18
  diagnostic imaging and
    templates   13–16, *15–16*, **15**
  guided surgery   16–17, *16–17*
  photographic records   18, 19–21,
    19–23
  template design   18–19
digital workflow in implant dentistry
    335–349
  advantages of full digital
    workflow   336
  cone beam computed tomography
    336, 337, *338*
  data acquisition for full arch
    cases   271–272, *272–273*
  diagnostic records   16, 18–19
  digital planning to manage
    aesthetics   268, *269–270*
  disadvantages and limitations of
    analogue system   335
  guided implant surgery   342–343, *342*
  implant treatment planning and
    placement   337–338, *339–340*
  impression taking   219, 225, 250,
    336–337, *336–337*, 343, *343–346*
  manufacturing the customised
    prosthesis   343–346, *346*
  pre-surgical fabricated temporary
    prosthesis   342
  shift from analogue to digital
    265, 335
  surgical guide   338–341, *341*
direct observation   379
drilling protocols   173, 176–177

e
ectopic eruption   124, *126*
edentulism
  abutments   246
  impression taking in implant
    dentistry   224, *224*
  loading protocols in implantology
    131, 133
  maxillary anatomical structures   54
  occlusion   300
  prosthodontic rehabilitation for fully
    edentulous patient   315–326
  tooth loss and implant placement
    32–33
edentulous space   230
elastomeric impression materials
    219–220
embedment relaxation   308
EMD *see* enamel matrix derivative
emergence profile *see* peri-implant
    emergence profile
EMP *see* enamel matrix proteins
enamel matrix derivative (EMD)
    74–78, *76*
enamel matrix proteins (EMP)   74–78
endodontic lesions   120, *120*
engaging impression copings   223, *223*
envelope flap   148–149, *149*
external hex feature   *91*, 96–97, *99*,
    309–310
extraction
  pre-surgical tissue evaluation
    167–169, *168–169*
  timing of implant placement
    110, *111*
  tooth loss and implant placement
    29–34, *30–31*, *33*

extraction ridge management   73–86
  biologically active materials   74–78,
    76–78, 82
  implant site preparation   124, *126*
  implant treatment in the aesthetic
    zone   230
  influence of buccal wall thickness
    79–81, 82
  osteoconductive materials
    74–76, 82
  pre-surgical tissue evaluation
    166–167, *167*, 170
  study findings   73–74
  suturing techniques   155
  timing of implant placement   106,
    107–108
  tooth loss and implant placement   34
extrusion   123–124, *125*, 170

f
facial bones   37
facial expression
  anatomic and biological principles
    for implant placement   41,
    44–45, *46*
  implant treatment in the aesthetic
    zone   227–230, *228*
FAIFDP *see* full arch implant-fixed
    dental prosthesis
FGG *see* free gingival graft
fibrous encapsulation   129, 177
fixed dental prostheses
  complications   373–374
  implant site preparation   117
  impression taking in implant
    dentistry   223
  occlusion   303–304, *304*
  prosthodontic rehabilitation for fully
    edentulous patient   319–320,
    319–320, 323–326, 324–325
flap design and management
    145–154
  apically repositioned flap   188–190,
    188, 190
  bone augmentation   213–214, *214*
  buccally repositioned flap   191–193,
    191–192

buccal roll   152, 183–186, *183–185*
  considerations for flap design and
    management   146
  envelope flap   148–149, *149*
  free gingival graft   195–196,
    195, 197
  neurovascular supply to implant site
    145–146
  Palacci flap   152, *153*
  papilla-sparing flap   151–152, *151*
  pouch roll   186–188, *186–187*
  pre-surgical tissue evaluation   169
  soft tissue augmentation   203–207,
    206–209
  surgical protocols for implant
    placement   173, 176–177
  suturing techniques   *149*, 155
  tissue punch   148, *148*
  triangular and trapezoidal
    flaps   150–151, *150*
  types of flap reflection
    146–148, *147*
flapless protocol
  digital workflow in implant
    dentistry   343
  surgical protocols for implant
    placement   173
  timing of implant placement
    111–112
framework misfit   380–381
free gingival graft (FGG)
  extraction ridge management
    73, 75
  maxillary anatomical structures   56
  peri-implant emergence
    profile   193–196, *193, 195, 197*
  soft tissue augmentation   200
fricative sounds   321
full arch implant-fixed dental prosthesis
    (FAIFDP)   303, *346*, 373
full arch restorations
  definitive prosthesis   290
  laboratory perspective on implant
    dentistry   271–274, *272–276*
  prosthodontic rehabilitation for fully
    edentulous patient   317–320,
    318–320, 323–326

full-thickness mucoperiosteal flap
    reflection 146–148, *147*
  bone augmentation 213–214, *214*
  peri-implant emergence profile
    187, 188
  surgical protocols for implant
    placement 173
  suturing techniques 155

g
GBR *see* guided bone regeneration
genial tubercles 63
gingival biotype
  flap design and management for
    implant placement 147–148,
    151–152
  implant site preparation 118
  implant treatment in the aesthetic
    zone 230, 232–233
gingival contours *105*, 107
gingival display 228–230, *228*
gingival fistula 381, *381*
gingival recession
  surgical protocols for implant
    placement 176, *176*
  timing of implant placement 107, 114
gingival zeniths 229–230
gingivectomy 122, *123*
gold abutments 247
GPA *see* greater palatine artery
GPF *see* greater palatine foramen
granulation tissue 29–31, *31*
graphene-strengthened polymer 274
greater palatine artery (GPA) 50,
  55–56, *56*, 200–201
greater palatine foramen (GPF)
  200–201
greater palatine nerve 55–56, *56*
guided bone regeneration (GBR) 50,
  212, 217
guided surgery
  diagnostic records 16–17, *16–17*
  digital workflow in implant
    dentistry 338–343, *341–342*
  surgical protocols for implant
    placement 173
gutta percha 16, 18

h
hard palate 200–201, *202–203*
hard tissue fillers 73, 108
HBO *see* hyperbaric oxygen therapy
HERS *see* Hertwig's epithelial root
  sheath
Hertwig's epithelial root sheath
  (HERS) 74–78
hexagonal anti-rotation feature *see*
  external hex feature
history taking *see* patient assessment
  and history taking
horizontal mattress sutures
  159–161, *160*
hybrid cement/screw restorations
  257–259, *258*
hyperbaric oxygen therapy (HBO) 9
hypertension 6

i
implant biomechanics 277–287
  application to materials and
    occlusion 279–280, *280*
  beams 280–281, *281*
  bone 283–284
  cantilevers 282–283, *283–285*
  compressive, tensile, and shear
    forces 279–280, *279*
  forces and their nature 277–280,
    278–281
  impulse 278–279
  incline plane mechanics 280, *281*
  levers 281–282, *282*
  pressure 278
  survival rates 277, *278*
implant materials, designs, and surfaces
  87–102
  body shape design *91*, 95–96
  bulk implant materials 87–92
  classification of implant surface
    treatments **93**
  complications 357
  connection design *91*, 96–101,
    98–100, **98**
  implant screw joint 308–310
  loading protocols in implantology
    130–131, 133

other bulk materials   92
pure titanium   88–90, *88–90*, 234
thread design   *91*, 96, *97–98*
titanium alloys   90, *91*
wettability   92–94, *93*
zirconia   90–92, *91*, 234
see also surface roughness
implantoplasty   359, *359*
implant placement
  anatomic and biological principles
    37–47
  complications   375, *375*
  digital workflow in implant dentistry
    337–338, *339–340*
  flap design and management   145–154
  surgical protocols   173–180
  timing   103–115
  tooth loss   29–35
implant screw joint   307–313
  abutment/implant interface design
    309–310
  abutment/implant interface misfit   309
  complications   375–377, *376*, 382
  effects of excessive external forces
    307, *308*
  embedment relaxation/settling
    effect   308
  factors affecting implant screw joint
    stability   308–310
  functional forces   310
  number of implants   310
  practical measures to limit screw
    loosening/fracture   **311**
  preload   307–308
  retrieving a fractured screw
    311–312, *312*
  screw design   309
  screw material and coating   308–309
  torque wrench   310
implant site preparation   117–127
  adjacent and opposing teeth
    121–122, **121**
  aesthetic assessment   119
  assessing implant sites and adjacent
    teeth   118–120, *118–120*
  crown lengthening and
    gingivectomy   122, *123*

  endodontic status of adjacent teeth
    120, *120*
  gingival biotype and attached
    mucosa   118
  grafting   121
  occlusal analysis   120
  occlusal failure   121
  options for patients in replacing
    missing teeth   117
  orthodontics   122–124, *124–126*
  peri-implant emergence profile   194
  periodontal charting   118
  photographic records   118–119, *118*
  pre-surgical tissue evaluation   166–
    167, *167*, 170
  provisional phase   124–125
  radiography   119–120, *119*, *124*
  surgical protocols for implant
    placement   174
implant stability quotient (ISQ)   131,
  131, 177
implant-supported restorations *see*
  cement-retained restorations;
  screw-retained restorations
implant treatment failure   1–3
impression taking   219–226
  abutment level impressions   220
  abutments   245, 250
  complications   381
  customised impression copings
    222, *222*
  digital impression techniques   219,
    225, 250
  digital workflow in implant dentistry
    336–337, *336–337*, 343, *343–346*
  elastomeric impression materials
    219–220
  implant level impressions   220–222,
    221, **221**, 224–225, *225*
  multiple unit impressions   222–224,
    223–224, 226
  prosthodontic rehabilitation for fully
    edentulous patient   322, 323
  provisionalisation in
    implantology   240
  techniques used in implant dentistry
    220–222, *221*, **221**

impulse   278–279
incisive foramen, canal and nerve
  anatomic and biological principles for
    implant placement   41
  mandibular anatomical
    structures   62
  maxillary anatomical structures
    49–50, *51*
incline plane mechanics   280, *281*
induced pluripotent stem cells
  (iPSC)   78
inferior alveolar canal and nerve   41,
  65–67, *66*
inflammation   3–4
  complications   351, 353–354
  implant materials, designs, and
    surfaces   98, *100*
  screw- versus cement-retained
    restorations   256
informed consent   25–26
infraorbital foramen   52, *52*
infraorbital nerve   40
INR *see* International Normalised Ratio
insertion torque value
  abutments   250–251
  definitive prosthesis   292,
    293–294, 298
  implant screw joint   307, 309–310
  loading protocols in
    implantology   134
  surgical instrumentation
    142–143, *142*
  surgical protocols for implant
    placement   177, 179
inter-arch space   256
internal conical connection   98–101,
  99–100
International Normalised Ratio
  (INR)   7
interocclusal space   315, *316*
interproximal bone height
  integrity   168, *168*
intra-oral periapical radiographs   13
intra-oral scanning
  diagnostic records   18–19
  digital workflow in implant dentistry
    336–337, *336–337*, 343, *343–346*

laboratory perspective on implant
  dentistry   268–274, *270–273*
ionising radiation dosage   14, **15**
iPSC *see* induced pluripotent stem cells
ISQ *see* implant stability quotient

k

keratinised tissue
  flap design and management for
    implant placement   146, 148–149
  peri-implant emergence profile
    188–194, *188, 191, 193*
  soft tissue augmentation   199–200,
    200, 203–207, *206–209*
  surgical protocols for implant
    placement   173
  timing of implant placement   107, 109

l

laboratory perspective on implant
  dentistry   265–275
  digital data acquisition for full arch
    cases   271–272, *272–273*
  digital planning to manage aesthetics
    268, *269–270*
  importance of implant planning
    267–268, *267–268*
  inserting full arch cases at surgery
    272–274, *274–276*
  scanning for implant restorations
    268–271, *270–271*
  shift from analogue to digital   265
  standards in manufacturing today
    265, *266*
laser therapy   359–360
lateral cephalometric radiographs   14
lateral set-screw   261–262, *261*
levers   281–282, *282*
lingual foramen   63, *64*
lingual inclination   262
lingual nerve   41, 67–68
lip contour and length   228
lip support   316, *317*
loading protocols in implantology   3,
  129–135
  assessing primary stability for
    immediate loading   134

conventional loading   129, 130

definitions   129, *130*

early loading   129, 130

immediate loading   129, 130–134, *131*

progressive loading   129, 130

selecting a loading protocol
131–134, *132*, **133**

lymph nodes   43

m

maintenance of dental implants   3–4,
327–334

bony changes/bone loss   329

oral hygiene   327–328, *328*, **328**,
330–333, *331*

radiographic imaging   328–330,
331–332, 332–333

survival rates   327

mandibular anatomical structures
59–72

genial tubercles   63

inferior alveolar canal and nerve
65–67, *66*

lingual and mylohyoid nerves   67–68

lingual foramen and accessory lingual
foramina   63, *64*

mandibular incisive canal and
nerve   62

mandibular ramus   69

mental foramen and nerve   59–62,
60–61

sublingual fossa   64–65

submandibular fossa   68–69, *68*

submental and sublingual
arteries   65

mandibular arch   41

mandibular dentition   40

mandibular incisal edge   317

mandibular nerve   40–41

mandibular occlusal plane   317

mandibular ramus   69

manufacturer rescue kits   312

mastication

anatomic and biological principles for
implant placement   41, 43, **44**, *46*

occlusion   299, 305

mattress sutures   159–161, *160–161*

maxillary anatomical structures   49–58

greater palatine artery and nerve   50,
55–56, *56*

infraorbital foramen   52, *52*

maxillary incisive foramen and canal
49–50, *51*

maxillary sinus   52–54, *53, 55*

nasal cavity   50–52

maxillary dentition   40

maxillary incisal edge   316

maxillary nerve   40, 49–54

maxillary occlusal plane   317

maxillary sinus   52–54, *53, 55*

maxillofacial anatomical structures   37

maxillo-mandibular relationship
(MMR)   17–18

maximum intensity projection
(MIP)   120

maximum intercuspal position (MIP)
278, 302–304

mechanostat   301

medical history   5–7, **6**

medications   6

medico-legal considerations and risk
management   25–28

checklists   *27*, 28

dental records   26–28

ethical and legal principles   25

informed consent   25–26

medio-distal position   174, *175*

membrane fixation systems   213

mental foramen and nerve   59–62,
60–61

microgap/micromotion   2–3

complications   353

implant materials, designs, and
surfaces   98, *100*

implant screw joint   307

loading protocols in implantology
131–133

surgical protocols for implant
placement   177

mid-crestal incision   149, *149*

middle superior alveolar nerve
(MSA)   40

MIP *see* maximum intensity projection;
maximum intercuspal position

MMR *see* maxillo-mandibular relationship

Morse/Morse-like taper connections 99–101, *99*, 309–310

MSA *see* middle superior alveolar nerve

M sound 321

mucosa thickness 234

multiple unit impressions 222–224, *223–224*, 226

multi-unit abutments 246–247, 322–323

muscular system 41–43, **44–45**, *46*

mylohyoid nerve 67–68

n

nasal cavity 50–52

nasal floor augmentation (NFA) 52

nasopalatine nerve 49–51

nervous system *see* neurovascular supply

neurapraxia 62

neurotmesis 62

neurovascular supply
  anatomic and biological principles for implant placement 40–41, *42–43*
  flap design and management for implant placement 145–146
  mandibular anatomical structures 59–69
  maxillary anatomical structures 49–56
  soft tissue augmentation 200
  timing of implant placement 108–109, 111

NFA *see* nasal floor augmentation

non-absorbable sutures 156–157

non-engaging impression copings 223, *223*

non-keratinised tissue 200

non-parallel implants 223

non-resorbable membranes 213–214, *214*

o

occlusal vertical dimension (OVD) 315–317, 320–321, **321**

occlusion 299–306
  balanced, group function, and mutually protected occlusion 302
  bone loss 299–301

bruxism 301–302, **302**
  clinical occlusal applications 303–304, *304*
  complications 374–375, 382
  definitive prosthesis 290, 294
  diagnostic records 14
  excessive forces on dental implants 301
  full arch implant-fixed dental prosthesis 303
  implant biomechanics 279–280, *280*, 283
  implant screw joint 310, 312
  implant site preparation 120, 121
  loading protocols in implantology 130, 133
  maintenance of dental implants 330, 332–333
  mastication 299, 305
  minimising forces on dental implants 302–303, *303*
  osseointegration 299–301
  overdentures 304
  overloading 300–301, **301**, 305
  peripheral afferent feedback 299–300, 305
  posterior fixed prostheses 304
  prosthodontic rehabilitation for fully edentulous patient 317, 323
  provisionalisation in implantology 237
  screw- versus cement-retained restorations 255, 256
  single-tooth implant restorations 304, *304*

one-screw test 380

one-stage protocols 177, 182–183

open tray impression techniques 220–222, *221*, **221**

OPG *see* orthopantomogram

opposing teeth 121–122, **121**

oral anatomical structures 37

oral hygiene
  complications 357, 359–361, 366, *366–367*
  definitive prosthesis 295, *295*

maintenance of dental implants
327–328, *328*, **328**, 330–333, *331*
prosthodontic rehabilitation for fully
edentulous patient 326
screw- versus cement-retained
restorations 255, *255*
orthodontics
implant biomechanics 283
implant site preparation 122–124,
124–126
pre-surgical tissue evaluation 170
orthopantomogram (OPG)
maintenance of dental
implants 329
prosthodontic rehabilitation for fully
edentulous patient *324*
surgical protocols for implant
placement 174
osseointegration 1
complications 351, 353, 357, 363,
371, 378–379
extraction ridge management 74
implant materials, designs, and
surfaces 92–95
loading protocols in implantology
129–133
occlusion 299–301
patient assessment and history
taking 7
peri-implant emergence profile
181–182
surgical protocols for implant
placement 177
timing of implant placement 108
osseoperception 300
osteoblasts 92
osteoconductive materials 74–76, 82
osteology 37, *38–39*, **38**
osteonecrosis 8
osteoplasty 63, 141, 143, 361
osteoporosis 8–9
osteotomy
implant materials, designs, and
surfaces 95
mandibular anatomical structures
60, 61, 63, 65, 67, 69
surgical instrumentation 143

surgical protocols for implant
placement 173, 176, 179
timing of implant placement 107,
110–111, *111*
OVD *see* occlusal vertical dimension
overdentures
implant treatment in the aesthetic
zone 231–232
occlusion 304
prosthodontic rehabilitation for fully
edentulous patient 315, 317–318,
318–319, 323
overloading
complications 374
occlusion 300–301, **301**, 305

p
Palacci flap 152, *153*
palatal bone height (PH) 74–75
palatal tissue graft 200–201, *202–203*
panoramic radiographs
diagnostic records 14
maintenance of dental implants 329
mandibular anatomical
structures 62
maxillary anatomical structures *55*
papilla fill
implant site preparation 121–122,
121, 124–125
implant treatment in the aesthetic
zone 229–230, *233*
provisionalisation in implantology
239–240, **240**
papilla-sparing flap 151–152, *151*
parallel implants 223–224, *225*
partial-thickness mucoperiosteal flap
reflection 146–148, *147*
peri-implant emergence profile *187*,
188–196, *190, 192, 195, 197*
suturing techniques 155, 189–190,
190, 192–193, *192*, 195–196,
195, 197
passivity
complications 378–380, *379*,
382, *382*
definitive prosthesis 289, 296
implant screw joint 312

passivity (*cont'd*)
   prosthodontic rehabilitation for fully
      edentulous patient   322–323
   screw- versus cement-retained
      restorations   254–255, 257–258
patient assessment and history
     taking   5–11
   age of patient   7
   anatomic and biological principles for
      implant placement   37, 43, 47
   dental history   9–10
   implant site preparation   117
   implant treatment in the aesthetic
      zone   227
   loading protocols in
      implantology   133
   medical history and contraindications
      5–6, **6**
   medications and allergies   6
   osteoporosis and bisphosphonate
      therapy   8–9
   past medical history   6–7
   provisionalisation in
      implantology   237
   radiotherapy   9
   smoking   7–8
   social history   10
   soft tissue augmentation   199
   tooth loss and implant placement   33
patient compliance   133, 134
PDT *see* photodynamic therapy
PEEK *see* polyetheretherketone
periapical radiographs
   definitive prosthesis   290
   implant site preparation   119, *119*
   impression taking in implant
      dentistry   224, *225*
   maintenance of dental implants   329
   mandibular anatomical
      structures   *61*
   surgical protocols for implant
      placement   174, 179
peri-implant emergence profile   181–198
   apically repositioned flap   188–190,
     188, 190
   buccally repositioned flap   191–193,
     191–192

buccal roll   183–186, *183–185*
   complications   356–357, *356*
   definitions   181–182, *182*
   definitive prosthesis   289–290, **291**
   free gingival graft   193–196, *193,*
     195, 197
   one-stage versus two-stage implant
     surgery   182–183
   pouch roll   186–188, *186–187*
   screw- versus cement-retained
     restorations   255, *255*
peri-implantitis/mucositis   3–4
   complications   351–357, **355**, *356*
   extraction ridge management   78
   implant biomechanics   283
   implant materials, designs, and
     surfaces   94, 98–99, *100*
   maintenance of dental implants
     327–328, *328*, **328**, 330–333, *331*
   occlusion   300
   prevalence of peri-implant
     disease   354
   prosthodontic rehabilitation for fully
     edentulous patient   326
   risk factors   354–357, **355**, *356*
   screw- versus cement-retained
     restorations   256
   supportive care   365–366
   timing of implant placement   107
   treatment of peri-implant
     disease   357–366, *358–359,*
     362–364, 366–367
periodontal charting   118
periodontal integrity   167–169,
   168–169
periodontal plastic surgery   201
periodontal probing depth   354, 366
periotest   134
peripheral afferent feedback
   299–300, 305
permanent luting agents   **294**
PH *see* palatal bone height
phonetics   321–322
photodynamic therapy (PDT)
   359–360
photogrammetry   271–272, *272,*
   343–344

photographic records
  diagnostic records   18, 19–21, *19–23*
  implant site preparation
    118–119, *118*
  implant treatment in the aesthetic
    zone   228, *228*
  maintenance of dental implants   *332*
pick-up impression copings   220–222,
    221, **221**
piezoelectric scalers   332
piezosurgery   143
pink aesthetics   163–165, *164*
  abutments   248
  complications   375, *376*
  definitive prosthesis   295, *295*
  implant treatment in the aesthetic
    zone   227, 229
  soft tissue augmentation   199
pink porcelain   295, *295*
plaque   330–332, 359–361
platelet-rich fibrin (PRF)   74, 215
platelet-rich plasma   74
platform switch   98, *100*
polyetheretherketone (PEEK)   92,
    246–247
pontics   124–125
posterior fixed prostheses   304
posterior superior alveolar nerve
    (PSA)   40
post-operative management protocols
    177, **178–179**
pouch roll   186–188, *186–187*
preload   279–280, *279*, 292, 307–308
pressure   278
pre-surgical fabricated temporary
    prosthesis   342
pre-surgical tissue evaluation
    163–171
  buccal plate integrity   169, *169*
  diagnosis of periodontal
    integrity   167–169, *168–169*
  essential criteria evaluation
    168–169, *169*
  interproximal bone height integrity
    168, *168*
  pre-operative implant site assessment
    166–167, *167*

tissue volume and peri-implant
    aesthetics   163–165, *164*
  tissue volume availability and
    requirements   165–166, *165–166*
PRF *see* platelet-rich fibrin
primary closure   217
primary stability
  laboratory perspective on implant
    dentistry   268
  loading protocols in implantology
    133, **133**, 134
  surgical protocols for implant
    placement   174, 177
primary wound healing   212
prosthetically driven approach   2
  digital workflow in implant
    dentistry   338
  provisionalisation in implantology
    237–240, *238*, **239–240**
  surgical protocols for implant
    placement   174–176, *175–176*
prosthodontic rehabilitation
  abutment selection   322–323
  complications   357–358
  dentofacial aesthetics   316–317, 322
  fixed implant-supported bridgework
    319–320, *319–320*, 323–326,
    324–325
  fully edentulous patient   315–326
  impression taking   322, 323
  interocclusal space   315, *316*
  maintenance of dental implants
    331–332
  occlusal vertical dimension
    315–317, 320–321, **321**
  occlusion   317, 323
  phonetics   321–322
  removable overdentures   315,
    317–318, *318–319*, 323
  swallowing   322
  transition line and lip support   316,
    317, 325
provisionalisation   237–242
  abutments   246
  aesthetics and oral hygiene
    241, *241*
  contour management   239, **239**

provisionalisation (*cont'd*)
  definitive prosthesis   289–290, **291**
  digital workflow in implant
      dentistry   342
  direct and indirect techniques
      240, *241*
  functions in implant dentistry   237
  implant site preparation   125
  implant treatment in the aesthetic
      zone   233–234
  loading protocols in
      implantology   *132*
  papilla fill   239–240, **240**
  prosthetically guided tissue healing
      237–240, *238*, **239–240**
  screw- versus cement-retained
      restorations   256
  surgical protocols for implant
      placement   177
  timing of implant placement   *105,*
      237–239, *238*
proximal contact loss,
    complications   374
PSA *see* posterior superior alveolar nerve
pterygoid plexus   40

r
radiographic imaging
  complications   351, *352*, 379, *379, 382*
  definitive prosthesis   290, 297–298
  developments   2
  diagnostic records   13–16, *15–16*, **15**
  implant screw joint   *308*
  implant site preparation   119–120,
      119, 124
  impression taking in implant
      dentistry   224, *225*
  maintenance of dental implants
      328–330, *331–332, 332–333*
  mandibular anatomical structures
      60–62, *61*
  maxillary anatomical structures   50,
      51, 55
  pre-surgical tissue evaluation   169
  surgical protocols for implant
      placement   174, 176, 179
  tooth loss and implant placement
      31, 34

radiotherapy   9
RANK-OPG-RANKL pathway   78
recombinant bone morphogenic
      protein 2   74
reconstructive surgery   361–363,
      363–364
rehabilitation *see* prosthodontic
      rehabilitation
removable prostheses
  implant site preparation   117
  implant treatment in the aesthetic
      zone   231–232
  prosthodontic rehabilitation for fully
      edentulous patient   315, 317–318,
      318–319, 323
resonance frequency analysis
      (RFA)   134
resorbable membranes   73, 212
restorative space   315, *316*
retention
  abutments   243, 250
  definitive prosthesis   292–297, **294**
  implant treatment in the aesthetic
      zone   231–232
  screw- versus cement-retained
      restorations   253–264
retrievability
  definitive prosthesis   292, 294–295
  screw- versus cement-retained
      restorations   253, 257–259, 261
RFA *see* resonance frequency analysis
ridge lap   255, *255*
root canal treatment   120, *120*
root coverage   202, *204*
rubber dam   *132*, 263

s
sandblasting and acid etching (SLA)
      93–95, *94*
scanning electron microscopy (SEM)
      94, 99
Schneiderian membrane   54
screwdriver technique   312
screw resistance test   380
screw-retained restorations   253–264
  aesthetics   254–255, *254–255*
  angle screw correction/bi-axial
      screws   262–263, *262–263*

clinical performance 256–257

complications 355–356, 375–380, *376*, *378–379*

definitive prosthesis 289, 294–295

health of peri-implant tissue 256

hygiene/emergence profile 255, *255*

inter-arch space 256

lateral set-screw/cross-pinning 261–262, *261*

occlusion 256

passivity 254–255, 257

procedures for screw retention 257–260, **257**, *258–259*

provisionalisation 256

reduced occlusal material fracture 255

retrievability 253, 257–259, 261

see also implant screw joint

SEM *see* scanning electron microscopy

semi-lunar vertical releasing incision 151–152, *151*, *153*

sessile water droplet test 92, *93*

settling effect 308

SFE *see* sinus floor elevation

shear forces 279–280, *279*

sibilant sounds 321

simple/interrupted sutures 158–159, *158*

single-tooth implant restorations 304, *304*, 372–373

sinus floor elevation (SFE) 54, *55*

sinus grafts 121

SLA *see* stereolithography

smile evaluation 227–230, *228*

smile line 228–229, *228*

smoking 7–8, 133

social history 10

socket morphology 110, *111*

soft tissue augmentation 199–210

anatomical considerations for harvesting autogenous grafts 200–201

definitive prosthesis 289–290, **291**

flap design and management for implant placement 146

gaining keratinised tissue 203–207, *206–209*

harvesting palatal tissue graft 201, *202–203*

implant site preparation 121

implant treatment in the aesthetic zone 230–231, *231*

loading protocols in implantology 130

peri-implant emergence profile 182

pre-surgical tissue evaluation 165–167, *166–167*, 170

prior to bone grafting 202–203, *205–206*

purpose of soft tissue graft 201

root coverage 202, *204*

soft tissue substitutes 201

timing of implant placement 106, 108, 112–113

types of oral soft tissue 199–200, *200*

see also extraction ridge management

soft tissue impingement 259

soft tissue punch 148, *148*

soft tissue substitutes 73

space maintenance 212, 217

SPIT *see* supportive peri-implant therapy

split-thickness crestal incision 191–192

stability

bone augmentation 212

implant materials, designs, and surfaces 97–98, *99*

provisionalisation in implantology 237

see also primary stability

stereolithography (SLA) 17

stripped screw head 377–378, *378*

sublingual artery 65

sublingual fossa 64–65

submandibular fossa 68–69, *68*

submental artery 65

supportive peri-implant therapy (SPIT) 365–366

supragingival margins 298

surface roughness 2–3

abutments 248

complications 357

implant materials, designs, and surfaces 89, 93–95, *94*

implant screw joint 308

surface roughness (*cont'd*)
  loading protocols in implantology
    130–131, 133
  screw- versus cement-retained
    restorations   259
  timing of implant placement   107
surgical instrumentation   137–144
  Anthogyr Torq Control   142–143, *142*
  Benex extraction system
    141–142, *141*
  bone harvesters   142, *142*
  curettes   138
  depth probe   139
  extraction forceps, periostomes and
    elevators   140
  grafting well   141
  kidney dish   140
  mirror, probe, and tweezers   137
  mouth props/bite blocks   140
  needle holders   138
  periosteal elevators   139
  piezosurgery   143
  retractors   139, *139*
  rongeurs   141
  scalpel blades   138, 198, *198*
  scalpel handles   137
  scissors   140
  surgical cassette   *143*, 144
  surgical kit, electric motor, 20:1
    handpiece, and consumables
    140–141
  tissue forceps/pliers   139–140
  types and uses for
    implantology   137, *138*
surgical protocols for implant
    placement   173–180
  flap design and management   173,
    176–177
  implant positioning   174–176,
    175–176
  implant site preparation   174
  one-stage versus two-stage
    protocols   177
  peri-implant emergence profile
    182–183
  post-operative management protocols
    177, **178–179**

survival rates
  complications   371
  definitive prosthesis   289
  implant biomechanics   277, *278*
  maintenance of dental implants   327
  screw- versus cement-retained
    restorations   256–257
suturing techniques   155–162
  absorbable sutures   156
  continuous/uninterrupted sutures
    159, *159*
  flap design and management for
    implant placement   *149*, 155
  implant treatment in the aesthetic
    zone   234
  mattress sutures   159–161, *160–161*
  non-absorbable sutures   156–157
  peri-implant emergence profile
    189–190, *190*, 192–193, *192*,
    195–196, *195*, *197*
  simple/interrupted sutures
    158–159, *158*
  sizes   157, *157*
  soft tissue augmentation
    207–208, 209
  surgical needles   157–158, *158*
  suture removal   162
  tissue adhesive   157
  types of sutures   155–157
swallowing   299, 317, 322

t
tactile sensation   379
tapered implant body
  implant materials, designs, and
    surfaces   *91*, 95–96
  Morse/Morse-like taper
    connections   99–101, *99*, 309–310
  timing of implant placement
    104, 107
β-TCP *see* tricalcium phosphate
templates   14–16, *15–16*, 18–19
temporary cylinders   *105*, *132*
temporary luting agents   **294**
temporary prosthesis *see*
    provisionalisation
temporomandibular joint (TMJ)   43

tensile forces   279–280, *279*, 292, 307–308

thread design

  implant materials, designs, and surfaces   *91*, 96, *97–98*

  surgical protocols for implant placement   177

  timing of implant placement   *104*, 107

three-dimensional (3D) printing   3

  diagnostic records   16–17

  digital workflow in implant dentistry   338–341

  laboratory perspective on implant dentistry   272, *273*

timing of implant placement   103–115

  adjunctive procedures   112–113

  biomaterials   109–110

  classification system   103–104, **104**

  clinician experience   112

  delayed placement   107–108, 113

  flapless protocol   111–112

  immediate placement   104–107, *104–106*, 108–114, 233–234, 237–239, *238*

  implant treatment in the aesthetic zone   233–234

  loading protocols in implantology   131–133, *132*

  local risk factors   108–109, *109–110*

  provisionalisation in implantology   237–239, *238*

  selecting appropriate treatment protocol   113, **113**

  socket morphology   110, *111*

  systemic risk factors   108

tissue adhesive   157

tissue blanching   259

tissue compression   250

tissue punch   148, *148*

tissue volume   163–166, *164–166*

titanium

  abutments   *244*, 247–248, 251

  bulk implant materials   88–90, *88–90*

  implant treatment in the aesthetic zone   234

laboratory perspective on implant dentistry   274

  screw- versus cement-retained restorations   257–259

titanium alloys   90, *91*

TMJ *see* temporomandibular joint

tooth characteristics   229

tooth display   228

tooth loss

  bone resorption   29, *30*

  implant placement   29–35

  individual level effects   32, *33*

  local site effects   29–32

  patient assessment and history taking   33

  population level effects   32–33

  tripartite effect of tooth loss   29, *30*

tooth resorption   *233*

torque *see* insertion torque value

trabecular bone   174, 179

transfer impression copings   220–222, **221**

transition line   316, *317, 325*

transmucosal abutments   96

trapezoidal flap   150–151, *150*

traumatic tooth loss   108

triangular flap   150–151, *150*

tricalcium phosphate (β-TCP)   74

trigeminal nerve   40–41

tuberosity   200–201

two-piece implants   96

two-stage protocols   177, 182–183

u

ultrasonic decontamination   358

ultrasonic scalers   311–312, *312, 332*

v

vascular system *see* neurovascular supply

veneering porcelain   255, *259*

vertical bitewing radiograph   *61*

vertical mattress sutures   159–161, *161*

vertical releasing incision   150–152, *150–151, 153, 154*

W

wettability   92–94, *93*
white aesthetics   163–165, *164*
  abutments   248
  implant treatment in the aesthetic
    zone   227
  provisionalisation in
    implantology   241, *241*
  soft tissue augmentation   199

X

xenografts   73–74, 201

Z

zirconia
  abutments   247–251, *248*
  bulk implant materials
    90–92, *91*
  implant treatment in the aesthetic
    zone   234
  laboratory perspective on implant
    dentistry   272
  screw- versus cement-retained
    restorations   259
zygomatic nerve   40